I0044381

Clinical Neuroendocrinology

Clinical Neuroendocrinology

Editor: Joy Foster

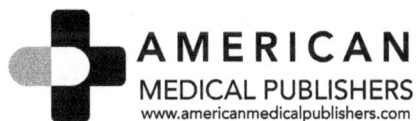

AMERICAN
MEDICAL PUBLISHERS
www.americanmedicalpublishers.com

AMERICAN
MEDICAL PUBLISHERS
www.americanmedicalpublishers.com

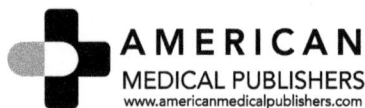

Cataloging-in-Publication Data

Clinical neuroendocrinology / edited by Joy Foster.
    p. cm.
Includes bibliographical references and index.
ISBN 978-1-63927-111-5
1. Neuroendocrinology. 2. Clinical medicine. 3. Endocrinology. 4. Neurology.
5. Neurohormones. I. Foster, Joy.
QP356.4 .C55 2022
612.8--dc23

© American Medical Publishers, 2022

American Medical Publishers,
41 Flatbush Avenue,
1st Floor, New York,
NY 11217, USA

ISBN 978-1-63927-111-5 (Hardback)

This book contains information obtained from authentic and highly regarded sources. Copyright for all individual chapters remain with the respective authors as indicated. All chapters are published with permission under the Creative Commons Attribution License or equivalent. A wide variety of references are listed. Permission and sources are indicated; for detailed attributions, please refer to the permissions page and list of contributors. Reasonable efforts have been made to publish reliable data and information, but the authors, editors and publisher cannot assume any responsibility for the validity of all materials or the consequences of their use.

Trademark Notice: Registered trademark of products or corporate names are used only for explanation and identification without intent to infringe.

Contents

Preface

Neuroendocrinology is the domain of biology that is concerned with the study of the interaction between the nervous system and the endocrine system. In the process of neuroendocrine integration, the nervous and endocrine systems act together in order to control the physiological processes of the human body. For understanding and treating neurobiological brain disorders, neuroendocrinology is used as an essential part. The neuroendocrine system is the tool through which the hypothalamus maintains homeostasis that helps in regulating metabolism, eating, reproduction, osmolarity, blood pressure and drinking behavior. The four main neuroendocrine systems are hypothalamic-pituitary-adrenal axis, hypothalamic-pituitary-thyroid axis, hypothalamic-pituitary-gonadal axis and hypothalamic-neurohypophyseal system. This book contains some path-breaking studies in the field of neuroendocrinology. It strives to provide a fair idea about this discipline and to help develop a better understanding of the latest advances within this field. This book is appropriate for students seeking detailed information in this area as well as for experts.

The information contained in this book is the result of intensive hard work done by researchers in this field. All due efforts have been made to make this book serve as a complete guiding source for students and researchers. The topics in this book have been comprehensively explained to help readers understand the growing trends in the field.

I would like to thank the entire group of writers who made sincere efforts in this book and my family who supported me in my efforts of working on this book. I take this opportunity to thank all those who have been a guiding force throughout my life.

Editor

Clinical, pathological and prognostic characteristics of gastroenteropancreatic neuroendocrine neoplasms in China

Xianbin Zhang[1†], Li Ma[2†], Haidong Bao[1], Jing Zhang[1], Zhongyu Wang[1] and Peng Gong[1*]

Abstract

Background: Gastroenteropancreatic neuroendocrine neoplasms (GEP-NENs) are rare neuroendocrine tumors, and lack of data in Asian populations especially in China. The aim of this retrospective study was to assess the clinical, pathological and prognostic characteristics of GEP-NENs in China.

Methods: We collected clinical and pathological data of 168 patients diagnosed with GEP-NENs and treated at the First and Second Affiliated Hospitals of Dalian Medical University between January 2003 and December 2012. Kaplan-Meier method and log rank analysis was used to analyze the prognostic significance of clinical and pathological characteristics.

Results: Mean age was 51.83 ± 14.03 and the male-to-female ratio was 1.5:1. Primary sites were the rectum (58.93%), pancreas (13.69%), stomach (9.52%), duodenum (5.36%), colon (4.76%), appendix (4.76%), ileum (2.38%) and jejunum (0.60%). Most patients (95.83%) presented non-functional tumors with non-specific symptoms such as abdominal or back pain (29.17%) and gastrointestinal bleeding (25.60%). Based on the 2010 World Health Organization (WHO) classification, patients were diagnosed with neuroendocrine tumor (NET) (24.40%) or neuroendocrine carcinoma (NEC) (7.14%). The estimated mean survival was 8.94 ± 0.28 years (95% CI: 8.40-9.48). Male gender, young age, small tumor size and NET tumor type were favorable prognostic factors.

Conclusion: Chinese GEP-NENs patients present characteristics that are similar to American and European patients. However, there is an urgent need to establish a national database for understanding the clinical and epidemiological features of GEP-NENs in China.

Keywords: Neuroendocrine neoplasms, Carcinoma, Epidemiology, China

Background

Neuroendocrine neoplasms (NENs) are epithelial tumors with a predominant neuroendocrine differentiation, and they can develop in most organs. This fairly rare neoplasms displays a large spectrum of clinical presentations [1]. According to the Surveillance, Epidemiology and End results (SEER) database, more than half of all NENs are gastroenteropancreatic NENs (GEP-NENs) (61%), with the highest frequency being observed in the rectum (17.7% of

NENs), small intestine (17.3% of NENs) and colon (10.1% of NENs), followed by the pancreas (7.0%), stomach (6.0%), and appendix (3.1%) [2]. The annual incidence of GEP-NENs is about 3.65-4.7 cases per 100,000 people in the United States (USA) [2,3]. African Americans show a higher incidence than Caucasians (6.46 vs. 4.60 per 100,000) [2]. The incidence is also slightly higher in men compared with women (4.97 vs. 4.49 per 100,000) [2]. Similar rates were reported in Sweden, Norway, Spain and England [4-7].

None of the published nomenclatures and classifications of NENs present a unified classification that is accepted by clinicians and pathologists [8,9]. In 2010, the WHO presented a new classification of NENs, in which

* Correspondence: gongpengdalian@163.com
†Equal contributors
[1]Department of Hepatobiliary Surgery, the First Affiliated Hospital of Dalian Medical University, Zhongshan Road No. 222, Dalian 116011, Liaoning Province, China
Full list of author information is available at the end of the article

the term NENs describes all tumors with a neuroendo-crine differentiation. GEP-NENs can be subdivided into two groups: the well-differentiated neuroendocrine tumors (NETs) and the poorly-differentiated neuroendocrine carcinomas (NECs) [10,11]. Furthermore, NETs and NECs are graded into three types, grades 1 (G1), 2 (G2) and 3 (G3), according to different definitions of proliferation using the mitotic count and/or the Ki-67 index [11]. In general, both G1 and G2 NENs are considered as NETs, and G3 NENs are considered as NECs [11].

Many studies reported the epidemiology, diagnosis, pathology and management of GEP-NENs in the American and the European populations [2,8,12-14], but there is a lack of data in Asian populations, especially in China. Therefore, the objective of the present study was to perform an epidemiological study of GEP-NENs in a Chinese population. The present study might provide new clues about the development and the management of these rare tumors.

Methods
Patients
We performed a retrospective analysis of all patients diagnosed with GEP-NENs according to the WHO 2000 classification [15,16] between January 2003 and December 2012 at the First and Second Affiliated Hospitals of Dalian Medical University.

All patients included in the present study had to have received a pathological diagnosis of GEP-NENs, and the original pathology report had to be available. Patients were excluded if they had received a diagnosis of primary NENs of any other site, or if the primary NEN site was unknown. In addition, patients with incomplete records (clinical and pathological), who were lost to follow-up, or who refused to participate in our study were also excluded. The ethics committee of the First Affiliated Hospital of Dalian Medical University approved the study protocol (LCKY 2012–32).

Data collection
At the Dalian Medical University, all cancer cases are prospectively collected into a database. Therefore, the following variables were collected and analyzed: clinical characteristics (gender, age, symptoms, signs), diagnostic procedures (imagery, pathology), tumor characteristics (primary site, size, stage, grading, World Health Organization (WHO) 2010 classification, WHO 2000 classification), treatments (surgery, hepatic artery interventional chemotherapy, pharmacotherapy), and follow-up (date of diagnosis, date of death and cause of death).

Cancer staging was performed using the usual tumor node metastasis (TNM) approach according to the anatomical sites of the tumors [11,17]. Grading was based on morphological criteria and tumor proliferative activity.

Tumors with a Ki-67 index of ≤ 2% were classified as G1, 3-20% as G2, and > 20% as G3. Similarly, tumors with a mitotic rate of < 2 per 10 high power fields (HPF) were classified as G1, 2-20/10 HPF as G2, and > 20/10 HPF as G3. GEP-NENs were further classified as NET (G1 and G2), or NEC (G3), according to the 2010 WHO classification [10,11].

We performed the final follow-up by telephone, mail or outpatient department visit in December 2012.

Statistical analysis
All statistical analyses were performed using SPSS 20.0 for Windows (IBM Corporation. Armonk, NY, USA). We tested continuous variables for normal distribution. Normally distributed continuous variables are expressed as mean and standard deviation, and were analyzed using independent samples t-tests. Categorical variables are expressed as frequencies and proportions, and were analyzed using the chi-square test or Fisher's exact test, as appropriate. We used the Kaplan-Meier method for survival analysis, log-rank tests were used for comparision among groups and post hoc analysis for pairwise comparisons between groups. We performed Cox proportional hazards model to identify independent factors associated with prognosis. The level of significance was set at $P < 0.05$.

Results
Patients' clinical characteristics
One hundred-sixty-eight patients were included in the present study. All were Han Chinese and Dalian natives; 102 (61.00%) patients were male, 66 (39.00%) female, and the male-to-female ratio was 1.5:1. Mean age was 51.83 ± 14.03. The most frequent initial symptoms and signs were abdominal or back pain (n = 49, 29.17%), followed by gastrointestinal bleeding (n = 43, 25.60%), dyspepsia (n = 24, 14.29%), and diarrhea (n = 21, 12.50%) (Table 1). Eight (4.76%) cases were incidental findings during routine health examinations; these patients were asymptomatic. Seven (4.16%) patients received a diagnosis of functional tumors: all of these were insulinomas, and the patients were hypoglycemic.

Diagnostic procedures
The following procedures were performed at least once during the diagnosis and management of these tumors: endoscopy (n = 133, 79.17%), ultrasound (n = 82, 48.81%), computed tomography (CT) scan (n = 96, 57.14%), and magnetic resonance imaging (MRI) (n = 17, 10.12%). The highest positive rate was 97.74% (130/133) for endoscopy, followed by endoscopic ultrasound (90.00%), MRI (70.59%), ultrasound (58.54%), and CT (54.17%). Positron emission computed tomography imaging using (^{18}F)-fluoro-deoxy-glucose as tracer (^{18}F-FDG-PET) was

Table 1 Patients' characteristics

	Male	Female	Total	P-value
N (%)	102 (61.00)	66 (39.00)	168 (100.00)	
Age (years)	52.91 ± 13.65	50.15 ± 14.56	51.83 ± 14.03	0.06
Primary tumor site				
Gastrointestinal tract	93 (55.36)	52 (30.95)	145 (86.31)	0.02*
Stomach	12 (7.14)	4 (2.38)	16 (9.52)	0.22
Duodenum	6 (3.57)	3 (1.79)	9 (5.36)	1.00
Jejunum	1 (0.60)	0(0.0)	1 (0.60)	1.00
Ileum	3 (1.79)	1 (0.60)	4 (2.38)	1.00
Colon	6 (3.57)	2 (1.19)	8 (4.76)	0.48
Appendix	4 (2.38)	4 (2.38)	8 (4.76)	0.71
Rectum	61 (36.31)	38 (22.62)	99 (58.93)	0.74
Pancreas	9 (5.36)	14 (8.33)	23 (13.69)	0.02*
Clinical Symptoms				
Abdominal or back pain	27 (16.07)	22 (13.10)	49 (29.17)	0.33
Gastrointestinal bleeding[a]	28 (16.67)	15 (8.93)	43 (25.60)	0.49
Dyspepsia[b]	16 (9.52)	8 (4.76)	24 (14.29)	0.52
Diarrhea	18 (10.71)	3 (1.79)	21 (12.50)	0.12
Tenesmus	13 (7.74)	6 (3.57)	19 (11.31)	0.47
Appetite loss	11 (6.55)	7 (4.17)	18 (10.71)	0.97
Constipation	3 (1.79)	5 (2.98)	8 (4.76)	0.27
Hypoglycemia[c]	5 (2.98)	2 (1.19)	7 (4.17)	0.71
Weight loss	4 (2.38)	1 (0.60)	5 (2.98)	0.65
Asthenia	1 (0.60)	1 (0.60)	2 (1.19)	1.00
Dysphagia	1 (0.60)	0(0)	1 (0.60)	1.00
Main Signs				
Abdominal mass	2 (1.19)	2 (1.19)	4 (2.38)	0.65
Jaundice[d]	1 (0.60)	1 (0.60)	2 (1.19)	1.00
Rash	1 (0.60)	2 (1.19)	3 (1.79)	0.56

[a]fecal occult blood, bloody stool, hematemesis.
[b]fullness, bloating, belching, nausea, vomiting.
[c]tremors, cold sweats, palpitations, hunger, irritability, headache, dizziness, blurred vision, disorientation, coma or seizures.
[d]skin or sclera.

performed in four patients, and detected the lesion in three of them, showing a detection rate of 75.00%. Chromogranin A, synaptophysin and neuronspecific enolase (NSE) are general neuroendocrine markers [18], and were positive in 72.62%, 76.19%, 32.74% of patients, respectively (Table 2).

Tumors' characteristics

As listed in Table 1, the rectum (n = 99, 58.93%) was the most frequent primary site, followed by the pancreas (n = 23, 13.69%), stomach (n = 16, 9.52%), duodenum (n = 9, 5.36%), colon (n = 8, 4.76%), appendix (n = 8, 4.76%), ileum (n = 4, 2.38%), and jejunum (n = 1, 0.60%). There was gender difference in primary tumor site (Table 1).

According to the pathology reports of the 168 tumors, 23 specimens were too small to be properly described (tumor size or extension). The mean size (longest diameter) of the remaining 145 tumors was 2.4 ± 2.3 cm.

At diagnosis, tumor spread was local in 64.29% (n = 108) of patients, loco-regional in 14.29% (n = 24), and metastatic in 8.33% (n = 14) (Table 3). The most common site of distant metastases was the liver (11/14, 78.57%), followed by the peritoneum (n = 2), and bones (n = 1). Two patients presented metastatic tumors in the liver accompanied with brain (n = 1) or ovary (n = 1) metastases. According to the 2000 WHO classification, 7.14% of GEP-NENs (n = 12) were classified as well-differentiated endocrine tumors, 4.17% (n = 7) were classified as well-differentiated

Table 2 Diagnostic procedures

	Cases tested, N (%)	Positive, N (%)
Imaging diagnosis		
Endoscopy	133 (79.17)	130 (97.74)
Gastroscopy	26 (15.48)	26 (100.00)
Small intestinal endoscopy	11 (6.55)	8 (72.73)
Proctoscopy	96 (57.14)	96 (100.00)
Ultrasound	82 (48.81)	48 (58.54)
Endoscopic ultrasound	20 (11.90)	18 (90.00)
CT	96 (57.14)	52 (54.17)
MRI	17 (10.12)	12 (70.59)
PET-CT	4 (2.38)	3 (75.00)
Immunohistochemistry		
Chromogranin A	168 (100)	122 (72.62)
Synaptophysin	168 (100)	128 (76.19)
NSE	168 (100)	55 (32.74)

CT, computed tomography scan; MRI, magnetic resonance imaging; PET-CT, positron emission computed tomography; NSE, neuron-specific enolase.

endocrine carcinomas, and 7.74% (n = 13) were classified as poorly differentiated endocrine carcinomas. Mitotic rates were missing in all pathology reports. Most reports (n = 115) did not present morphological criteria and the Ki-67 index. According to the available Ki-67 indexes, 20.23% of tumors were G1, 4.17% were G2, and 7.14% were G3. The most common tumor type was NET (n = 41), followed by NEC (n = 12) (Table 3).

Treatment

Table 4 presents the treatment modalities: 86.90% of patients underwent surgery. The surgical approach in each patient was the most optimal one, tailored to each patient's disease. Sixteen patients underwent conversion to radical resection after endoscopic resection. Seven patients had postoperative complications (intestinal fistula, seroperitoneum, anastomotic stricture, intestinal obstruction, incision fat necrosis, and anastomotic fistula), and five patients had to be reoperated for their complications.

Only 1.79% (n = 3) of patients underwent hepatic transcatheter arterial chemoembolization (TACE) to treat liver

Table 3 Tumors' characteristics

	Stomach n = 16	Duodenum n = 9	Jejunum n = 1	Ileum n = 4	Colon n = 8	Appendix n = 8	Rectum n = 99	Pancreas n = 23	Total N = 168 (%)
Size									
<1 cm	2	0	0	0	1	0	39	2	44 (26.19)
1-2 cm	1	4	0	2	1	3	31	8	50 (29.76)
>2 cm	9	5	1	2	5	1	15	13	51 (30.36)
Unclear	4	0	0	0	1	4	14	0	23 (13.69)
Stage									
$T_1N_0M_0$	4	0	0	0	1	2	43	5	55 (32.74)
$T_2N_0M_0$	1	3	0	0	0	1	17	5	27 (16.07)
$T_3N_0M_0$	2	1	0	1	2	4	2	7	19 (11.31)
$T_4N_0M_0$	1	2	0	0	0	0	0	4	7 (4.17)
$T_{any}N_1M_0$	5	1	1	3	3	0	10	1	24 (14.29)
$T_{any}N_{any}M_1$	2	2	0	0	2	1	6	1	14 (7.74)
Unclear	1	0	0	0	0	0	21	0	22 (13.69)
WHO 2010									
NET/G1	0	2	0	0	1	0	26	5	34 (20.23)
NET/G2	0	1	0	0	1	0	3	2	7 (4.17)
NEC/G3	1	0	0	0	2	0	4	5	12 (7.14)
Unclear	15	6	1	4	4	8	66	11	115 (68.45)
WHO 2000									
WDET	0	2	1	0	0	0	5	4	12 (7.14)
WDEC	0	2	0	0	0	0	5	0	7 (4.17)
PDEC	1	2	0	0	0	0	4	6	13 (7.74)
Unclear	15	3	0	4	8	8	85	13	136 (80.95)

TNM: tumor-node-metastasis approach [11]; NET, neuroendocrine tumor; NEC, neuroendocrine carcinoma; G1, grade 1; G2, grade 2; G3, grade 3; WDET, well differentiated endocrine tumour; WDEC, well differentiated endocrine carcinoma; PDEC, poorly differentiated endocrine carcinoma.

Table 4 Treatment modalities

	Male	Female	Total	P-value
	N = 102	N = 66	N = 168	
Surgery	89 (52.98)	57 (33.93)	146(86.90)	0.87
Laparotomy	69 (41.07)	36 (21.43)	105 (62.50)	0.09
Laparoscopic	3 (1.79)	1 (0.60)	4 (2.38)	1.00
Endoscopic	17 (10.12)	20 (11.90)	37 (22.02)	0.04
TACE	2 (1.19)	1 (0.60)	3 (1.79)	1.00
Pharmacotherapy				
Chemotherapy	14 (8.33)	4 (2.38)	18 (10.71)	0.12
Octreotide	12 (7.14)	12 (7.14)	24 (14.29)	0.25

TACE, transcatheter arterial chemoembolization.

metastases. Chemotherapy was the only intervention treatment in five patients with inoperable tumors, and 13 patients underwent chemotherapy as postoperative adjuvant therapy (Table 4). The most commonly used regimen was FOLFOX4 (oxaliplatin, leucovorin and 5-fluorouracil, n = 7), followed by oxaliplatin and capecitabine (n = 5), oxaliplatin and fluoropyrimidine (n = 1), paclitaxel and carboplatin (n = 1), docetaxel and gemcitabine (n = 1), cisplatin and 5-fluorouracil (n = 1), streptozotocin and 5-fluorouracil (n = 1), and taxane and platinum (n = 1). Twenty-four patients (14.29%) received octreotide, a somatostatin analogue, as a biological therapy combined with surgery or chemotherapy. Except for endoscopic therapy, the treatment modality distribution showed no difference in gender for any other therapies.

Follow-up
The median follow-up was 2.67 years (range: 0.01-10.00 years). Because of the short follow-up period, the GEP-NENs' median survival time was not attained during the study. At the last follow-up, 14 patients had died from their GEP-NENs, and 16 patients had died from accidents or other diseases (cerebral thrombosis, lung cancer, myocardial infarction, etc.). The estimated mean overall survival was 8.94 ± 0.28 years (95% confidence interval (CI): 8.40-9.48). We analyzed potential independent survival factors, such as age, gender, primary tumor site, tumor size, and tumor type (NET or NEC). As shown in Table 5, survival was significantly better in young patients, male patients, patients with small tumor and the NET subtype (Figure 1). Multivariate

Table 5 Overall survival

	Number	Mean survival times (years)	95% CI	χ^2	P-value
All	168	8.94 ± 0.28	8.40-9.48		
Age				4.33	0.04*
≤ 50	76	9.50 ± 0.29	8.92-10.07		
> 50	92	7.46 ± 0.38	6.73-8.20		
Gender				4.25	0.04*
Male	102	9.31 ± 0.27	8.78-9.84		
Female	66	7.71 ± 0.61	6.52-8.91		
Site				4.40	0.11
Rectum	99	9.40 ± 0.27	8.88-9.92		
Pancreas	23	4.09 ± 0.48	3.14-5.03		
Others[a]	46	7.59 ± 0.57	6.47-8.72		
Size				18.485	<0.01*
< 1 cm	44	9.84 ± 0.16	9.53-10.15		<0.01[c]
1-2 cm	50	8.88 ± 0.28	8.34-9.42		0.01[c]
> 2 cm	51	5.06 ± 0.51	4.07-6.06		
Unclear[b]	23	8.50 ± 0.39	7.74-9.26		0.01[c]
Tumor type				58.840	<0.01*
NET	41	7.35 ± 0.63	6.13-8.58		<0.01[c]
NEC	12	2.80 ± 0.87	1.09-4.50		
Unclear	115	9.80 ± 0.14	9.53-10.08		

[a]others represent stomach, duodenum, jejunum, ileum, colon, appendix.
[b]specimens too small to be properly described tumor size.
[c]log-rank test (pairwise over strata) according to size and tumor type; the P-values of tumor size 1 cm vs. > 2 cm, 1–2 cm vs. > 2 cm, Unclear vs. > 2 cm and NET vs. NEC were < 0.05.
*P <0.05.
NET, neuroendocrine tumor; NEC, neuroendocrine carcinoma.

analysis confirmed that age and tumor type were the only independent prognostic factors for overall survival (Table 6).

Discussion

The aim of this retrospective study was to assess the clinical, pathological and prognosis characteristics of GEP-NENs in China. The rectum, pancreas, stomach and duodenum were the most frequent primary sites. The majority of patients presented non-functional tumors with non-specific symptoms such as abdominal or back pain and gastrointestinal bleeding. Based on the 2010 WHO classification, most patients suffered from NET. The estimated mean survival was relatively short, with 8.94 ± 0.28 years (95% CI: 8.40-9.48). Male gender, young age, small tumor and NET tumor type were favorable prognostic factors.

NENs may develop anywhere in the body, but most of them do in the gastrointestinal tract [1]. A large-scale analysis of GEP-NENs (n = 29,664) from the SEER database revealed that the highest GEP-NENs frequency was in the rectum, followed by the small intestine, colon, pancreas, stomach, and appendix, and that the incidence increased with years at all primary sites, especially in the rectum and small intestine [3]. Similarly, we observed that the rectum

Table 6 Multivariate Cox proportional hazards model

Variable	Hazard ratio	95% CI	P-value
Age	2.01	1.14-3.56	0.02*
Site	2.94	0.82-10.53	0.10
Size	3.55	0.82-15.47	0.09
Tumor type	2.10	1.02-4.31	0.04*

*$P < 0.05$.

was the most frequent site of GEP-NENs, followed by the pancreas, and stomach; however, the small intestine only accounted for a small proportion of our cases. Nevertheless, primary tumor site distribution in the present study was similar to that of the Korean and Japanese populations [13,19], suggesting that the distribution of GEP-NENs' primary sites may be different between the Asian and the American populations. However, these observations might not reflect the true situation. Indeed, guidelines recommend that patients over 50 years undergo colonoscopy when they receive health check at our institutions, which should increase the early diagnosis rate of the disease. Meanwhile, with diagnostic improvements, more and more patients received a diagnosis of appendix NEN because of an incidental finding of the surgery for an

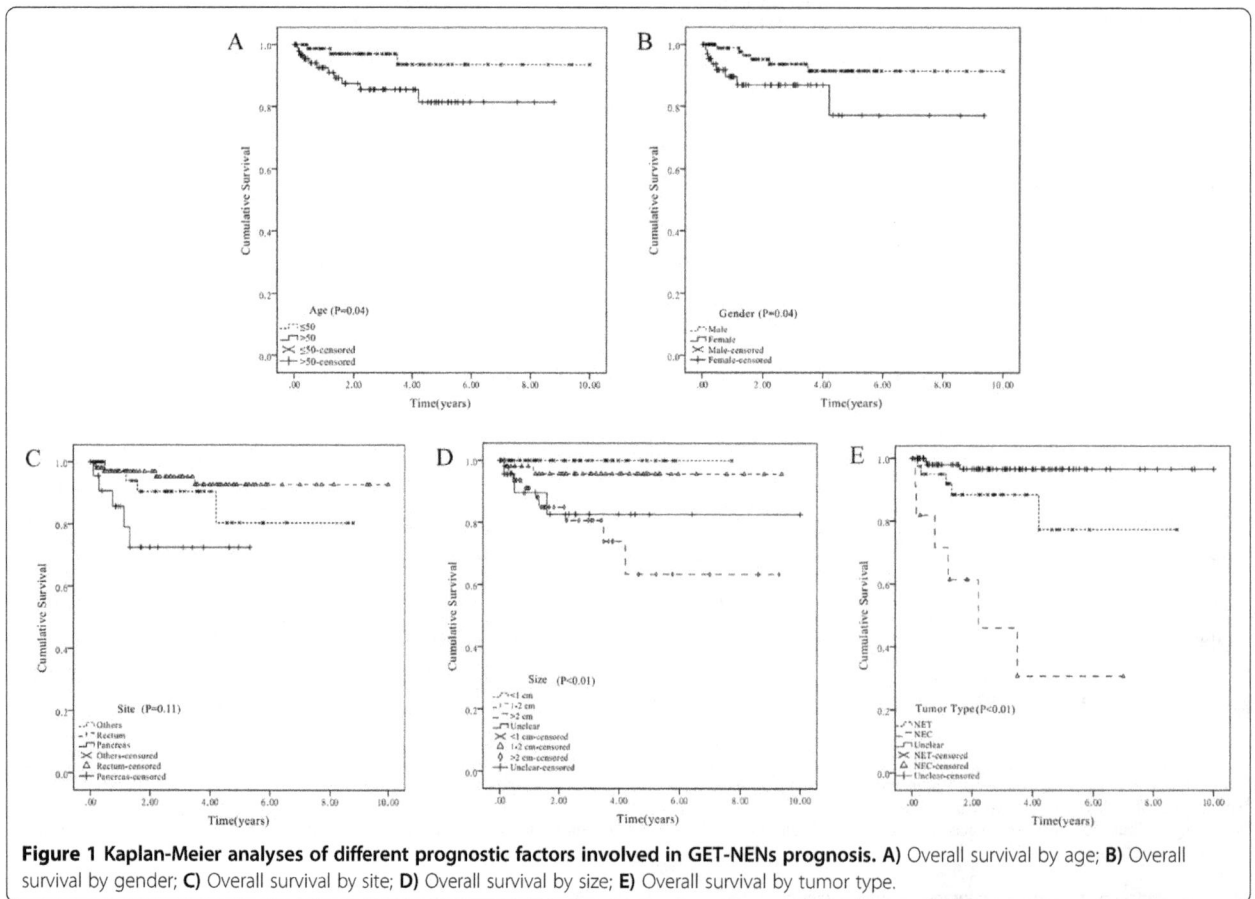

Figure 1 Kaplan-Meier analyses of different prognostic factors involved in GET-NENs prognosis. A) Overall survival by age; **B)** Overall survival by gender; **C)** Overall survival by site; **D)** Overall survival by size; **E)** Overall survival by tumor type.

acute appendicitis. All of these might create a false impression that the incidence of GEP-NENs is increasing.

NENs can be classified into functional or nonfunctional tumors according to the symptoms associated with peptides and hormones overproduction [20]. The present study showed that most GEP-NENs in the Chinese population were nonfunctional tumors. Carcinoid syndrome, Zollinger-Ellison syndrome, Whipple triad, Verner-Morrison syndrome and glucagonoma syndrome are typical symptoms of functional NENs [21], but no patient showed these symptoms in the present study. This might be due to two reasons: 1) clinicians may not pay enough attention to these symptoms; or 2) NENs were diagnosed at the early stages, before being symptomatic.

The lack of a uniform nomenclature and classification system of GEP-NENs prevent the physicians from diagnosing and treating these tumors. The WHO updated its classification in 2010 and accepted the term "GEP-NENs" [22]. We reviewed the diagnosis process in our participating institutions. Unfortunately, but as expected, it was not standardized. The "gold standard" in our participating institutions was the use of general neuroendocrine markers, such as chromogranin A, synaptophysin or NSE [23]. We reviewed the pathology reports of our patients according to the new WHO 2010 diagnosis and classification criteria, and we observed that 24.40% patients suffered from NET (n = 41) and 7.14% from NEC (n = 12). Fourteen patients presented metastases at diagnosis. The total metastasis rate was 8.33%, which was lower than what was previously reported [24]. The reasons may be responsible for regional difference. Unlike other solid tumors, there is a wide array of therapeutic options, such as surgery, interventional radiology, systemic therapy, somatostatin analogues, interferon, peptide-receptor radionuclide therapy, chemotherapy, and targeted agents (sunitinib, everolimus, bevacizumab) to palliate symptoms and extend survival in patients with GEP-NENs [25]. As for other tumors, surgery is an essential treatment in many GEP-NENs and is usually the only way to cure patients. The extent of surgical resection depends on the extent of the disease (local, regional or distant metastases). Cytoreductive surgery is recommended for palliation and to increase survival for patients with advanced disease [26]. In the present study, most patients underwent surgery, and only two patients who underwent surgery died during follow-up.

Chemotherapy is the first treatment option for inoperable or metastatic GEP-NENs. The cisplatin and etoposide combination is the most widely used chemotherapy regimen for GEP-NENs [27]. In our cohort, 18 patients received chemotherapy. The most frequently used chemotherapy regimen was the oxaliplatin, leucovorin and 5-fluorouracil combination.

More and more studies report that biological and targeted therapies show great promises against NENs. Somatostatin analogues can reduce the hormone-related symptoms, and they are an effective therapeutic option for functional neuroendocrine tumors [28]. Sunitinib and everolimus may be used for patients with inoperable locally advanced or metastatic, progressive, well differentiated pancreatic NENs [2,29,30]. In the present study, 24 patients underwent somatostatin analogues treatment, seven of them suffering from functional tumors (insulinoma).

The present study suffered from some limitations. The population's characteristics (age and gender) presented in our study are similar to those reported in other studies of Asian populations [13,19,24,31,32]. However, they are different from those previously published using the SEER database or European populations [12,14,33]. Selection biases among races, populations and hospitals may be responsible for these differences. Second, the follow-up of the present study did not reach the median survival time previously reported. Indeed, our mean survival was 8.94 ± 0.28 years, and was shorter than the 9.5 years reported by other investigators [24]. This is due to a short follow-up time and to the slow growing rate of the disease. Third, the small sample size might have been responsible for some bias in the multivariate and prognosis analyses. Fourth, the retrospective nature of the study prevented us from obtaining some information, such as the Ki-67 index. In addition, our follow-up system only contains data about the vital status (alive or not), and not about progression, preventing us to determine the progression-free survival. Finally, tumors in the rectum are more easily found at their early stages by endoscopic examination, while tumors at other sites (e.g. in the pancreas) necessitate examinations that are not routinely performed, which might affect the incidence.

Conclusion

In our study, non-specific clinical symptoms were the most common symptoms in patients with GEP-NENs. Diagnosis was mainly based on clinical manifestation, endoscopy and imagery, as well as on pathology. However, the recommended morphological criteria and proliferative activity of the tumor were not commonly used in pathological diagnosis. Surgery was the most common intervention. Male gender, young age (≤ 50 years), tumor size (< 2 cm) and NET diagnosis might be favorable prognostic factors. A national database of GEP-NENs should be established for studying the clinical and epidemiological features of these tumors, and to help physicians taking better clinical decisions.

Consent

Written informed consents were obtained from the patient for the publication of this report and any accompanying images.

Competing interests
All authors declare that they have no competing interests.

Authors' contribution
XZ: conception and design, acquisition of data, writing the manuscript. LM: analysis and interpretation of data. HB: acquisition of data. JZ: acquisition of data, analysis and interpretation of data. ZW: acquisition of data. PG: revising the manuscript. All authors read and approved the final manuscript.

Acknowledgements
This study was funded by the Specialized Research Fund for the Doctoral Program of Higher Education (No. 20122105110009) and the China National Natural Science Foundation (No.81200989). The funders had no role in study design, data collection and analysis, decision to publish, or preparation of the manuscript.

Author details
[1]Department of Hepatobiliary Surgery, the First Affiliated Hospital of Dalian Medical University, Zhongshan Road No. 222, Dalian 116011, Liaoning Province, China. [2]Department of Epidemiology, Dalian Medical University, Dalian 116044, Liaoning Province, China.

References

1. Modlin IM, Oberg K, Chung DC, Jensen RT, de Herder WW, Thakker RV, Caplin M, Delle Fave G, Kaltsas GA, Krenning EP, Moss SF, Nilsson O, Rindi G, Salazar R, Ruszniewski P, Sundin A: **Gastroenteropancreatic neuroendocrine tumours.** *Lancet Oncol* 2008, **9**(1):61–72.
2. Yao JC, Hassan M, Phan A, Dagohoy C, Leary C, Mares JE, Abdalla EK, Fleming JB, Vauthey JN, Rashid A, Evans DB: **One hundred years after "carcinoid": epidemiology of and prognostic factors for neuroendocrine tumors in 35,825 cases in the United States.** *J Clin Oncol* 2008, **26**(18):3063–3072.
3. Lawrence B, Gustafsson BI, Chan A, Svejda B, Kidd M, Modlin IM: **The epidemiology of gastroenteropancreatic neuroendocrine tumors.** *Endocrinol Metab Clin North Am* 2011, **40**(1):1–18. vii.
4. Hemminki K, Li X: **Incidence trends and risk factors of carcinoid tumors: a nationwide epidemiologic study from Sweden.** *Cancer* 2001, **92**(8):2204–2210.
5. Hauso O, Gustafsson BI, Kidd M, Waldum HL, Drozdov I, Chan AK, Modlin IM: **Neuroendocrine tumor epidemiology: contrasting Norway and North America.** *Cancer* 2008, **113**(10):2655–2664.
6. Ploeckinger U, Kloeppel G, Wiedenmann B, Lohmann R, representatives of 21 German NETC: **The German NET-registry: an audit on the diagnosis and therapy of neuroendocrine tumors.** *Neuroendocrinology* 2009, **90**(4):349–363.
7. Lepage C, Rachet B, Coleman MP: **Survival from malignant digestive endocrine tumors in England and Wales: a population-based study.** *Gastroenterology* 2007, **132**(3):899–904.
8. Pape UF, Jann H, Muller-Nordhorn J, Bockelbrink A, Berndt U, Willich SN, Koch M, Rocken C, Rindi G, Wiedenmann B: **Prognostic relevance of a novel TNM classification system for upper gastroenteropancreatic neuroendocrine tumors.** *Cancer* 2008, **113**(2):256–265.
9. Kloppel G, Rindi G, Perren A, Komminoth P, Klimstra DS: **The ENETS and AJCC/UICC TNM classifications of the neuroendocrine tumors of the gastrointestinal tract and the pancreas: a statement.** *Virchows Arch* 2010, **456**(6):595–597.
10. Bosman FT, Carneiro F, Hruban RH, Theise ND: *WHO classification of tumours of the digestive system.* 4th edition. Lyon: International Agency for Research on Cancer; 2010.
11. Bosman FT, Carneiro F, Hruban RH, Theise ND: *WHO classification of tumours of the digestive system.* Geneva, Switzerland: World Health Organization; 2010.
12. Niederle MB, Hackl M, Kaserer K, Niederle B: **Gastroenteropancreatic neuroendocrine tumours: the current incidence and staging based on the WHO and European Neuroendocrine Tumour Society classification: an analysis based on prospectively collected parameters.** *Endocr Relat Cancer* 2010, **17**(4):909–918.
13. Ito T, Sasano H, Tanaka M, Osamura RY, Sasaki I, Kimura W, Takano K, Obara T, Ishibashi M, Nakao K, Doi R, Shimatsu A, Nishida T, Komoto I, Hirata Y, Nakamura K, Igarashi H, Jensen RT, Wiedenmann B, Imamura M: **Epidemiological study of gastroenteropancreatic neuroendocrine tumors in Japan.** *J Gastroenterol* 2010, **45**(2):234–243.
14. Garcia-Carbonero R, Capdevila J, Crespo-Herrero G, Diaz-Perez JA, Martinez Del Prado MP, Alonso Orduna V, Sevilla-Garcia I, Villabona-Artero C, Beguiristain-Gomez A, Llanos-Munoz M, Marazuela M, Alvarez-Escola C, Castellano D, Vilar E, Jimenez-Fonseca P, Teule A, Sastre-Valera J, Benavent-Vinuelas M, Monleon A, Salazar R: **Incidence, patterns of care and prognostic factors for outcome of gastroenteropancreatic neuroendocrine tumors (GEP-NETs): results from the National Cancer Registry of Spain (RGETNE).** *Ann Oncol* 2010, **21**(9):1794–1803.
15. KLÖPPEL G, PERREN A, HEITZ PU: **The gastroenteropancreatic neuroendocrine cell system and its tumors: the WHO classification.** *Ann N Y Acad Sci* 2004, **1014**(1):13–27.
16. Niederle MB, Niederle B: **Diagnosis and treatment of gastroenteropancreatic neuroendocrine tumors: current data on a prospectively collected, retrospectively analyzed clinical multicenter investigation.** *Oncologist* 2011, **16**(5):602–613.
17. Oberg K: **Diagnostic work-up of gastroenteropancreatic neuroendocrine tumors.** *Clinics (Sao Paulo)* 2012, **67**(Suppl 1):109–112.
18. Strosberg JR, Nasir A, Hodul P, Kvols L: **Biology and treatment of metastatic gastrointestinal neuroendocrine tumors.** *Gastrointest Cancer Res* 2008, **2**(3):113–125.
19. Gastrointestinal Pathology Study Group of Korean Society of P, Cho MY, Kim JM, Sohn JH, Kim MJ, Kim KM, Kim WH, Kim H, Kook MC, Park do Y, Lee JH, Chang H, Jung ES, Kim HK, Jin SY, Choi JH, Gu MJ, Kim S, Kang MS, Cho CH, Park MI, Kang YK, Kim YW, Yoon SO, Bae HI, Joo M, Moon WS, Kang DY, Chang SJ: **Current Trends of the Incidence and Pathological Diagnosis of Gastroenteropancreatic Neuroendocrine Tumors (GEP-NETs) in Korea 2000–2009: Multicenter Study.** *Cancer Res Treat* 2012, **44**(3):157–165.
20. Metz DC, Jensen RT: **Gastrointestinal neuroendocrine tumors: pancreatic endocrine tumors.** *Gastroenterology* 2008, **135**(5):1469–1492.
21. Oberg K, Akerstrom G, Rindi G, Jelic S, Group EGW: **Neuroendocrine gastroenteropancreatic tumours: ESMO Clinical Practice Guidelines for diagnosis, treatment and follow-up.** *Ann Oncol* 2010, **21**(Suppl 5):v223–227.
22. Stoyianni A, Pentheroudakis G, Pavlidis N: **Neuroendocrine carcinoma of unknown primary: a systematic review of the literature and a comparative study with other neuroendocrine tumors.** *Cancer Treat Rev* 2011, **37**(5):358–365.
23. Kuiper P, Verspaget HW, Overbeek LI, Biemond I, Lamers CB: **An overview of the current diagnosis and recent developments in neuroendocrine tumours of the gastroenteropancreatic tract: the diagnostic approach.** *Neth J Med* 2011, **69**(1):14–20.
24. Wang YH, Lin Y, Xue L, Wang JH, Chen MH, Chen J: **Relationship between clinical characteristics and survival of gastroenteropancreatic neuroendocrine neoplasms: A single-institution analysis (1995–2012) in South China.** *BMC Endocr Disord* 2012, **12**:30.
25. Ramage JK, Ahmed A, Ardill J, Bax N, Breen DJ, Caplin ME, Corrie P, Davar J, Davies AH, Lewington V, Meyer T, Newell-Price J, Poston G, Reed N, Rockall A, Steward W, Thakker RV, Toubanakis C, Valle J, Verbeke C, Grossman AB, Uk, Ireland Neuroendocrine Tumour S: **Guidelines for the management of gastroenteropancreatic neuroendocrine (including carcinoid) tumours (NETs).** *Gut* 2012, **61**(1):6–32.
26. Garcia-Carbonero R, Salazar R, Sevilla I, Isla D: **SEOM clinical guidelines for the diagnosis and treatment of gastroenteropancreatic neuroendocrine tumours (GEP NETS).** *Clin Transl Oncol* 2011, **13**(8):545–551.
27. Sun W, Lipsitz S, Catalano P, Mailliard JA, Haller DG, Eastern Cooperative Oncology G: **Phase II/III study of doxorubicin with fluorouracil compared with streptozocin with fluorouracil or dacarbazine in the treatment of advanced carcinoid tumors: Eastern Cooperative Oncology Group Study E1281.** *J Clin Oncol* 2005, **23**(22):4897–4904.
28. Rinke A, Muller HH, Schade-Brittinger C, Klose KJ, Barth P, Wied M, Mayer C, Aminossadati B, Pape UF, Blaker M, Harder J, Arnold C, Gress T, Arnold R, Group PS: **Placebo-controlled, double-blind, prospective, randomized study on the effect of octreotide LAR in the control of tumor growth in patients with metastatic neuroendocrine midgut tumors: a report from the PROMID Study Group.** *J Clin Oncol* 2009, **27**(28):4656–4663.
29. Raymond E, Dahan L, Raoul JL, Bang YJ, Borbath I, Lombard-Bohas C, Valle J, Metrakos P, Smith D, Vinik A, Chen JS, Horsch D, Hammel P, Wiedenmann B,

Van Cutsem E, Patyna S, Lu DR, Blanckmeister C, Chao R, Ruszniewski P: Sunitinib malate for the treatment of pancreatic neuroendocrine tumors. *N Engl J Med* 2011, **364**(6):501–513.

30. Yao JC, Shah MH, Ito T, Bohas CL, Wolin EM, Van Cutsem E, Hobday TJ, Okusaka T, Capdevila J, de Vries EG, Tomassetti P, Pavel ME, Hoosen S, Haas T, Lincy J, Lebwohl D, Oberg K, Rad001 in Advanced Neuroendocrine Tumors TTSG: **Everolimus for advanced pancreatic neuroendocrine tumors.** *N Engl J Med* 2011, **364**(6):514–523.

31. Lim T, Lee J, Kim JJ, Lee JK, Lee KT, Kim YH, Kim KW, Kim S, Sohn TS, Choi DW, Choi SH, Chun HK, Lee WY, Kim KM, Jang KT, Park YS: **Gastroenteropancreatic neuroendocrine tumors: incidence and treatment outcome in a single institution in Korea.** *Asia Pac J Clin Oncol* 2011, **7**(3):293–299.

32. Li AF, Hsu CY, Li A, Tai LC, Liang WY, Li WY, Tsay SH, Chen JY: **A 35-year retrospective study of carcinoid tumors in Taiwan: differences in distribution with a high probability of associated second primary malignancies.** *Cancer* 2008, **112**(2):274–283.

33. Yao JC, Phan AT, Chang DZ, Wolff RA, Hess K, Gupta S, Jacobs C, Mares JE, Landgraf AN, Rashid A, Meric-Bernstam F: **Efficacy of RAD001 (everolimus) and octreotide LAR in advanced low- to intermediate-grade neuroendocrine tumors: results of a phase II study.** *J Clin Oncol* 2008, **26**(26):4311–4318.

2

Post-partum pituitary insufficiency and livedo reticularis presenting a diagnostic challenge in a resource limited setting in Tanzania

Faheem G Sheriff*, William P Howlett and Kajiru G Kilonzo

Abstract

Background: Pituitary disorders following pregnancy are an important yet under reported clinical entity in the developing world. Conversely, post partum panhypopituitarism has a more devastating impact on women in such settings due to high fertility rates, poor obstetric care and scarcity of diagnostic and therapeutic resources available.

Case presentation: A 37 year old African female presented ten years post partum with features of multiple endocrine deficiencies including hypothyroidism, hypoadrenalism, lactation failure and secondary amenorrhea. In addition she had clinical features of an underlying autoimmune condition. These included a history of post-partum thyroiditis, alopecia areata, livedo reticularis and deranged coagulation indices. A remarkable clinical response followed appropriate hormone replacement therapy including steroids. This constellation has never been reported before; we therefore present an interesting clinical discussion including a brief review of existing literature.

Conclusion: Post partum pituitary insufficiency is an under-reported condition of immense clinical importance especially in the developing world. A high clinical index of suspicion is vital to ensure an early and correct diagnosis which will have a direct bearing on management and patient outcome.

Keywords: Post partum panhypopituitarism, Lymphocytic hypophysitis, Sheehan's syndrome, Livedo reticularis, Africa

Background

The pituitary gland undergoes major anatomic, physiologic and immunologic changes during pregnancy. Its enlargement is chiefly attributed to lactotroph hyperplasia [1]. These changes then predispose the pregnant woman to a spectrum of pituitary disorders in the intra-partum and post-partum periods. These include Sheehan's syndrome which is by far the commonest, lymphocytic hypophysitis and rarely, apoplexy of pituitary adenomas [1,2].

Sheehan's syndrome (SS) is becoming increasingly rare in the developed world due to improved standards of obstetric care; the same is not yet true for the developing world. The prevalence of women of reproductive age with suspected SS in the Kashmir valley (Indian subcontinent) was estimated at 3.2% [3]. Similar cross-sectional studies are virtually non-existent for Africa but a couple of case series have appeared in the literature. Cénac et al reported 40 cases of SS within a 5-year period at a hospital in Niger. All their patients were black African women living in rural areas and had no medical assistance during the last delivery [4]. Another group of researchers from Senegal noted that the main risk factors were traditions of home delivery and lack of obstetric care [5]. In addition, they observed a long latency period before the disease manifestations became overt [5]. Not surprisingly, lymphocytic adenohypophysitis with an estimated annual incidence in the UK of one case per 9 million [6], is even less commonly reported in sub-Saharan Africa with only a couple of isolated case reports till date from South Africa [7,8].

* Correspondence: fsheriff.md@gmail.com
Kilimanjaro Christian Medical Centre, Moshi, Tanzania

Case presentation

History

ZM, a 37 year old multiparous woman from Northern Tanzania, presented with complaints of generalized body swelling associated with progressive weight gain for ten years. The onset coincided with her last child birth which was complicated by mild post-partum haemorrhage following which she failed to lactate. She also experienced cold intolerance, loss of libido and a complete cessation of her menses. Four years prior admission she had had a serious febrile illness following which she experienced a brief period of altered level of consciousness and transient aphasia; since then she noted slowing of speech. As part of her systems review, she reported an anterior neck swelling which increased during her last pregnancy then gradually subsided a few months later. She also reported headaches of moderate intensity but no gross visual changes; she suffered from occasional rashes in sunlight exposed areas but no mucosal ulceration. Her past medical history revealed no previously diagnosed chronic illnesses; she was sero-negative for HIV and syphilis. Her obstetric history revealed she had a parity of five with four living children (one still birth at term with no obvious congenital malformations noted). Since she had received no formal antenatal care, there were no records of blood pressure measurements during pregnancy. All were home deliveries in the absence of a qualified birth attendant.

Physical examination

Vitals: Pulse: 70/min; BP: 102/68 mm Hg; Temp: 36.2 degrees C; Respiratory rate 14/min. Orthostatics: Supine BP 110/80 mm Hg, standing BP 95/60 mm Hg. **General/ endocrine:** overweight woman (BMI 29. 1 kg/m^2), looking younger than her stated age. She was pale with generalized, non-pitting edema involving face and extremities. Of note she had no oral ulcers and her thyroid gland was not palpable. She had "alabaster" skin with patchy hair loss over scalp; sparse axillary and pubic hair. **Cardiovascular:** Regular rate and rhythm with distant heart sounds. **Respiratory/Abdominal exams** were unremarkable. **Neurologic Exam:** *Higher centres*: Fully oriented to time, place and person but with marked slowing of speech and mentation. *Cranial nerves*: Optic nerve- Visual acuity 20/30 both eyes; gross visual fields normal at bedside. Fundoscopy: no papilledema noted. Extra-ocular movements were intact. *Motor*: Limbs hypotonic; power reduced to grade 4/5 MRC (Medical Research Council grade) with proximal weaker than distal muscle groups. *Reflexes*: Ankle jerks were delayed and plantar responses flexor. *Sensation* was normal for all modalities tested.

Investigations

Labs

Please see Table 1.

Table 1 Relevant laboratory results

CBC/ESR	Hb = 96.6 g/L (121–153), MCV = 83.3 fL (82–103), ESR = 60 mm/hr (0–10)
Coagulation panel	International Normalized Ratio (INR): 2.06 (1.0-1.5). The patient was not on any oral anti-coagulants; this had normalized on a follow-up exam. Activated Partial Thromboplastin Time(APTT): 31.15 sec (20–35)
Chemistry panel	Fasting blood glucose: 3.2 mmol/L (3.6 -6.3), Na$^+$: 113.9 mmol/L (137–147), K$^+$: 3.4 mmol/L (3.4-5.3), aspartate aminotransferase (AST): 83.6 IU/L (11–47); creatinine: 67 mcmol/L (44–150)
Dipstick urinalysis	proteinuria 2+, specific gravity: 1.030 (1.010-1.025)
Endocrine panel	T4: 38 ng/mL (60–160), T3: 0.8 ng/mL (1.0-3.1), TSH: 0.0 uIU/ml (0.4-6.2); LH, FSH, ACTH, GH, prolactin and cortisol could not be tested due to lack of reagents
Autoimmune panel	ANA (anti-nuclear antibody) titres less than 1:40; Anti-cardiolipin and anti-B2-glycoprotein IgM / IgG were all within normal limits. Thyroid auto-antibodies and angiotensin converting enzyme (ACE) levels could not be tested.

Computerized visual perimetry

Minor field defects were noted in both temporal fields.

Radiology

Chest X-ray: cardiomegaly, small left sided pleural effusion; Echo: 15 mm pericardial effusion, normal left ventricular function; X-ray of Sella: no evidence of mass lesion, symmetric floor (Figure 1); Non-contrast axial head CT scan: possible asymmetric density within the sella turcica (but no 'empty sella' sign); dorsum sellae poorly visualized (Figure 2).

Management and progress in wards

The patient was started on hormone replacement therapy including thyroxine 50 mcg daily, prednisone 5 mg AM and 2.5 mg PM and a combined oral contraceptive. During her stay in the wards the patient's condition deteriorated abruptly due to an adrenal crisis probably precipitated by the vigorous thyroid hormone replacement. The dose of thyroxine was lowered to 25 mcg daily and the patient kept on normal saline and IV hydrocortisone 100 mg 6hourly. In addition, severe hyponatremia should be managed with water restriction and hypertonic saline infusion; the latter was avoided because of the difficulty monitoring Na$^+$ levels and the associated risk of osmotic demyelination syndrome. Upon discharge three weeks later her rate of speech, mentation and exercise tolerance was significantly better compared to admission. On a two-month follow-up visit, there was a marked reduction in the generalised edema. The thyroxine dosage was subsequently increased gradually to 100 mcg daily. Her hair pattern had normalized in three months. At her five-month follow up visit, it

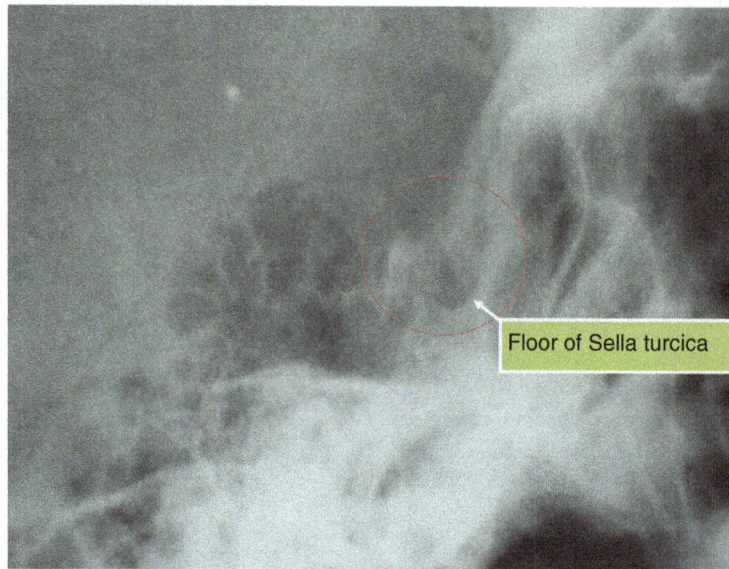

Figure 1 *Sella turcica X-ray* **(lateral view).** Legend: No evidence of mass lesion seen, symmetric floor with no erosion or `double floor` sign.

was noted that she had developed livedo reticularis over her lower extremities bilaterally. (Figure 3) She was subsequently started on anti platelet therapy (junior aspirin 75 mg daily) and the oral contraceptive stopped. The livedo reticularis had disappeared on a subsequent visit. At 16 months, the patient was in good general health except for a headache and occasional palpitations. At this juncture, the thyroxine dose was lowered to 75 mcg daily.

Differential diagnosis
This patient has anterior pituitary insufficiency beginning in the post partum period. Neurohypophyseal involvement is unlikely given the persistently elevated urine specific gravity even post steroid therapy which essentially rules out diabetes insipidus. The most likely differentials are lymphocytic hypophysitis (LyHy) and Sheehan's syndrome. An underlying co-morbid auto-immune condition such as systemic lupus erythematosus (SLE) or anti-phospholipid syndrome is a relevant clinical consideration but is made less likely given her negative antibody screens. Neoplasms and other granulomatous disorders of the hypophysis (tuberculosis, syphilis, sarcoidosis and histiocytosis X) are also possibilities but would be lower on the list of

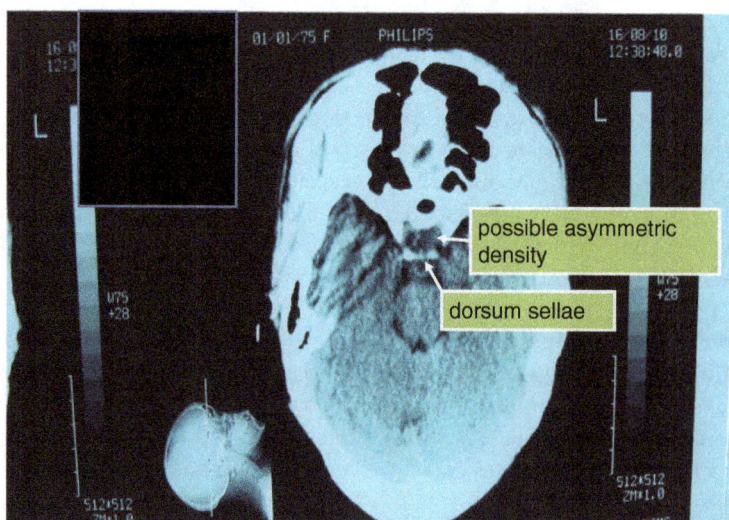

Figure 2 *Non-contrast axial head CT scan* **(at the level of sella).** Legend: Possible asymmetric density within the pituitary gland on the left (but no 'empty sella' sign); dorsum sellae poorly visualized.

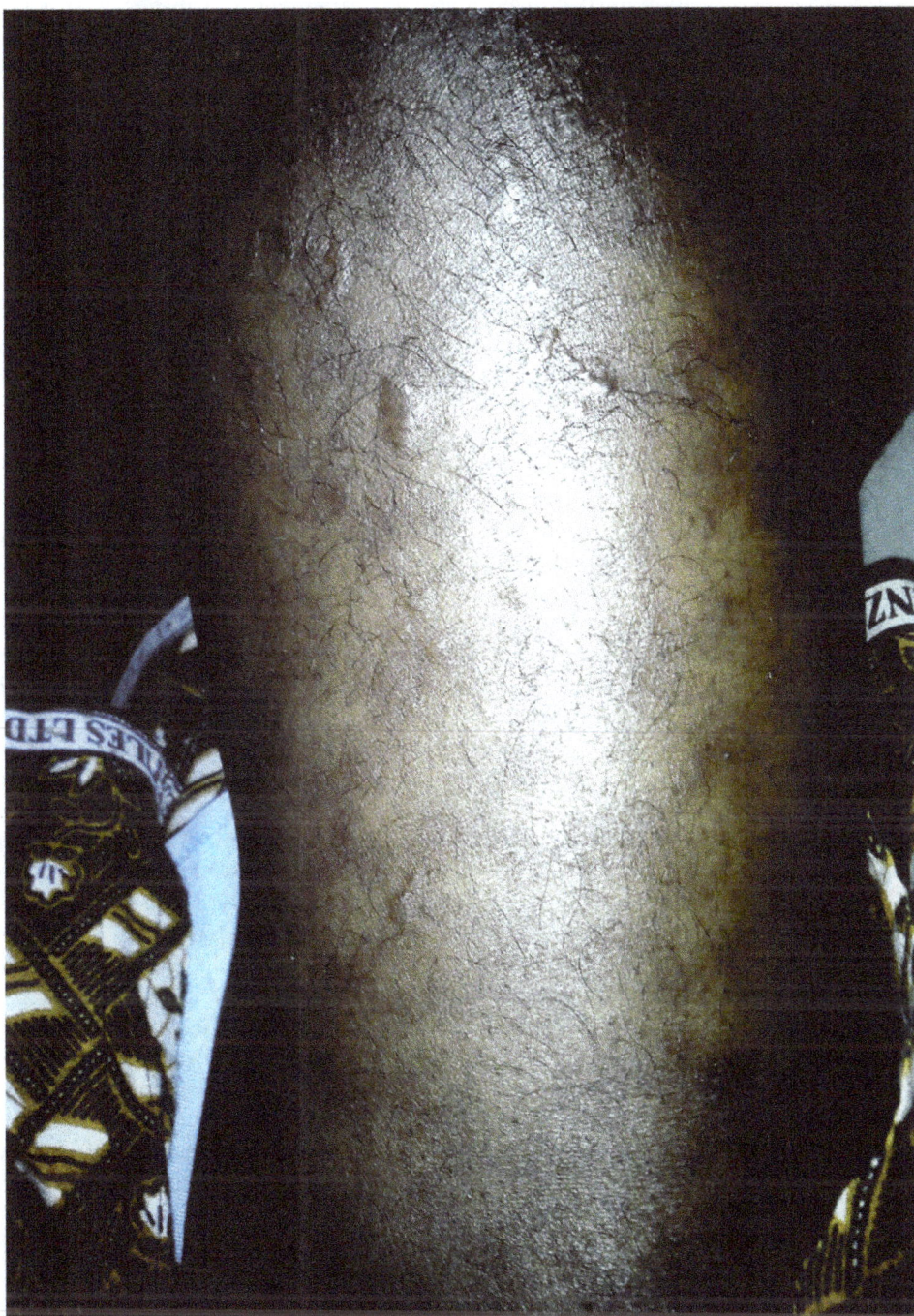

Figure 3 Photograph of proximal left lower extremity at five-month follow up visit. Legend: appearance of diffuse reticular rash consistent with livedo reticularis.

differentials in the absence of appropriate clinical and laboratory evidence.

Discussion

In this patient, the diagnosis of anterior pituitary insufficiency is evident from the constellation of secondary hypothyroidism, secondary amenorrhoea and the clinical manifestations of secondary adrenocortical insufficiency (hypoglycaemia, orthostatic hypotension and marked hyponatremia with low normal K^+ levels). Interestingly, her TSH levels were undetectable which is quite rare in panhypopituitarism but has been previously reported [9]. Also noteworthy in this case is the severe hyponatremia which is likely multifactorial. In secondary adrenal insufficiency, one accepted explanation is that hypocortisolism leads to failure of inhibition of vasopressin secretion. In addition severe secondary hypothyroidism, which this patient also had, leads to a syndrome of inappropriate secretion of ADH (SIADH)-like picture [10-12].

Arriving at an etiologic diagnosis is more challenging. The history of post-partum hemorrhage albeit mild, and lactation failure may favor Sheehan's syndrome (SS) over lymphocytic hypophysitis (LyHy) which is another recognized, but less common cause of post-partum pituitary insufficiency [1,2]. However in light of a history suggestive of painless post-partum thyroiditis, a physical exam which revealed signs of co-existing autoimmune conditions such as alopecia areata and the elevated ESR, the latter provides a better diagnostic fit [2,9,13,14]. While LyHy often presents with hyperprolactinemia from stalk dysfunction leading to galactorrhoea in a quarter to one-third of cases [1,6], agalactia has been reported in 11% of patients [6].

Although, thyroid auto-antibodies could not be tested and her antinuclear antibody and antiphospholipid antibodies were negative, a comprehensive retrospective analysis of 379 patients with lymphocytic hypophysitis (LyHy) by Caturgeli et al found that the prevalence of auto-antibodies for Hashimoto's and SLE was only 7.4% and 1.3% respectively [6]. Similarly; anti-pituitary antibodies could not be assayed however these are considered of limited sensitivity and specificity in the diagnosis of lymphocytic hypophysitis since they are present in other autoimmune conditions and several non-immune pituitary disorders (including Sheehan's syndrome) [6]. In the latter, post partum hemorrhage may trigger pituitary autoimmunity by the release of sequestered antigens following necrosis of the gland [15].

Assessment of visual fields is a simple but very useful diagnostic test. The minor defect in the patient's temporal visual fields detected bilaterally upon visual perimetry may signify an ischemic process secondary to a mass effect at the optic chiasm – this could indicate a pituitary macroadenoma or an infiltrative process such as LyHy. The normal size sella on skull X-ray and CT scan might argue against a large tumor.

MRI is the imaging study of choice for the pituitary [16], the lack of which makes it difficult to accurately diagnose pituitary disease in most hospitals in the developing world. In any case, up to 9% of patients suffering from LyHy have normal imaging findings on CT/MRI. More common presentations include symmetric enlargement of sellar content (66%), thickening of the pituitary stalk (56%), homogenous enhancement (51%) and occasionally asymmetry of the enlarged sellar content (18%) [17]. This differs from the imaging findings in Sheehan's syndrome which almost always results in a partially or completely empty sella that may be normal or reduced in size [18,19].

A definitive diagnosis usually requires a tissue biopsy often obtained via the endonasal transsphenoidal approach which was not possible in this case. Molitch et al have suggested criteria for making a strong presumptive clinical diagnosis non-invasively. These are as follows: a history of gestational / postpartum hypopituitarism, a contrast-enhancing sellar mass with MRI features characteristic of LyHy, a pattern of endocrine deficiency with early loss of adrenocorticotrophic hormone and thyroid-stimulating hormone unlike that found with macroadenomas and pituitary failure disproportionate to size of the mass [20].

Of note, livedo reticularis has never been reported before in patients with a clinical or histopathologic diagnosis of lymphocytic hypophysitis and may be unrelated. However, an association is not inconceivable particularly if the patient were to have an underlying co-morbidity such as SLE, since both LyHy and livedo reticularis have independently been documented in lupus [21,22]. This patient likely meets four (4) of the eleven (11) criteria required for a diagnosis of lupus namely photosensitivity, proteinuria, serositis (pleural and pericardial effusions) and hematologic abnormalities (normocytic anemia) [23]. However her ANA was negative and more specific tests such as anti-ds DNA or anti-Sm antibodies to rule out antinuclear-antibody negative disease were not available.

Finally, does a definitive diagnosis necessarily influence management in post-partum panhypopituitarism? The simple answer is yes - while hormone replacement is often all that is necessary for Sheehan's syndrome, additional measures may be required for patients with LyHy presenting with symptoms of sellar compression. While surgery or pituitary radiotherapy may eventually be needed, in the absence of urgent visual symptoms it is reasonable to advocate using high dose glucocorticoids as first line therapy for LyHy under imaging surveillance if possible; decrease in volume of the pituitary mass and improving hormone status helps to confirm the diagnosis retrospectively [6,17]. Methotrexate and azathioprine can be used for poor responders [24-26]. Among the 320 patients with LyHy followed by Caturgeli, 73% required long term hormone replacement therapy, 16% recovered following mass-reduction without need for hormone-replacement, 8% died probably from irreversible adrenal insufficiency and 3% experienced spontaneous resolution without treatment [6].

Conclusion

In the developing world, post-partum pituitary insufficiency is not altogether a rare clinical entity. The differential diagnosis becomes more challenging if clinical features suggestive of an auto-immune condition are also present. An accurate history and a keen physical exam become indispensable in correctly diagnosing and appropriately managing such patients especially in resource limited settings. A specific diagnosis may allow effective use of pharmacologic therapy before resorting to more invasive measures. There is a dire need for educating health care professionals and the general public since the disorder left undiagnosed has a devastating impact on maternal morbidity and mortality; properly designed epidemiologic studies to quantify the exact magnitude of the problem will be a necessary step towards the solution.

Consent

The patient has provided explicit informed consent for publication of this case report and all accompanying images in a scientific journal.

Abbreviations

ACTH: Adrenocorticotrophic hormone; ANA: Anti-nuclear antibody; BMI: Body mass index; ESR: Erythrocyte sedimentation rate; FSH: Follicle stimulating hormone; GH: Growth hormone; LH: Luteinizing hormone; LyHy: Lymphocytic hypophysitis; MCV: Mean corpuscular volume; SLE: Systemic lupus erythematosus; SS: Sheehan's syndrome; TSH: Thyroid stimulating hormone.

Competing interests

The authors declare that they have no competing interests.

Acknowledgements

We wish to sincerely thank the patient and her family; special thanks to D Gibbs M.D., Ph. D. for proof reading the manuscript and providing valuable insight into the diagnostic process. He is a consultant neurologist at Oregon Health and Science University, Portland OR. Prof Gibbs has completed a research fellowship in neuroendocrinology at UCSD and has over thirty publications in this area of research. We would also like to acknowledge the contributions of the following individuals: H Diefenthal, M.D., Ph.D. (Professor in Diagnostic Radiology Kilimanjaro Christian Medical Centre (KCMC), Tanzania); M Jaffer, M.D. (Physician, Nairobi Kenya); V Maro, M.D. (Head of department, Internal medicine KCMC, Tanzania) and Mr C Mataro (Lab technologist KCMC, Tanzania). Personal funds were utilized during the entire process of patient work up – no external funding was made use of.

Authors' contributions

FGS, WPH and KGK were involved in the initial case diagnosis. FGS and WPH were involved with revising the manuscript for publication. KGK continues clinical follow up of the patient to date. All authors read and approved the final manuscript.

References

1. Karaca Z, Tanriverdi F, Unluhizarci K, Kelestimur F: Pregnancy and pituitary disorders. Eur J Endocrinol 2010, 162(Suppl 3):453–475.
2. Gutenberg A, Hans V, Maximilian J: Primary hypophysitis: clinical-pathological correlations. Eur J Endocrinol 2006, 155(Suppl 1):101–107.
3. Zargar AH, Singh B, Laway BA, Masoodi SR, Wani AI, Bashir MI: Epidemiologic aspects of postpartum pituitary hypofunction (Sheehan's syndrome). Fertil Steril 2005, 84(Suppl 2):523–528.
4. Cénac A, Soumana I, Develoux M, Touta A, Bianchi G: Sheehan's syndrome in Sudano-Sahelian Africa 40 observations. Bull Soc Pathol Exot 1991, 84(Suppl 5):686–692.
5. Sidibe EH: Sheehan's syndrome: experience in Africa. Ann Med Interne (Paris) 2000, 151(Suppl 5):345–351.
6. Caturegli P, Newschaffer C, Olivi A, Pomper M, et al: Autoimmune hypophysitis. Endocr Rev 2005, 26:599–614.
7. Ouma JR, Farrell VJ: Lymphocytic infundibulo- neurohypophysitis with hypothalamic and optic pathway involvement: report of a case and review of the literature. Surg Neurol 2002, 57(Suppl 1):49–53.
8. Castle D, De Villiers JC, Melvill R: Lymphocytic adenohypophysitis. Report of a case with demonstration of spontaneous tumour regression and a review of the literature. Br J Neurosurg 1988, 2(Suppl 3):401–405.
9. Ozawa Y, Shishiba Y: Recovery from lymphocytic hypophysitis associated with painless thyroiditis: clinical implications of circulating antipituitary antibodies. Acta Endocrinol 1993, 128:493–498.
10. Diederich S, Franzen N, Bahr V, Oelkers W: Severe hyponatremia due to hypopituitarism with adrenal insufficiency: report on 28 cases. Eur J Endocrinol 2003, 148:609–617.
11. Raff H: Glucocorticoid inhibition of neurohypophysial vasopressin secretion. Am J Physiol 1987, 252:635–644.
12. Erkut ZA, Pool C, Swaab DF: Glucocorticoids suppress corticotropin-releasing hormone and vasopressin expression in human hypothalamic neurons. J Clin Endocrinol Metab 1998, 83:2066–2073.
13. Ajith C, Gupta S, Bhansali A, Radotra B, Kanwar A, Kumar B: Alopecia areata associated with idiopathic primary hypophysis. Clin Exp Dermatol 2005, 30:250–252.
14. Honegger J, Fahlbusch, Bornemann: Lymphocytic and granulomatous hypophysitis: experience with nine cases. Neurosurgery 1997, 40(Suppl 4):713–722.
15. Goswami R, Kochupillai N, Crock PA, et al: Pituitary autoimmunity in patients with Sheehan's syndrome. J Clin Endocrinol Metab 2002, 87(Suppl 9):4137–4141.
16. Errarhay S, Kamaoui I, Bouchikhi C, et al: Sheehan's Syndrome: A case report and literature review. doi:10.4176/081201 http://www.ncbi.nlm.nih.gov/pmc/articles/PMC3066722/pdf/LJM-4-081.pdf.
17. Kristof RA, Van Roost D, Klingmüller D, et al: Lymphocytic hypophysitis: non-invasive diagnosis and treatment by high dose methylprednisolone pulse therapy? Neurol Neurosurg Psychiatry 1999, 67:398–402.
18. Lee HC, Lee EJ, Lee KW, Ahn KJ, Jung TS, Kim DI, Huh KB: Computed tomographic correlation with pituitary function in Sheehan's syndrome. Korean J Intern Med 1992, 7(Suppl 1):48–53.
19. Bakiri F, Bendib SE, Maoui R, Bendib A, Benmiloud M: The sella turcica in Sheehan's syndrome: computerized tomographic study in 54 patients. J Endocrinol Invest 1991, 14(Suppl 3):193–196.
20. Molitch ME, Gillam MP: Lymphocytic Hypophysitis. Horm Res 2007, 68(Suppl 5):145–150.
21. Ji JD, Lee SY, Choi SJ, et al: Lymphocytic hypophysitis in a patient with systemic lupus erythematosus. Clin Exp Rheumatol 2000, 18(Suppl 1):78–80.
22. Golden R: Livedo reticularis in systemic lupus erythematosus. Arch Dermatol 1963, 87:299–301.
23. Tan EM, Cohen AS, Fries JF, Masi AT, McShane DJ, Rothfield NF, et al: The 1982 revised criteria for the classification of systemic lupus erythematosus. Arthritis Rheum 1982, 25:1271–1277.
24. Leung GK, Lopes MB, Thorner MO, Vance ML, Laws ER Jr: Primary hypophysitis: a single-center experience in 16 cases. J Neurosurg 2004, 101:262–271.
25. Tubridy N, Saunders D, Thom M, Asa SL, Powell M, Plant GT, Howard R: Infundibulohypophysitis in a man presenting with diabetes insipidus and cavernous sinus involvement. J Neurol Neurosurg Psychiatry 2001, 71:798–801.
26. Lecube A, Francisco G, Rodriguez D, Ortega A, Codina A, Hernandez C, Simo R: Lymphocytic hypophysitis successfully treated with azathioprine: first case report. J Neurol Neurosurg Psychiatry 2003, 74:1581–1583.

3

Neurological symptoms in a patient with isolated adrenocorticotropin deficiency

Yukihiro Goto[*], Kazunori Tatsuzawa, Kazuyasu Aita, Yuichi Furuno, Takuya Kawabe, Kei Ohwada, Hiroyasu Sasajima and Katsuyoshi Mineura

Abstract

Background: Isolated adrenocorticotropic hormone (ACTH) deficiency is a pituitary disorder characterized by reduction only in the secretion of ACTH. Although the underlying mechanism remains to be elucidated, numbers of cases with this entity have been increasing. We experienced a case presenting with gait disturbance necessitating differential diagnosis from idiopathic normal pressure hydrocephalus (iNPH).

Case presentation: A 69-year-old female with a complaint of difficulty walking and suspected to have iNPH at a prior hospital was referred to our department. For the prior three years, she had suffered from a progressive gait disturbance. Magnetic resonance imaging (MRI) revealed global ventricular dilatation. The typical features of the gait in iNPH cases were all identifiable. Neuropsychological dementia scale tests showed deterioration. However, the major feature of a disproportionately enlarged subarachnoid-space on MRI was not obvious. The patient developed progressively worsening fatigue during hospitalization. Her symptoms resembled those of hypothalamic-pituitary tumor patients. Serum ACTH and cortisol levels were low. While corticotrophin releasing hormone stress tests showed no response, other stress tests using thyrotropin releasing hormone, luteinizing hormone releasing hormone, and growth hormone releasing hormone yielded normal responses, indicating a diagnosis of isolated ACTH deficiency. We initiated corticosteroid therapy, and her gait disturbance improved promptly.

Conclusion: Isolated ACTH deficiency may have major significance to the differential diagnosis of iNPH. Early consideration of this entity is anticipated to facilitate making an early diagnosis.

Keywords: Isolated ACTH deficiency, Neurological symptom, Gait disturbance, Idiopathic normal pressure hydrocephalus

Background

Isolated adrenocorticotropic hormone (ACTH) deficiency causes adrenal insufficiency as a result of impaired secretion of ACTH but no other anterior pituitary gland hormones. ACTH secretory cell damage, resulting from neurohypophysitis and an autoimmune mechanism, has been implicated in the etiology of this disorder [1]. Definitive diagnosis is relatively simple using serum ACTH measurement and pituitary stimulation tests [2], however, early diagnosis is not always easy because symptoms of adrenal insufficiency such as hypoglycemia and depressive state are nonspecific, and can be misdiagnosed as mental disorders [3]. The number of reports regarding isolated ATCH deficiency has increased along with the popularization of ACTH measurement, and in the field of cerebral/ neurological medical treatment, this disorder should be kept in mind when making a differential diagnosis. We experienced a case of isolated ATCH deficiency presenting with gradually progressive gait disturbance that needed to be distinguished from other forms of idiopathic normal pressure hydrocephalus (iNPH). We describe this case herein, with a review of the relevant literature.

* Correspondence: yoursongmysong@hotmail.com
Department of Neurosurgery, Kyoto Prefectural University Graduate School of Medicine, Kawaramachi-Hirokoji, Kamigyo-ku, Kyoto 602-8566, Japan

Case presentation

The patient was a 65-year-old woman who had undergone surgery at 19 years of age for appendicitis. Her medical history was otherwise unremarkable. Starting 3 years prior to the current presentation, the patient had gradually developed a gait disturbance, for which she consulted a local orthopedic surgery department, and upon diagnosis of knee osteoarthrosis received conservative therapy. At approximately 1 week before admissions, she had begun to experience loss of appetite and vomiting, and consulted a local physician. On suspicion of gastrointestinal disease, a thorough examination of the gastrointestinal tract was performed, but no organic disease was identified. Although the loss of appetite and vomiting resolved spontaneously, the gait disturbance gradually worsened, and magnetic resonance imaging (MRI) of the head revealed ventricular enlargement. The patient was thus referred to our department for suspected iNPH related to the gait disturbance.

Her height of 148.3 cm, weight of 54.4 kg, and body mass index of 24.8 were all within standard ranges.

There was no medical history that could have led to secondary hydrocephalus. There were no abnormalities in vital signs with body temperature 36 °C, blood pressure 110/63 mm/Hg, and heart rate 83 beats per minute. Although the patient's consciousness was clear, 15 on the Glasgow Coma Scale (GCS), and there was no muscle weakness, she walked with her legs apart in short quick steps, and required a walking aid. While muscle tonus was normal, the patient complained of mild pain when extending the knee. As to higher order brain functions, mini mental state examination (MMSE) results were 24/30, and the frontal assessment battery (FAB) results were 9/18. Blood test findings at the time of admission were within normal range apart from mild hypoalbuminemia (total protein 4.6 g/dL, albumin 2.7 g/dL, total cholesterol 147 mg/dL, and LDL cholesterol 100 mg/dL), and elevated thyroid free T3 (TSH 4.333 μIU/mL, free T3 3.78 pg/mL, free T4 1.16 ng/dL). There were no blood-sugar or electrolyte (Na 140 mmol/L, Cl 106 mmol/, K 4.1 mmol/L, serum glucose 73 mg/dL) abnormalities. Head MRI revealed enlargement of all cerebral

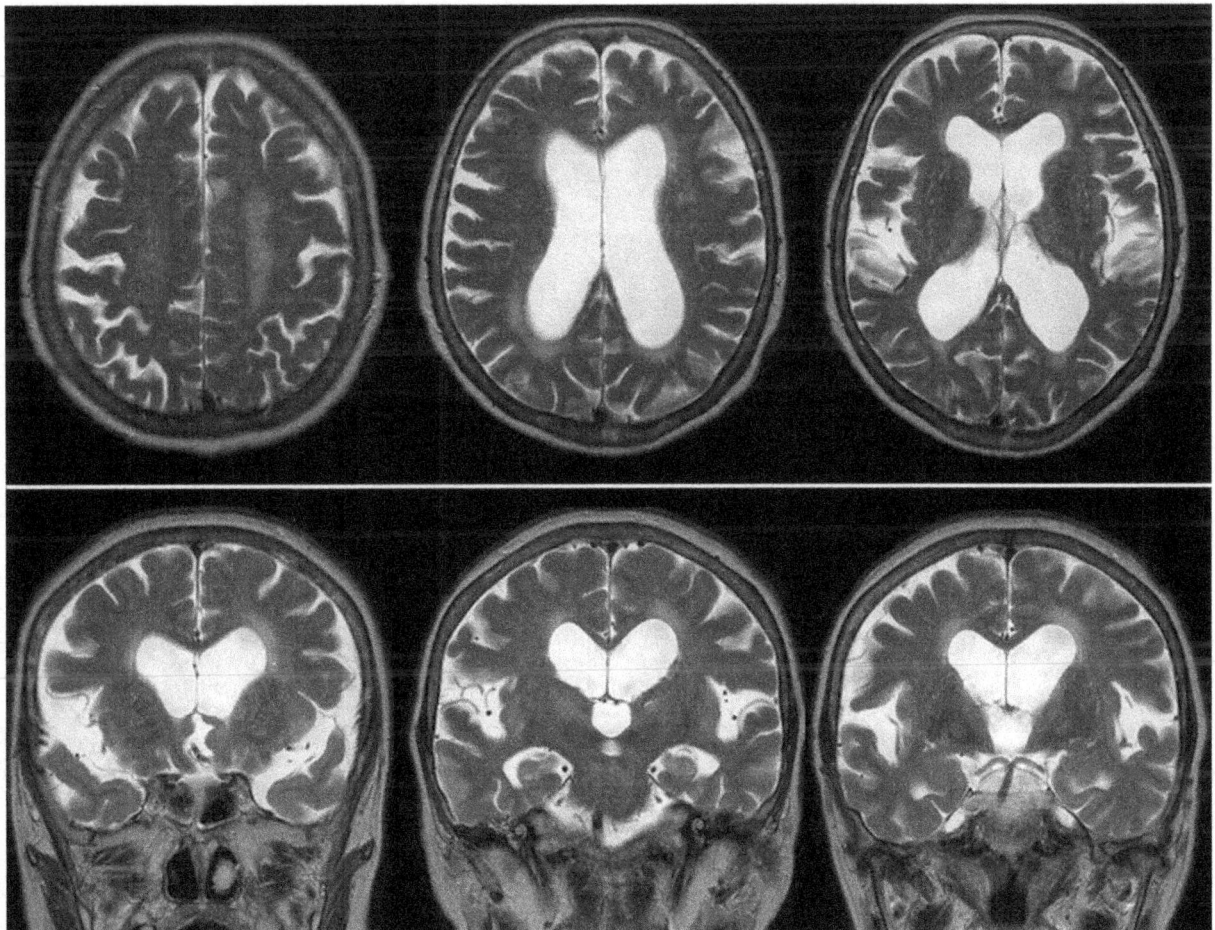

Fig. 1 Upper: T2-weighted axial MRI revealed enlarged ventricles. Lower: In T2-weighted coronal MRI also showed enlarged ventricles, however, the major feature of disproportionately enlarged subarachnoid-space was not obvious

ventricles, with an Evan's index of 0.4, and the Sylvian fissure appeared wide open consistent with iNPH. However, the specific feature of narrowing of the sulci at the high convexity area was not obvious (Fig. 1). Single-photon emission computed tomography revealed reduced cerebral blood flow (CBF) surrounding the Sylvian fissure, with relatively increased CBF in the convexity, which was consistent with the pattern for iNPH (Fig. 2). Findings for the sulci at the high convexity area were inconsistent with typical iNPH, however, and we thus reconsidered the possibility of other diseases that may have caused the gait disturbance.

Detailed tests were ultimately performed after hospital admission including a spinal tap. Following admission, the patient gradually became less active, and tended to stay in bed. Re-examination revealed blood sugar levels of 40 mg/dL and systolic blood pressure of 90 mm/Hg. On suspicion of impaired anterior pituitary function, scans were performed of the pituitary in the diencephalon, and baseline pituitary hormone levels were verified.

The spinal tap results were negative. On MRI, pituitary gland was normal measuring 12 mm in maximum diameter with no enlargement or deviation of stalk, and there were no neoplastic lesions, inflammatory lesions in the pituitary area of the diencephalon, or changes suggesting that surgery had been performed in all sequences including contrast-enhanced dynamic images (Fig. 3). Table 1 presents baseline hormone levels, and Table 2 the results of the anterior pituitary gland hormone loading test using corticotrophin releasing hormone, thyrotropin releasing hormone, luteinizing hormone releasing hormone, and growth hormone releasing hormone. Pituitary hormone results included ACTH <1.0 pg/ml (normal range: 7.2–63.3), and cortisol levels <1.0 μ/dL (normal range: 4.0–18.3), indicating pituitary adrenal insufficiency. There were no decreases in other hormone levels, with relatively mild elevations of growth hormone, prolactin and free T3 levels. We checked carefully again the medical history of the patient, but there were no recent history of exogenous glucocorticoid treatment.

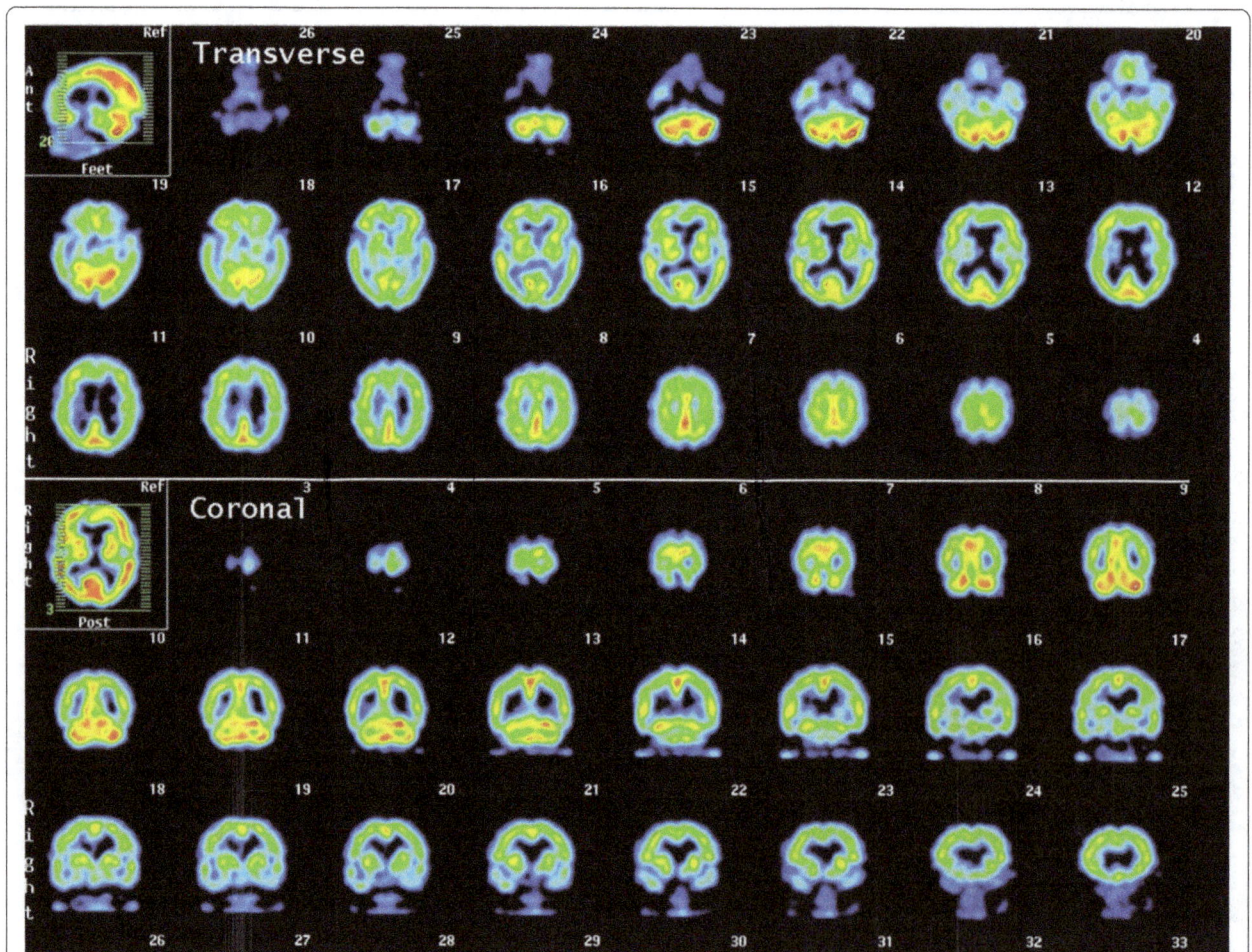

Fig. 2 Single-photon emission computed tomography revealed areas of relatively decreased blood perfusion around the Sylvian fissure, while increased blood perfusion in the external layer around the convexity side

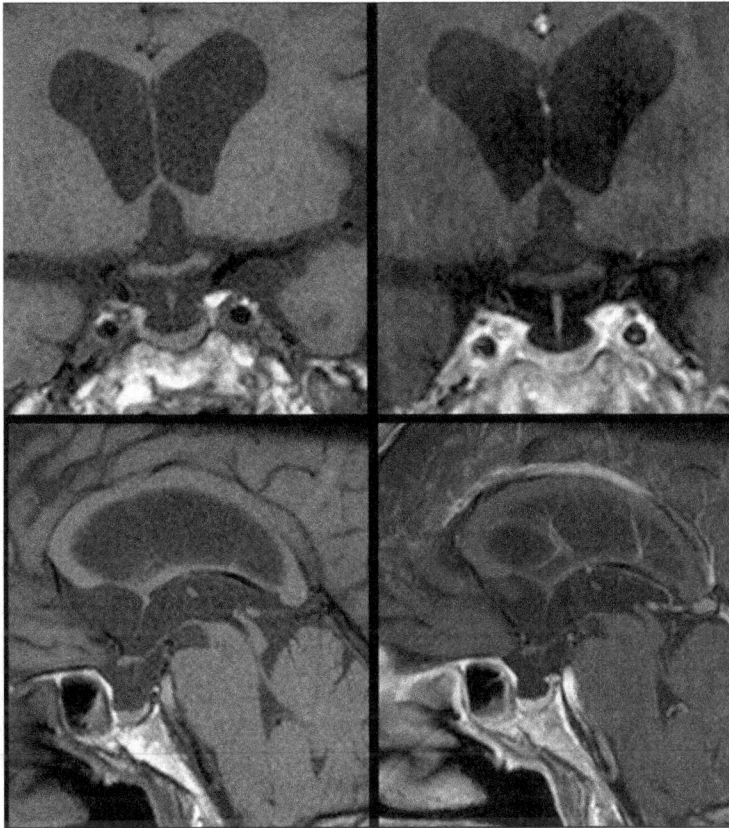

Fig. 3 MRI showed normal pituitary gland measuring 12 mm in maximum diameter with no deviation of stalk, and there is no tumor or inflammatory lesion around the hypothalamic-pituitary area. (Upper left: T1 coronal MRI, Upper right: T1 gadolinium coronal MRI, Upper right: T1 gadolinium sagittal MRI, lower left: T1 gadolinium sagittal MRI)

An additional pituitary stimulation test was performed, in which ACTH and cortisol responses only were found to have disappeared, and isolated ACTH deficiency was thus diagnosed (Fig. 4). After initiation of hydrocortisone supplements, her gait quickly improved. While observing the clinical symptoms, hydrocortisone (Cortril ®) was adjusted to a daily dose of 15 mg, and after instructing the patient as to how to respond on sick days, she was discharged to return home. At approximately 6 months after discharge, although the ventricular enlargement on MRI was same as before, the patient scored 27/30 points on the MMSE and 15/18 points on the FAB.

Table 1 Endocrinogical findings about basal level of anterior pituitary hormone

TSH	4.333μIU/mL (0.350–4.940)
freeT3	3.78 pg/mL (1.71–3.71)
freeT4	1.16 ng/dL (0.70–1.48)
GH	1.85 ng/mL (0.28–1.64)
IGF-1	40 ng/mL (57–175)
LH	17.19 mIU/mL (5.72–64.31)
FSH	48.20 mIU/mL (<157.79)
PRL	34.61 ng/mL (4.91–29.32)
ACTH	<1.0 pg/mL (7.2–63.3)
Cortisol	≤1.0 μg/dL (4.0–18.3)

TSH thyroid stimulating hormone, *IGF* insulin-like growth factor, *LH* luteinizing hormone, *FSH* follicle stimulating hormone, *PRL* prolactin
(): Normal range of each test

Discussion

Isolated ACTH deficiency is caused by damage to the ACTH-producing cells of the pituitary gland and can lead to secondary adrenocortical insufficiency. In 1954, Steinberg and colleagues were the first to report a patient presenting with general fatigue, weight loss, and hypoglycemia which improved after ACTH administration and their case was described as having true pituitary Addison's disease [4]. This disorder has been called isolated ACTH deficiency. With the development and popularization of endocrine tests, the number of such reports has increasing in number.

The mean age at disease onset of patients withisolated ACTH deficiency is 50 years and the male to female is 1.2–3.6: 1, with the disease being slightly more common in men. In some instances, isolated ACTH deficiency is

Table 2 Endocrinogical findings about pituitary function test using CRH, TRH, LHRH and GRH

Time(min)	LH (mIU/mL)	FSH (mIU/mL)	GH (ng/mL)	TSH (µIU/mL)	ACTH (pg/mL)	Cortisol (µg/dL)	PRL (ng/mL)
0	17	58.35	4.77	1.563	<1.0	≤1.0	23.79
30	64.72	79.98	32.9	14.168	<1.0	≤1.0	154.7
60	77.72	88.88	45	11.643	<1.0	≤1.0	108
90	76.4	100.67	21.1	9.143	<1.0	≤1.0	82.13

CRH corticotropin-releasing hormone, *TRH* thyrotropin-releasing hormone, *LHRH* luteinizing hormone-releasing hormone, *GRH* growth hormone releasing hormone

concurrent with primary hypothyroidism and Hashimoto's disease. Furthermore, some cases may also be positive for anti-thyroglobulin antibodies and anti-pituitary antibodies [1], which implies the involvement of an autoimmune mechanism, though the details remain unclear. There have also been a few reports of cases associated with lymphocytic neurohypophysitis [5]. Other reported cases have presented with general fatigue, weight loss, and hyponatremia along with loss of olfaction following head trauma [6].

Isolated ACTH deficiency primarily presents with symptoms of adrenal insufficiency due to lack of ACTH secretion, along with general fatigue, loss of appetite, nausea, vomiting and skin dryness. However, when patients have psychological symptoms such as apathy and depression in addition to the above, the condition can be mistakenly diagnosed as a mental disorder. Thus, diagnosis on the basis of clinical symptoms is not necessarily easy [2]. Our case had symptoms resembling those experienced by patients with pituitary gland lesions of the diencephalon, which allowed us to make an early diagnosis.

In the presence of isolated ACTH deficiency, if low serum ACTH levels are confirmed, then a pituitary

stimulation test will specifically exhibit the disappearance of ACTH only. Serum ACTH levels are usually below the sensitivity threshold of 5.0 pg/ml, though this may vary among reported cases. It is assumed that reported cases with ACTH deficiency also include patients with limited ACTH reserves, i.e. partially impaired ACTH secretion, which would be regarded as ACTH deficiency syndrome based on reports classifying disease severity [2].

Reported cases presenting with neurological symptoms of ACTH deficiency, excluding those in adrenal crisis with induced disturbance of consciousness and psychological symptoms, are relatively rare. There are reported cases presenting with elevated creatinine kinase and predominant proximal muscle weakness that required differential diagnosis from neuromuscular diseases, and that 2 years elapsed between the initial examination, prompted by serum ACTH levels measured incidentally, and definitive diagnosis [7]. The improvements of gait disturbance and cognitive dysfunction in this case are not interpreted in detail. It can be inferred that the replacement therapy cause any metabolic or circulating change as morphological change had not seem in this case. There are case reports describing isolated ACTH deficiency associated with dementia, in which CBF increased on positron emission tomography following hormone replacement therapy, while at the same time cognitive function improved [8].

Treatment for isolated ACTH deficiency involves replacement therapy, and as with more common forms of hypoadrenocorticism, a fixed amount of cortisol, a physiological glucocorticoid, is generally provided as a supplement. As with other adrenal insufficiency replacement therapies, it is vital to instruct patients that the medication dose should be increased at times of stress such as fever and infection.

The symptoms of isolated ACTH deficiency are nonspecific, and diagnosis can be challenging. Cases have been reported in which diagnosis, including differential diagnosis from mental disorders, was difficult. In individuals age 60 years and older, iNPH presents with a triad of symptoms, i.e. gait disturbance, dementia, and urinary incontinence. Gait disturbance, which is a major cause of reduced activities of daily living, can be improved by shunt implantation and is a rare type of

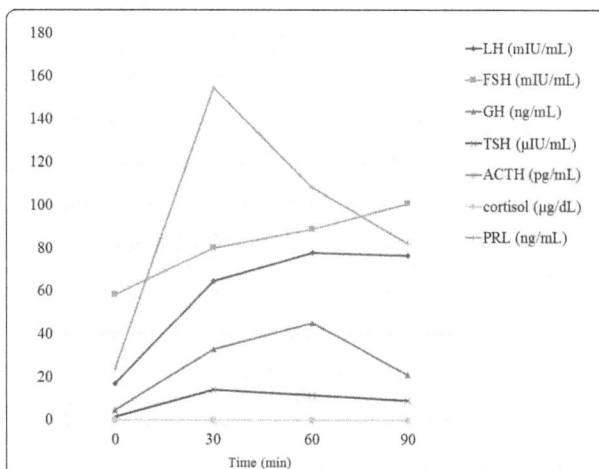

Fig. 4 Pituitary stimulation test using corticotropin-releasing hormone, thyrotropin-releasing hormone, luteinizing hormone-releasing hormone and growth hormone releasing hormone showed no response in plasma cortisol level and ACTH level, while other hormones showed adequate response

treatable dementia. However, gait disturbance and dementia are not limited to iNPH, instead being common in elderly individuals. Furthermore, iNPH is a disease in which caution is essential when differentiating the imaging findings occasionally seen in elderly individuals, such as ventricular enlargement due to atrophy of the cerebrum and cerebrovascular changes that develop with aging.

In the iNPH treatment guidelines, ventricular enlargement is defined by an Evan's index of 0.3 or above, and although this is one criterion required to make the diagnosis of this disorder, an Evan's index greater than 0.3 is seen in 3–4 % of healthy elderly individuals, and thus cannot be called a specific finding [9]. Characteristic findings of iNPH include a wide-open Sylvian fissure and narrowing of the sulci at the high convexity. In the present case, although iNPH was suspected on the basis of ventricular enlargement, no narrowing of the sulci was observed at the high convexity area. When the typical diagnostic findings of iNPH are not present, it is vital to keep isolated ACTH deficiency in mind when performing the differential diagnosis.

Conclusion

Isolated ATCH deficiency can cause a variety of clinical symptoms. Hormone replacement therapy improves symptoms, and early diagnosis is closely related to patient prognosis. In patients suspected of having iNPH with an atypical clinical presentation and imaging findings, isolated ACTH deficiency should be considered early.

Consent

Written informed consent was obtained from the patient for publication of this case report and any accompanying images. A copy of the written consent is available for review by the Editor of this journal.

Abbreviations

CBF: cerebral blood flow; FAB: frontal assessment battery; GCS: Glasgow coma scale; iNPH: idiopathic normal pressure hydrocephalus; MMSE: mini mental state examination; MRI: magnetic resonance imaging.

Competing interests

The authors declare that they have no competing interests.

Authors' contributions

YG and KT treated the patient and drafted the article. YF and KO did the spinal tap test. TK and KI did the pituitary stimulation test. KM and HS analyzed the data and critically revised the manuscript. All authors read and approved the final manuscript.

Acknowledgments

We thank Dr Kei Yamada (MD, PhD, Department of Radiology, Kyoto Prefectural University Graduate School of Medicine) for supply the MR images.

References

1. Murakami T, Wada S, Katayama Y, Nemoto Y, Kugai N, Nagata N. Thyroid dysfunction in isolated adrenocorticotropic hormone (ACTH) deficiency: case report and literature review. Endocr J. 1993;40:473–8. PubMed Abstract: http://www.ncbi.nlm.nih.gov/pubmed/7920902. Publisher Full Text: https://www.jstage.jst.go.jp/article/endocrj1993/40/4/40_4_473/_article.

2. Stacpoole PW, Interlandi JW, Nicholson WE, Rabin D. Isolated ACTH deficiency: a heterogeneous disorder. Critical review and report of four new cases. Medicine. 1982;61:13–24. PubMed Abstract: http://www.ncbi.nlm.nih.gov/pubmed/6276646.

3. Morigaki Y, Iga J, Kameoka N, Sumitani S, Ohmori T. Psychiatric symptoms in a patient with isolated adrenocorticotropin deficiency: case repor t and literature review. Gen Hosp Psychiatry. 2014;36:449 e3-5. PubMed Abstract: http://www.ncbi.nlm.nih.gov/pubmed/24725972 Publisher Full Text: http://www.sciencedirect.com/science/article/pii/S0163834314000620

4. Steinberg A, Shechter FR, Segal HI. True pituitary Addison's disease, a pituitary unitropic deficiency; fifteen-year follow-up. J Clin Endocrinol Metab. 1954;14:1519–29. Publisher Full Text: http://press.endocrine.org/doi/pdf/10.1210/jcem-14-12-1519.

5. Richtsmeier AJ, Henry RA, Bloodworth Jr JM, Ehrlich EN. Lymphoid hypophysitis with selective adrenocorticotropic hormone deficiency. Arch Intern Med. 1980;140:1243–5. PubMed Abstract: http://www.ncbi.nlm.nih.gov/pubmed/6250507 Publisher Full Text: http://archinte.jamanetwork.com/article.aspx?articleid=600261.

6. Scoble JE, Havard CW. Anosmia and isolated ACTH deficiency following a road traffic accident. Case report. J Neurosurg. 1990;73:453–4. PubMed Abstract: http://www.ncbi.nlm.nih.gov/pubmed/2166780 Publisher Full Text: http://thejns.org/doi/pdf/10.3171/jns.1990.73.3.0453.

7. Kubo N, Itokazu N, Inoue S. A case of isolated ACTH deficiency with neuromuscular symptoms. No to Hattatsu. 1997;29:67–72. Publisher Full Text: https://www.jstage.jst.go.jp/article/ojjscn1969/29/1/29_1_67/_pdf.

8. Nagai Y, Shimizu H, Sato N, Mori M. A case of isolated ATCH deficiency. Folia Endocrinol. 1994;70:989–94. Publisher Full Text: https://www.jstage.jst.go.jp/article/endocrine1927/70/9/70_989/_pdf.

9. Mori E, Ishikawa M, Kato T, Kazui H, Miyake H, Miyajima M, et al. Guidelines for management of idiopathic normal pressure hydrocephalus: second edition. Japanese Society of Normal Pressure Hydrocephalus. Neurol Med Chir. 2012;52:775–809. PubMed Abstract: http://www.ncbi.nlm.nih.gov/pubmed/23183074. Publisher Full Text: https://www.jstage.jst.go.jp/article/nmc/52/11/52_2012-0247/_article.

4

Clinical experiences and success rates of acromegaly treatment: the single center results of 62 patients

Mehtap Evran[*], Murat Sert and Tamer Tetiker

Abstract

Background: This study aimed to report the clinical and outcome data from a large cohort of patients diagnosed with acromegaly and treated at our institution over a 20-year period.

Methods: Sixty-two acromegaly patients (32 women and 30 men) treated and monitored at the endocrinology polyclinic between 1984 and 2013 were enrolled in this retrospective study. Clinical features and patients' treatment outcomes were evaluated. A level of growth hormone (GH) of <2.5 ng/ml was considered as the criterion for remission, and the normal insulin-like growth factor (IGF) range was based on gender and age.

Results: The mean age at the time of diagnosis was 38.8 ± 1.4 years, the time to diagnosis was 4.5 ± 0.3 years, and the follow-up duration was 7.3 ± 0.8 years. Among patients' symptoms, growth in hands and feet and typical facial dysmorphism were the most prominent (92%). The number of patients with diabetes mellitus, hypertension and hyperprolactinemia were 22 (35%), 13 (21%) and 13 (21%), respectively. Microadenomas and macroadenomas were found in eight and 54 patients, respectively. A significant correlation was found between the initial tumor diameters and GH levels ($p = 0.002$). The mean GH and IGF-1 levels were 39.18 ± 6.1 ng/ml and 993.5 ± 79 ng/ml, respectively. Visual field defect was found in 16 patients (32%). Thirty-one patients were treated by transsphenoidal surgery. Four of these were cured, 10 patients developed postoperative anterior pituitary hormone deficiency, and one patient developed diabetes insipidus. Twenty patients were treated by transcranial surgery, of which two were cured, while 17 patients developed postoperative anterior pituitary hormone deficiency. In total, five of the patients who were not cured after surgery were given conventional radiotherapy, of which two were cured. Four of 15 patients, on whom Gamma Knife radiosurgery was performed, were cured. Biochemical remission was achieved in 32 of 52 patients who received octreotide treatment, and in two of five patients who received lanreotide treatment.

Conclusions: The rate of surgical success in our patients was found to be low. This could be explained by an absence of experienced pituitary surgical centers or surgeons in our region, and the fact that most patients presented late at the macroadenoma stage.

Keywords: Acromegaly, Diagnosis, Treatment, GH, IGF-1, Pituitary hormone deficiency

Background

Acromegaly is a rare condition with a prevalence of around 60 in 1,000,000 [1]. The cause in most patients is a pituitary adenoma that produces growth hormone (GH). Serum insulin-like growth factor 1 (IGF-1) concentration increases when its production is stimulated by GH over-secretion. The clinical features of the disease occur because of the peripheral effects of excessive GH and IGF-1, as well as tumor pressure. Diagnosis is made based on increased serum basal GH level, an IGF-1 level higher than normal limits for gender and age, and an absence of suppression in serum GH levels (>1.0 ng/ml) by the oral glucose tolerance test (OGTT). In acromegaly, progressive deformations occur in the body, especially in the face and extremities, the severity of which are associated with the time to diagnosis. The condition may also cause other morbidities such as arterial hypertension,

* Correspondence: mehtap.evran@hotmail.com
Department of Internal Medicine, Division of Endocrinology, Balcali Hospital, Cukurova University Medical Faculty, 01330 Adana, Turkey

cardiomyopathy, sleep apnea syndrome, diabetes mellitus (DM), menstrual irregularities, arthropathy, and peripheral neuropathy. Sometimes acromegaly occurs together with hyperprolactinemia [2]. The risk of malignancy, particularly colon cancer, is increased in acromegalic patients [3,4]. The first treatment option for acromegaly is removal of the pituitary adenoma by an experienced surgeon at a specialist center for pituitary surgery. If surgery is unsuccessful, treatment using somatostatin analogs (SA), dopamine agonists, GH antagonist and/or Gamma Knife radiosurgery can be used [5]. For the disease to be considered under control, the basal GH level should be <2.5 ng/ml, GH levels should be <1.0 ng/ml by the OGTT, and the IGF-1 levels should be within normal limits based on the patient's age and gender [6,7].

In this study, we report the clinical and outcome data from a large cohort of acromegalic patients who were diagnosed and followed up over a 20-year period at our institution.

Methods
Patients
Sixty-two acromegaly patients (32 women and 30 men) diagnosed, treated and monitored at our endocrinology polyclinic between 1984 and 2013 were enrolled in this retrospective study. The files of the patients diagnosed before 2007 were reviewed, and their details were evaluated. Patients diagnosed after 2007 were included in the 62 patients and were followed prospectively in this study. In addition to the demographics of the patients, we reviewed time to diagnosis, age at the time of diagnosis, clinical examination findings, assessment of field of vision, follow-up time, treatment approach (surgical, radiotherapy, drug treatment and/or their combination) and the outcomes of these treatments. Postoperative pituitary hormone deficiency, tumor diameter, serum GH and IGF-1 levels based on age and gender, and GH response to oral glucose challenge were assessed. IGF-1 levels could not be measured before 2001 at our center; consequently, 21 of our patients did not have IGF-1 levels available at the time of diagnosis. This paper is undertaken in accordance with the ethical standards laid down in the 1964 Declaration of Helsinki and its later amendments. The local ethical committee of Cukurova University approved the study.

Hormone assays
A chemiluminescence immunoassay was used to measure patients' serum GH and IGF-1 levels (Immulite 2000, Siemens; ng/ml), and prolactin levels (DxI 800, Beckman Coulter; ng/ml). For imaging of the pituitary gland, pituitary CT was used in 10 patients, and pituitary MRI was used in 52 patients.

In our study, biochemical remission was defined as a basal GH <2.5 ng/ml, post-OGTT GH <1 ng/ml and IGF-1 level within normal limits based on age and gender [8]. Cases that showed permanent remission after a successful surgery or radiotherapy (conventional radiotherapy or Gamma Knife) were considered cured.

Statistical analysis
Statistical analyses using the Shapiro–Wilk, Mann–Whitney U and Chi-squared tests were performed. For correlations between the groups, the Pearson correlation was used for the parameters that fitted normal distribution, and Spearman's tests were used for the parameters that did not the fit normal distribution. The results were expressed as n (%) and SE ± mean and a p value of less than 0.05 was considered significant. SPSS-19 software was used for all statistical analyses.

Results
Characteristics of patients
Demographic and clinical characteristics of the patients are shown in Table 1. The most common symptoms, seen in 55/62 (92%) of patients, were transversal growth-thickening in hands and feet and facial dysmorphism (such as prominent forehead, separation of teeth, prognathism, and growth of cartilage). Additionally, hyperprolactinemia was found in 13/62 patients at the time of diagnosis, with four of these patients also presenting with galactorrhea. Visual field defect was found in 16/50 patients who underwent visual field examinations. The most common conditions that coexisted with acromegaly in patients were DM (35%) and hypertension (21%).

Laboratory and imaging findings of patients
Patients' GH and IGF-1 levels before treatment are shown in Table 1 and Figure 1. The patients' pituitary CT/MRI images revealed microadenomas (<10 mm) in eight patients, and macroadenomas (>10 mm) in 54/62 (86%) patients. The tumor diameter of the patients with macroadenomas was 10–20 mm in 16 patients (25.8%), and >20 mm in 31 patients (50%). Cavernous sinuous invasion was found in 25 patients. There was a significant correlation between the initial tumor diameters and preoperative GH levels ($p = 0.002$).

Surgical treatment methods and outcomes
Treatment methods and outcomes are summarized in Table 2. Thirty-four patients underwent surgery in our center performed by one of two surgeons, six patients underwent surgery in another center performed by the same surgeon, four patients underwent surgery in different centers by the same surgeon and the remaining 12 patients underwent surgery in four other centers performed by different surgeons. Thirty-one patients (50%) underwent transsphenoidal surgery, with four attaining postoperative cure. Three of these latter patients had microadenoma,

Table 1 Demographic and clinical characteristics of acromegaly patients at the time of diagnosis

	SE ± mean (Range)		n	(%)
Age (years)	46.2 ± 1.4 (18–75)	Number of microadenomas	8/62	(13%)
Age at the time of diagnosis (years)	38.2 ± 1.4 (8–65)	Number of macroadenomas	54/62	(87%)
Time to diagnosis (years)	4.5 ± 0.3 (1–14)	Hyperprolactinemia	13/62	(21%)
Follow-up duration	7.3 ± 0.8 (1–29)	Hypertension	13/62	(21%)
GH level (ng/ml); (n = 54)	39.18 (2.1–179)	Diabetes Mellitus	22/62	(35%)
#IGF-1 level (ng/ml); (n = 41)	993.5 ± 79 (262–3000)	Carpal Tunnel Syndrome	2/62	(3.2%)
IGF-1 level (n = 1)*	1700 ± 0	Menstrual irregularity	4/32	(12.5%)
IGF-1 levels (n = 4)**	1318 ± 788	Loss of libido	2/62	(3.2%)
IGF-1 levels (n = 17)***	770.5 ± 694	Galactorrhea	4/62	(6.5%)
IGF-1 levels (n = 19)****	1078 ± 1249	Headache	4/62	(6.5%)
		Typical facial findings and growth in hands and feet	55/62	(92%)

#IGF-1 levels (based on age and gender).
*Male, for 6–8 years; normal range of IGF-1: 110-565 ng/ml.
**Female and male, for 16–25years; normal range of IGF-1: 182-780 ng/ml.
***Female, for > 25 years; normal range of IGF-1: 123-463 ng/ml.
****Male, for > 25 years; normal range of IGF-1: 123-463 ng/ml.

and one had macroadenoma. Two of the 20 patients who underwent transcranial surgery attained postoperative cure. One of these had macroadenoma, and one had microadenoma. Four of the patients who did not attain cure after transsphenoidal surgery underwent transcranial surgery again. None of these patients attained postoperative cure after the second surgery. Within the patients who could not be cured following pituitary surgery, eight underwent surgery a second time, two received surgery three times and one seven times.

Pituitary deficiency rates
Pituitary hormones were evaluated prior to transsphenoidal surgery in only one patient, which revealed evidence of preoperative pituitary hormone deficiency in this patient. The other 61 patients were evaluated postoperatively only. In the postoperative period, one or more anterior pituitary hormone deficiencies were found in 10 patients,

and permanent diabetes insipidus (DI) was found in one patient. One patient, who underwent transcranial surgery after transsphenoidal surgery, developed hypothyroidism.

In the 17 patients who underwent transcranial surgery, one or more anterior pituitary hormone deficiencies were detected during the postoperative period.

Outcomes of radiotherapy and gamma knife radiosurgery
Conventional radiotherapy was performed on only five patients, two of whom attained cure (their durations to cure were 5 and 10 years). These five patients also received postoperative octreotide treatment. Four of the 15 patients who received Gamma Knife treatment attained cure (the duration to cure was 5 years for two patients, 4 years for one patient, and 3 years for one patient). Seven of the remaining 11 patients achieved biochemical remission with postoperative octreotide treatment. Further treatment of the patients who did not enter remission is ongoing.

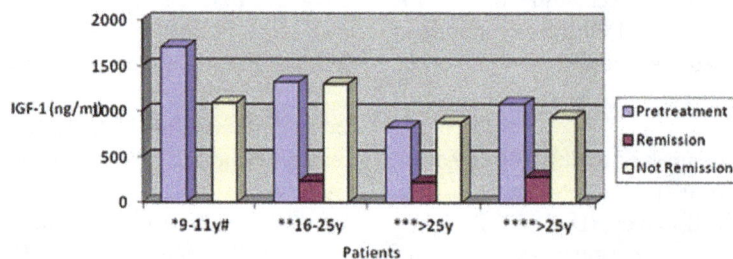

Figure 1 Before and after treatment IGF-1 levels of the patients (normal range is given according to age and gender). # y: years *Male; normal range of IGF-1: 110-565 ng/ml (n = 1), **Female and Male; normal range of IGF-1: 182-780 ng/ml (pretreatment n: 4, posttreatment n:5; remission:3) ***Female; normal range of IGF-1: 123-463 ng/ml (prereament n:17, posttreatment n:26; remission:21) **** Male; normal range of IGF-1: 123-463 ng/ml (pretreatment n:19, posttreatment n:23; remission:13).

Table 2 Rate of treatment response for different disease subtypes and treatment strategies in acromegaly patients

	Number of patients		Number of patients responded to treatment	
	n	(%)	n	(%)
Microadenomas	8	(13%)	4	(50%)
Macroadenomas	54	(87%)	8	(15%)
Transsphenoidal surgery	31	(52%)	4	(12.9%)
Transcranial surgery	20	(32.3%)	2	(10%)
Multiple surgery	11	(17.7%)		
Radiotherapy	20	(32.2%)	6	(30%)*
Only drug treatment	6	(9.6%)	3	(50%)**
Octreotide LAR	52	(84%)	32	(61.5%)**
Lanreotide	5	(8%)	2	(40%)**
Conventional radiotherapy + ocreotide LAR	5	(8%)	2	(40%)**
Gamma Knife + octeotide LAR	11	(17.7%)	7	(63%)**

*The number of patients who achieved cure by Gamma Knife and conventional radiotherapy.
**Biochemical remission.

Drug treatment and outcomes

SA treatment without surgery was administered in six patients owing to the lack of eligibility or consent for surgery. Four of these patients received primary octreotide LAR, while the remaining two were given primary lanreotide. The treatment dose of octreotide was 20–30 mg/month, and normalization was achieved in serum GH and IGF-1 levels in three of the four patients. The biochemical remission durations with medication of these three patients were 6, 8 and 11 years, respectively. No remission could be achieved in two patients who received primary lanreotide treatment (90–120 mg/month).

Forty-eight of the 62 patients who did not achieve postoperative success were given octreotide LAR treatment, and 29 of these 48 patients (60.2%) achieved remission. Likewise, a further three patients who did not achieve postoperative success were given lanreotide treatment and two of these (66.6%) achieved remission. The drug dose was increased to 120 mg for these patients (Figure 2). In total, 32 of the 52 patients (61.5%)

who were given octreotide treatment, and two of the five patients (40%) who were given lanreotide treatment, achieved GH levels of <2.5 ng/ml, and IGF-1 levels within normal limits based on age (Figure 1).

Tumor reduction

In two of the four patients who received octreotide treatment without surgery, the tumor diameter did not change (3- and 8-year follow-ups, respectively). In the other two patients, a reduction in tumor diameter was detected (from 8 to 7 mm after 6 years and from 15 to 12 mm after 12 years, respectively). In one of the two patients who received 60 mg/month of lanreotide treatment without surgery, a marked reduction in tumor diameter was observed after 6 months (from 33 to 20 mm), while in the other patient, a smaller reduction was observed after 1 year (from 11 to 9 mm).

Of the 32 patients in whom a reduction in tumor size was observed, only 20 achieved biochemical remission. Indeed, there was no significant relationship between tumor diameter and achievement of cure (p = 0.06). Interestingly, anterior pituitary hormone deficiency was found in three of eight patients with microadenoma (37.5%) and in 25 of 54 patients with macroadenoma (46.3%); this difference was statistically significant (p = 0.005; Table 3).

Discussion

Our study has made it possible to review the most important findings and challenges in managing a large cohort of acromegaly patients over a 20-year period. Although acromegaly can be seen in all ages, the average age of onset is 32 years. However, as it progresses subclinically, the diagnosis is delayed by between 4 and 10 years [1,2]. This duration has decreased recently, for example, in a study of 100 patients, the delay in diagnosis was found to be 3.2 years [9]. More frequent MRI performed for different reasons may be one explanation for earlier incidental diagnosis of acromegaly [10]. In our patients, the age average at the time of diagnosis was found to be 38.8 ± 1.4 years, and the time to diagnosis was found to be 4.5 ± 0.3 years.

The typical features of acromegaly develop over time, and their severity is associated with a patient's age, GH

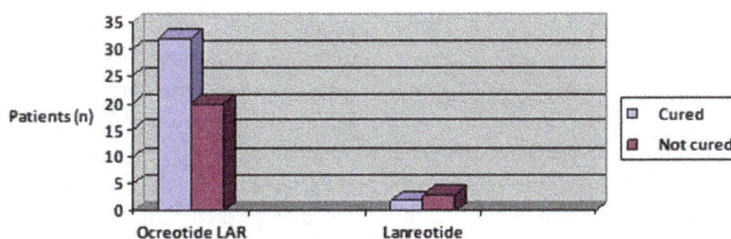

Figure 2 According to pharmacotherapy remission rates of the patients.

Table 3 Frequency of pituitary hormone deficiency in the postoperative period by disease subtype

Deficient hormones	Microadenomas (n)	Macroadenomas (n)
TSH		8
ACTH	2	
TSH + ACTH		6
FSH + LH		3
TSH + ACTH + FSH + LH		6
TSH + FSH + LH	1	2
ADH	1	
Total*	4	25

*Transsphenoidal: Anterior pituitary hormone deficiency in 10 patients, and DI in one patient.
TSH deficiency in one patient who underwent transcranial surgery after transsphenoidal surgery.
Transcranial: Anterior pituitary hormone deficiency in 17 patients.

and IGF-1 levels, tumor diameter and delay in diagnosis. Indeed the delay in diagnosis can be explained, in part, by the fact that any facial changes are often attributed to aging; old photographs of the patient are therefore a useful diagnostic tool. Skeletal and soft tissue changes, organomegaly and typical facial changes are also common [11]. The most common symptoms of our patients, seen in 92%, were growth in hands and feet, and facial dysmorphism. Additionally, acromegaly patients have an increased incidence of DM, hypertension, cardiovascular diseases, breathing problems, osteoporosis and osteoarticular dysfunctions compared with the normal population. The incidence of glucose intolerance is 16–46%, and the incidence of DM is 19–56% [12,13]. The anti-insulinergic effects of GH are considered to be responsible for the pathogenesis of acromegaly. In many cases, when acromegaly is cured, DM is also cured [14]. The most common conditions that coexisted with acromegaly in our patients were DM (35%) and hypertension (20.9%), in keeping with the literature.

The incidence of hyperprolactinemia in pituitary acromegaly patients is approximately 30–40%. The reasons for hyperprolactinemia are pressure on the pituitary stalk or simultaneous secretion of prolactin from tumor cells [15-17]. Incidence of simultaneous secretion of GH and prolactin is around 25% [18]. In our cohort, 13 patients (21%) were found to have hyperprolactinemia at the time of diagnosis, a significantly higher rate than that described in the study by Moyes et al. (13%) [19].

Around 40% of patients are diagnosed in clinics other than endocrinology for symptoms and findings of increased cranial pressure. For instance, neurological symptoms and vision problems may occur because of growth of a pituitary adenoma [11]. The incidence of visual field defect owing to increased pressure is around 19–20% in the literature [20]. The rate of visual field

defect in our patients was 32%. In keeping with the published literature, imaging detected macroadenomas in 54 of our patients (87%) [7,21].

In acromegaly, serum basal GH measurement, post-OGTT GH measurement and IGF-I levels measurement are the gold standard assays for measuring disease activity and monitoring the effectiveness of treatment. While GH measurement has become more sensitive in the recent decades, IGF-1 measurements can be misleading in situations such as malnutrition, liver disease and kidney failure [22,23]. In particular, inconsistencies between GH and IGF-1 measurements can be seen throughout SA treatment [17]. Our patients usually showed a positive correlation between the average GH levels and IGF-1 levels at the time of diagnosis and during SA treatment.

The first treatment option in acromegaly is transsphenoidal tumor excision, particularly for intrasellar microadenomas and noninvasive macroadenomas. In situations such as patient non-consent, existence of serious cardiomyopathy and respiratory disease or absence of an experienced surgeon, then other treatment options are considered. The finding of visual field defect or neurological deficit is almost always an urgent surgical indication [24,25]. We also apply transsphenoidal surgery as the first treatment option for many of our patients.

In a previous retrospective study of 100 patients who underwent transsphenoidal surgery with a remission criterion of GH <5 mU/l, 42% of the patients achieved postoperative remission. In this study, the remission rates were associated with tumor diameter and preoperative GH levels, and 21 patients were found to have pituitary hormone deficiency [26]. The postoperative cure rate of patients who underwent transsphenoidal surgery was 12.9%. In studies where remission criteria were considered to be either GH <2.5 ng/ml, post-OGTT GH <2 ng/ml or IGF-1 within normal limits based on age and gender, the remission rates after transsphenoidal surgery were found to be 38, 57 and 37%, respectively, and the anterior pituitary hormone deficiency rates were found to be 35, 8 and 10%, respectively [7,27,28]. Currently, the reported success of intrasellar surgery varies between 75 and 95% for intrasellar microadenomas, and between 45 and 68% for noninvasive macroadenomas, if undertaken by experienced surgeons who perform at least 50 case surgeries per year [24,29]. When our patients were evaluated, four of 31 patients who were operated transsphenoidally attained postoperative cure. Three of these patients had microadenoma, and one had macroadenoma. While anterior pituitary hormone deficiency was found only in one patient before surgery, it was found in 37% of the patients after surgery. The rate of post-operative pituitary hormone deficiency was found to be lower in our cohort compared with the study by Sheaves et al., but higher than that observed by Swearingan et al. [26,27].

Although the first approach in treatment is transsphenoidal surgery, a transcranial approach is required in some situations such as suprasellar tumor expansion. In another study with remission criteria similar to ours with a follow-up period of 19 years, 26 of 668 acromegaly patients underwent transcranial surgery. The postoperative remission rate of these was 7.7%, the anterior pituitary hormone deficiency rate was 5%, and the rate of permanent DI was 11.5%. In the latter series, 140 patients were re-operated, and the remission rate increased to 27.1% [30]. In our study, two of the 20 patients who were operated on transcranially attained postoperative cure, one of whom had macroadenoma and the other microadenoma. In the patients who did not achieve cure after transsphenoidal surgery and then underwent transcranial surgery, none attained cure, with only one developing secondary hypothyroidism. Although our data on pituitary hormone deficiency before transcranial surgery was insufficient, the rate of patients with anterior pituitary hormone deficiency after transcranial surgery was 85%, a markedly higher rate compared with similar published cohorts. Additionally, the rate of anterior pituitary hormone deficiency in our patients who underwent transcranial surgery was significantly higher than in the patients who underwent transsphenoidal surgery (p < 0.001).

The success of treatment in acromegaly is negatively correlated with tumor diameter and basal GH levels and positively correlated with the experience of the surgeon. Additionally, if the tumor is invasive, this decreases the likelihood of successful surgery [24,31]. Indeed, when we assessed our results based on tumor size, 50% of those with microadenoma and 15% of those with macroadenoma were cured. Unfortunately, owing to small sample numbers, assessment of significance was not feasible. Precise tumor diameter was significantly associated with GH level (p = 0.002), but did not correlate with cure rate (p = 0.06). Additionally, only 20 of 32 patients whose tumor diameters reduced developed biochemical remission. Twenty-five of our patients also had cavernous sinuous invasion.

Another important factor that affects success rate is the number of surgeons who can perform this surgery, and the number of pituitary surgeries performed by the surgeons. Additionally, a greater number of years of surgical experience also increases the surgical success rate [25]. Our cure rate after transsphenoidal and transcranial surgery was very low compared with the literature. More than half of our patients (n = 34) were operated on in our center by one of two surgeons while the others were operated on in several external centers. The lack of experience of our surgeons in pituitary surgery, the absence of a single specialist operating center and the existence of macroadenoma or cavernous sinuous invasion at the time of diagnosis are therefore likely contributors to our low surgical success rate.

Radiotherapy is preferred in situations where surgery is contraindicated or unsuccessful, or when medical treatment is insufficient in controlling GH secretion [32]. An average of 60% of patients who receive conventional radiotherapy attain GH and IGF-1 normalization, but the maximum response is seen after 10–15 years [24,33]. While conventional radiotherapy is preferred in large recidive tumors or in tumors close to the optical nerve, Gamma Knife radiosurgery is preferred in smaller tumors. The 5-year remission rates following Gamma Knife is between 29 and 60% [34]. The incidence of pituitary deficiency for both methods is similar [28,31]. Some of our patients who did not achieve cure after surgery received radiotherapy. Thirty percent of the patients who received conventional radiotherapy or Gamma Knife attained cure, and a further 50% entered biochemical remission. The time to cure was 5–10 years for the two patients who received conventional radiotherapy, and 3–5 years in the four patients who received Gamma Knife. Thus, our rate of cure with surgical treatment and radiotherapy was 19.3% (12 patients), which is in keeping with the literature.

It has been shown in vitro that natural somatostatin inhibits GH secretion in many GH-secreting tumors. For this reason, SAs have been developed for treating acromegaly. Somatostatin analogs work by activating somatostatin receptors. There are, however, major gastrointestinal side effects associated with these drugs. Long-lasting forms of somatostatin analogs are preferred, and octreotide LAR and lanreotide autogel are in current clinical use in Turkey, but not pasireotide. Pegvisomant is a GH receptor antagonist, which can be used alone or in combination with SAs [17]. Somatostatin analogs can be used for situations when there is little possibility of surgical cure such as large extrasellar tumors without pressure effect, in patients who cannot be controlled biochemically with surgery, and to provide biochemical control while waiting for the effect of radiotherapy. Although there are data that show that preoperative SA use has benefits on GH and IGF-1 normalization and on postoperative hospitalization, some studies have concluded that it does not [24,35]. Some studies have shown that with use of somatostatin analogs, biochemical remission is attained, and tumors become smaller in size [36,37]. Several long-term retrospective studies have reviewed the effects of SA given postoperatively and/or primarily, and have reported a wide variation of biochemical remission rates of between 34 and 95% [38,39]. Investigations comparing efficacy of lanreotide and octreotide treatments have reported a similar rate of cure of symptoms and biochemical cure for both agents [40-42].

It should be kept in mind that our study is not a study for evaluating response to primary SA treatment. In our study, we used serum GH <2.5 ng/ml and IGF-1 normalization as biochemical remission criterion, and the serum

GH and IGF-1 levels of our patients who received drug treatment decreased significantly compared with the baseline (p < 0.001). When we review all our patients with regards to biochemical remission, we see that 32/52 patients (61.5%) who received octreotide treatment and 2/5 patients (40%) who received lanreotide treatment are in biochemical remission. However, it should be noted that 10 of the patients who achieved biochemical remission received Gamma Knife, and five received conventional radiotherapy; therefore, the cause of remission may be multifactorial in these patients.

In a recent study by Coloa et al., which followed up 45 acromegalic patients, no improvement in glucose intolerance or DM prevalence was seen [37]. However, we observed improvement in DM in four of the 22 patients in our cohort who were initially diagnosed with DM. Two of these patients, whose blood glucose levels improved were in remission and one of them was cured.

A notable restriction of our study was that the file archiving system was more irregular and insufficient in previous years, and therefore we did not have access to a full range of data for all patients. For example, the initial IGF-1 level was the most important predictor of adequate response to treatment [43]; however, this measurement was not available for some patients. Furthermore, we did not have access to data concerning presence or absence of pituitary hormone deficiency before treatment. Additionally, the majority of our patients were operated on in different centers by different surgeons and some patients did not attend our hospital for assessment with optimum regularity. Indeed, infrequent monitoring may be an additional contributing factor to the low rate of cure in our cohort compared with the literature.

In conclusion, we believe the rate of successful treatment of acromegaly will increase with earlier diagnosis, greater surgical experience and regular and appropriate follow-up after surgery. Future prospective studies of large cohorts will help to provide further information on appropriate treatment strategies in this disease.

Competing interests

The authors declare that they have no competing interests. The authors declare that they have no a relationship with the organization that sponsored the research.

Authors' contributions

ME, MS and TT carried out the endocrinological studies, participated in the sequence alignment and drafted the manuscript. All authors read and approved the final manuscript.

Acknowledgements

We thank the local biochemistry laboratory staff and the nurses of endocrinology departmant for their help.

References

1. Holdaway IM, Rajasoorya C: Epidemiology of acromegaly. Pituitary 1999, 2:29–41.
2. Colao A, Ferone D, Marzullo P, Lombardi G: Systemic complications of acromegaly: epidemiology, pathogenesis and management. Endocr Rev 2004, 25:102–152.
3. Rokkas T, Pistiolas D, Sechopoulos P, Margantinis G, Koukoulis G: Risk of colorectal neoplasm in patients with acromegaly: a meta-analysis. World J Gastroenterol 2008, 14:3484–3489.
4. Orme SM, McNally RJ, Cartwright RA, Belchetz PE: Mortality and cancer incidence in acromegaly; a retrospective cohort study. United Kingdom acromegaly study group. J Clin Endocrinol Metab 1998, 83:2730–2734.
5. Melmed S, Casanueva FF, Cavagnini F, Chanson P, Frohman L, Grossman A, Ho K, Kleinberg D, Lamberts S, Laws E, Lombardi G, Vance ML, Werder KV, Wass J, Giustina A: Guidelines for acromegaly management. J Clin Endocrinol Metab 2002, 87:4054–4058.
6. Giustina A, Chanson P, Bronstein MD, Klibanski A, Lamberts S, Casanueva FF, Trainer P, Ghigo E, Ho K, Melmed S, Acromegaly Consensus Group: A consensus on criteria for cure of acromegaly. J Clin Endocrinol Metab 2010, 95:3141–3148.
7. Krzentowska-Korek A, Golkowski F, Baldys-Waligorska A, Hubalewska-Dydejczyk: A Efficacy and complications of neurosurgical treatment of acromegaly. Pituitary 2011, 14:157–162.
8. In From TIETZ's fundamentals of clinical chemistry. 6th edition. Edited by Burtis CA, Ashwood ER, Bruns DE. Philadelphia: Saunders Elsevier; 2007.
9. Nachtigall L, Delgado A, Swearingen B, Lee H, Zerikly R, Klibanski A: Changing patterns in diagnosis and therapy of acromegaly over two decades. J Clin Endocrinol Metab 2008, 93(Suppl 6):2035–2041.
10. Bengtsson BA, Edén S, Ernest I, Odén A, Sjögren B: Epidemiology and long-term survival in acromegaly. A study of 166 cases diagnosed between 1955 and 1984. Acta Med Scand 1988, 223(Suppl 4):327–335.
11. Lugo G, Pena L, Cordido F: Clinical manifestations and diagnosis of acromegaly. Int J Endocrinol 2012, 10.
12. Kreze A, Kreze-Spirova E, Mikulecky M: Risk factors for glucose intolerance in active acromegaly. Braz J Med Biol Res 2001, 34(Suppl 11):1429–1433.
13. Biering H, Knappe G, Gerl H, Lochs H: Prevalence of diabetes in acromegaly and Cushing syndrome. Acta Med Austriaca 2000, 27(Suppl 1):27–31.
14. Colao A, Baldelli R, Marzullo P, Ferretti E, Ferone D, Gargiulo P, Petretta M, Tamburrano G, Lombardi G, Liuzzi A: Systemic hypertension and impaired glucose tolerance are independently correlated to the severity of the acromegalic cardiomyopathy. J Clin Endocrinol Metab 2000, 85(Suppl 1):193–199.
15. Melmed S, Kronenberg HM: In Anterior pituitary from Wiiliams textbook of endocrinology. 11th edition. Edited by Kronenberg HM, Melmed S, Polonsky KS, Larsen PR. Philadelphia: Saunders Elsevier; 2008:209–223.
16. Barkan AL, Stred SE, Reno K: Increased growth hormone pulse frequency in acromegaly. J Clin Endocrinol Metab 1989, 69(Suppl 6):1225–1233.
17. Andersen M: GH excess: diagnosis and medical therapy. Eur J Endocrinol 2014, 170:31–41.
18. Chanson P, Salenave S: Acromegaly. Orphanet J Rare Dis 2008, 3:1–17.
19. Moyes V, Metcalfe K, Drake W: Clinical use of cabergoline as primary and andjunctive treatment for acromegaly. Eur J Endocrinol 2008, 159(Suppl 5):541–545.
20. AACE Acromegaly Guidelines Task Force: AACE medical guidelines for clinical practice for the diagnosis and treatment of acromegaly. Endocr Pract 2004, 10:213–225.
21. Daud S, Hamrahian AH, Weil RJ, Hamaty M, Prayson RA, Olansky L: Acromegaly with negative pituitary MRI and no evidence of ectopic source: the role of transphenoidal pituitary exploration? Pituitary 2011, 14(Suppl 4):414–417.
22. Giustina A, Barkan A, Casanueva FF, Cavagni F, Frohman L, Ho K, Veldhuis J, Wass J, Von Werder K, Melmed S: Criteria for cure of acromegaly: a consensus statement. J Clin Endocrinol Metab 2000, 85(Suppl 2):526–529.
23. Cordero RA, Barkan AL: Current diagnosis of acromegaly. Rev Endocrine Metab Dis 2008, 9(Suppl 1):13–19.
24. Melmed S, Colao A, Barkan A, Molitch M, Grossman AB, Kleinberg D, Clemmons D, Chanson P, Laws E, Schlechte J, Vance ML, Ho K, Giustina A: Guidelines for acromegaly management: an update. J Clin Endocrinol Metab 2009, 94:1509–1517.
25. Gittoes NJL, Sheppard MC, Johnson AP, Stewart PM: Outcome of surgery for acromegaly—the experience of a dedicated pituitary surgeon. QJM 1999, 92(Suppl 12):741–745.

26. Sheaves R, Jenkins P, Blackburn P, Huneidi AH: **Outcome of transsphenoidal surgery for acromegaly using strict criteria for surgical cure.** *Clin Endocrinol (Oxf)* 1996, **45**(Suppl 4):407–413.

27. Swearingen B, Barker FG, Katznelson L, Biller BM, Grinspoon S, Klibanski A, Moayeri N, Black PM, Zervas NT: **Long-term mortality after transsphenoidal surgery and adjunctive therapy for acromegaly.** *J Clin Endocrinol Metab* 1998, **83**(Suppl 10):3419–3426.

28. Erturk E, Tuncel E, Kiyici S, Ersoy C, Duran C, Imamoglu S: **Outcome of surgery for acromegaly performed by different surgeons: importance of surgical experience.** *Pituitary* 2005, **8**(Suppl 2):93–97.

29. Bates PR, Carson MN, Trainer PJ: **Wide variation in surgical outcomes for acromegaly in the UK.** *Clin Endocrinol* 2008, **68**(Suppl 1):136–142.

30. Nomikos P, Buchfelder M, Fahlbusch R: **The outcome of surgery in 668 patients with acromegaly using current criteria of biochemical 'cure'.** *Eur J Endocrinol* 2005, **152**:379–387.

31. Cozzi R, Montini M, Attanasio R, Albizzi M, Lasio G, Lodrini S, Doneda P, Cortesi L, Pagani G: **Primary treatment of acromegaly with octreotide LAR: a long-term (up to nine years) prospective study of its efficacy in the control of disease activity and tumor shrinkage.** *J Clin Endocrinol Metab* 2006, **91**:1397–1403.

32. Powell JS, Wardlaw SL, Post KD, Freda PU: **Outcome of radiotherapy for acromegaly using normalization of insulin-like growth factor I to define cure.** *J Clin Endocrinol Metab* 2000, **85**(Suppl 5):2068–2071.

33. Minniti G, Jaffrain-Rea ML, Osti M, Esposito V, Santoro A, Solda F, Gargiulo P, Tamburrano G, Enrici RM: **The long-term efficacy of conventional radiotherapy in patients with GH-secreting pituitary adenomas.** *Clin Endocrinol (Oxf)* 2005, **62**:210–216.

34. Pollock BE, Jacob JT, Brown PD, Nippoldt TB: **Radiosurgery of growth hormone-producing pituitary adenomas: factors associated with biochemical remission.** *J Neurosurg* 2007, **106**:833–838.

35. Carlsen SM, Lund-Johansen M, Schreiner T, Aanderud S, Johannesen O, Svartberg J, Cooper JG, Hald JK, Fougner SL, Bollerslev J: **Preoperative octreotide treatment in newly diagnosed acromegalic patients with macroadenomas increases cure short-term postoperative rates: a prospective, randomized trial.** *J Clin Endocrinol Metab* 2008, **93**:2984–2990.

36. Cozzi R, Attanasio R, Montini M, Pagani G, Lasio G, Lodrini S, Barausse M, Albizzi M, Dallabonzana D, Pedroncelli AM: **Four-year treatment with octreotide-long-acting repeatable in 110 acromegalic patients: predictive value of short-term results?** *J Clin Endocrinol Metab* 2003, **88**(Suppl 7):3090–3098.

37. Colao A, Renata SA, Galdiero M, Lombardi G, Pivonello R: **Effects of initial therapy for five years with somatostatin analogs for acromegaly on growth hormone and insulin-like growth factor-I levels, tumor shrinkage, and cardiovascular disease: a prospective study.** *J Clin Endocrinol Metab* 2009, **94**(Suppl 10):3746–3756.

38. Ayuk J, Stewart SE, Stewart PM, Sheppard MC: **Long-term safety and efficacy of depot long-acting somatostatin analogs for the treatment of acromegaly.** *J Clin Endocrinol Metab* 2002, **87**(Suppl 9):4142–4146.

39. Bhayana S, Booth GL, Asa SL, Kovacs K, Ezzat S: **The implication of somatotroph adenoma phenotype to somatostatin analog responsiveness in acromegaly.** *J Clin Endocrinol Metab* 2005, **90**(Suppl 11):6290–6295.

40. Al-Maskari M, Gebble J, Kendall-Taylor P: **The effect of a new slow-release, long-acting somatostatin analogue, lanreotide in acromegaly.** *Clin Endocrinol* 1996, **45**:415–421.

41. Turner HE, Vadivale A, Keenan J, Wass JAH: **A comparison of Lanreotide and Octreotide LAR for treatment of acromegaly.** *Clin Endocrinol* 1999, **51**:275–280.

42. Ozturk FY, Cil E, Ozderya A, Karaman O, Zuhur SS, Altuntas Y: **Unsatisfied treatment outcomes of acromegaly patients: a single center experience in Turkey.** *Endocrin Abstract 12th Eur Cong Endocrinol* 2010, **22**:569.

43. Espinosa-de-los-Monteros AL, Gonzalez B, Vargas G, Sosa E, Mercado M: *Ocreotide LAR treatment of acromegaly in "real life":longterm outcome at tertiary care center.* Publishing Springer; 2014. onlineservice@springer.com. Pituitary, Published Online: 30 April.

5

Novel MEN 1 gene findings in rare sporadic insulinoma

Viveka P. Jyotsna[1*], Ekta Malik[2], Shweta Birla[2] and Arundhati Sharma[2]

Abstract

Background: Insulinomas, which are rare tumors causing hyperinsulinemic hypoglycemia are usually sporadic but may also occur in association with multiple endocrine neoplasia type 1 (MEN-1) syndrome an autosomal dominant disorder caused by MEN1 gene mutations. MEN1 encodes a nuclear protein Menin, a tumor suppressor which acts as an adapter and interacts with partner proteins involved in crucial activities like transcriptional regulation, cell division, proliferation and genome stability.
This study reports on clinical findings and mutation screening in sporadic insulinoma patients.

Methods: Seventeen patients diagnosed with insulinoma were recruited along with 30 healthy volunteers who acted as controls for the present study. The patients presented with symptoms of sweating, tremors, drowsiness, palpitations, loss of consciousness, abnormal behavior, seizures and weight gain. Detailed clinical and family history was collected from all the participants along with 5 ml of blood sample after taking informed consent.
Genomic DNA isolated from blood was subjected to MEN1 gene amplification followed by direct sequencing. Nucleotide sequences obtained were compared with published MEN1 cDNA sequences. Prediction of functional effects of novel changes was done using various bioinformatics algorithms.

Results: Molecular analysis revealed presence of three novel exonic mutations (M561K, Q192K and Q261Q), two novel intronic variations c.445-44G → A and c.913-42G → C in introns two and six respectively and three reported exon SNPs; H433H (rs540012), D418D (rs2071313), A541T (rs2959656) and one intronic SNP (rs669976).

Conclusions: The study identified presence of novel pathogenic MEN1 mutations in sporadic cases of insulinoma. The new mutations identified were in regions involved in defective binding of menin to proteins implicated in genetic and epigenetic mechanisms. The outcome of the study extends the growing list of MEN1 pathogenic mutations even in sporadic cases providing consequential insight into phenotypic heterogeneity and in the expression of individual mutations.

Background

Insulinomas are neuroendocrine tumors of the pancreas with an incidence of 0.4 % [1] and present clinically with hypoglycemia [2]. They are usually benign solitary tumours [3] but 5–12 % of the cases have distant metastasis at diagnosis. Most of the insulinomas arise sporadically, but 5–8 % may develop as part of the hereditary multiple endocrine neoplasia type 1 (MEN1) syndrome [4, 5]. Insulinoma is the second most common

hormone secreting pancreatic neuroendocrine tumor in MEN1. Other pancreatic neuroendocrine tumors are gastriomas, glucagonomas, vasoactive intestinal polypeptidomas and their occurrence is 40–70 % in MEN1 patients [6]. Most of the insulinomas are small in size (<2 cm) and over 99 % of them originate in the pancreas with rare cases derived from ectopic pancreatic tissue [7]. Surgical removal is the main treatment and the neurological sequelae of hypoglycemia after surgery have been shown to revert [8].

MEN 1(OMIM 613733) located on chromosome 11q13.1, consists of ten exons spanning a region of >9 Kb of genomic DNA [9] and encodes a 621 amino acid protein 'menin', a putative tumor suppressor gene associated

* Correspondence: vivekapjyotsna@gmail.com
[1]Department of Endocrinology and metabolism, All India Institute of Medical Sciences, Room No. 305, Third Floor, Biotechnology Building, New Delhi, India
Full list of author information is available at the end of the article

with insulinoma [10]. Menin acts as an adapter and interacts with partner proteins involved in crucial activities like transcriptional regulation, cell division, proliferation and genome stability. Although located predominantly in the nucleus, in the non dividing cells it is found in the cytoplasm also [11]. We report here the results of MEN 1 screening in 17 sporadic insulinoma patients along with their clinical findings.

Methods

The study protocol adhered to the tenets of the Declaration of Helsinki and was approved by the Institutional Ethics Committee of All India Institute of Medical Sciences, New Delhi. Written informed consent was obtained from each patient for publication of individual clinical details.

A total of 17 patients diagnosed with insulinoma from the department of Endocrinology and Metabolism and 30 healthy volunteers as controls were recruited for the present study. Insulinoma was suspected when a patient presented with recurrent hypoglycemia and a diagnosis of insulinoma was made when during spontaneous or fast induced hypoglycemia plasma glucose was <45 mg/dl, serum insulin was > 6 μU/ml and C peptide was > 2.5 ng/ml [2]. After a biochemical diagnosis of hyperinsulinomic hypoglycemia was confirmed, localization of insulinoma was done by various imaging modalities like multiphasic CT, MRI, arterial calcium stimulation and venous sampling, endoscopic ultrasound and intraoperative ultrasound. After localization, the tumor was removed and location and size of the tumor intraoperatively was noted. From all the participants detailed family history was noted and peripheral blood drawn in EDTA vials for DNA extraction.

Mutation analysis

Genomic DNA was isolated from peripheral blood leukocytes using standard protocol and subjected to PCR amplification of all the MEN1 coding exons using 80–100 ng DNA, 1.25 mM MgCl2, 0.25 mM of each of the dNTPs (Invitrogen, Carlsbad, CA, USA), 20pM of each primer and 0.5 units of Taq Polymerase (Invitrogen, Carlsbad, CA, USA) in a 25 ul volume mixture using thermocycler ABI 9700 (Applied Biosystems, Foster City, CA).

All the amplified products were purified using Qiagen kits (Qiagen, GmbH, Hilden, Germany) and were then sequenced using ABI-3100 Genetic Analyzer (ABI).

Nucleotide sequences were compared with the published cDNA sequences of MEN1 gene (GenBank accession number ENST00000312049). Prediction of functional effects of the novel variations was done using algorithms Mutation Taster, SIFT and PROVEAN.

Results

Out of 17 patients, ten were males and seven were females. Main presenting symptoms were recurrent hypoglycemia, seizures, confusion and excessive weight gain. History of sweating, tremors and drowsiness was present in all (100 %) the patients, 13 (76.47 %) patients had palpitations, weakness and weight gain whereas only 12 (70.59 %) patients had loss of consciousness, abnormal behavior and seizures. Out of all, 15 (88.24 %) patients had been to the neurologist and/or psychiatrist for treatment before a diagnosis of insulinoma was made. The mean age at presentation was 35 ± 13 years. The mean duration of symptoms was 3.56 years (range 1 to 15 years) before diagnosis of insulinoma was established. The mean levels of insulin was 17.36 μU/ml (range 6.5 to 153), C peptide was 5.05 ng/ml (range 0.88 to 11.90) and mean plasma glucose of 32.86 mg/dl (range 18 to 45 mg/dl).

Other components of MEN1 syndrome were ruled out by taking history of symptoms, noting sign and laboratory tests. Clinical features of anterior pituitary tumors asked for were irregular periods, galactorrhoea, and infertility in females, erectile dysfunction in males, headache, visual impairment, central obesity and proximal muscle weakness in both. Signs looked for were presence of violaceous stria, buffalo hump, acral enlargement, prognathism, frontal bossing, thyroid enlargement. Clinical features of hyperparathyroididm asked for were bone pain, history of fractures, renal stones and abdominal pain. Laboratory testes performed to rule out pituitary or parathyroid tumors were serum fasting prolactin, ACTH, cortisol, growth hormone and insulin like growth factor1, T4, TSH, intact PTH, calcium and phosphorus. These symptoms/signs were absent and tests were normal in all the patients.

There was no history of consanguinity in any of the families. Only one patient (6 %) had malignant insulinoma and rests were benign. Insulinomas were found located in different parts of the pancreas and the sites of the primary tumors were junction of neck and body in one patient (6 %), uncinate process in two patients (12 %) and in seven patients each (41 %) it was located in head and tail of the pancreas (Table 1). All the patients (100 %) underwent surgery as curative procedure. Only one patient underwent resection twice because of recurrence of the tumor at different times.

MEN1 screening revealed presence of novel changes which include two non-synonymous missense mutations; M561K in which a nucleotide changes from T to A resulted in amino acid methionine being replaced by lysine at codon 561 in exon ten and Q192K resulting due to sequence variation C > A leading to amino acid change from Glutamine to Lysine at codon 192.

Table 1 Tumor characteristics and MEN1variations in insulinoma patients

ID.	Age/Sex	Tumour characteristics			MEN1 variations found
		Location	Size	Nature	
M1	35/M	3	2.0 [a]2.0 cm	B	Q260R[a]
					A541T (rs2959656)[d]
					H433H (rs 540012)[d]
M2	38/M	3	4.8[a]5.9 cm	M	H433H (rs 540012)[d]
M3	23/M	3	1.0[a]0.8 cm	B	H433H (rs 540012)[d]
					D418D (rs2071313)[d]
M4	34/M	3	0.8[a]0.9 cm	B	H433H (rs 540012)[d]
					A541T (rs2959656)[d]
M5	42/M	3	1.0 x 0.8 cm	B	H433H (rs 540012)[d]
					D418D (rs2071313)[d]
M6	35/F	2	2.0 [a]2.0 cm	B	Q260R[a]
					H433H (rs 540012)[d]
					D418D (rs2071313)[d]
					A541T (rs2959656)[d]
M7	65/F	2	1.5[a]1.2 cm	B	M561K[a]
					H433H (rs 540012)[d]
					D418D (rs2071313)[d]
					A541T (rs2959656)[d]
					Intronic rs 669976 [e]
M8	50/F	2	3.0[a]2.0 cm	B	H433H (rs 540012)[d]
					D418D (rs2071313)[d]
					A541T (rs2959656)[d]
M9	25/M	4	4.0[a]5.0 cm	B	H433H (rs 540012)[d]
					A541T (rs2959656)[d]
M10	29/F	4	1.0[a]0.5 cm	B	H433H (rs 540012)[d]
					A541T (rs2959656)[d]
M11	16/M	3	1.0 x 1.0 cm	B	H433H (rs 540012)[d]
					A541T (rs2959656)[d]
M12	18/F	3	2.0 x 1.0 cm	B	H433H (rs 540012)[d]
					Intronic rs 669976 [e]
					A541T (rs2959656)[d]
M13	17/M	4.	2.0 [a]2.0 cm	B	Q192K [a]
					H433H (rs 540012)[d]
M14.	45/F	1	3.0[a]2.0 cm	B	Q261Q[b]
					H433H (rs 540012)[d]
					D418D (rs2071313)[d]
					A541T (rs2959656)[d]
M15.	46/M	4	1.0[a]1.0 cm	B	H433H (rs 540012)[d]
					A541T (rs2959656)[d]

Table 1 Tumor characteristics and MEN1variations in insulinoma patients *(Continued)*

M16.	30/M	4	1.0[a]1.0 cm	B	Intronic c.913-42G → C[c]
					H433H (rs 540012)[d]
					D418D (rs2071313)[d]
M17	41/F	4	0.85[a]0.65 cm	B	Intronic c.445-44G → A[c]
					H433H (rs 540012)[d]
					A541T (rs2959656)[d]

Legend: *M* male, *F* female, *B* benign, *M* malignant, 1-junction of neck and body of the pancreas, 2-uncinate process of the pancreas, 3-head of the pancreas, 4-tail of the pancreas. [a] - novel non synonymous exonic mutations, [b]- novel synonymous exonic mutation, [c] novel intronic variations, [d] -reported exonic polymorphisms, [e]- reported intronic polymorphisms

A novel synonymous mutation (Q261Q) resulting in a nucleotide change from G to A at codon 261 was also identified with no change in the amino acid glutamine (Q).

Three reported exonic polymorphisms were identified: H433H (rs540012) in all patients and controls, D418D (rs2071313) in 8 (47 %) patients; none of the controls and A541T (rs2959656) in 11 (65 %) patients and in all the controls.

A reported intronic polymorphism rs669976 was identified in two (12 %) patients and was absent in all the controls. Two novel intronic variations c.445-44G → A in intron 2 and c.913-42G → C located in intron six were also identified (Table 1).

Assessment for pathogenicity using MutationTaster, PROVEAN and SIFT predicted all the novel exonic mutations and novel intronic variation (c.913-42G → C) to be deleterious and disease causing alterations.

To confirm the findings from genetic screening and bioinformatics analysis, 30 healthy controls were screened to check for the presence of the novel variations. The changes were not identified in any of them eliminating their possibility of being polymorphisms.

Discussion

In the present study we report clinical and genetic findings of 17 patients diagnosed with insulinoma. Clinical presentations of insulinomas are diverse and heterogeneous. Hypoglycaemia results in various neuroglycopenic and adrenergic symptoms. Neuroglycopenic symptoms include many psychiatric and neurological manifestations like behavioural changes, confusion, agitation, blurred vision and finally seizures [12, 13]. All the 17 patients (100 %) in the present report had hypoglycemia with neurological manifestations like confusion and seizures.

Pancreatic islet cell tumors can be the first manifestation in 15 % of all the MEN1 cases [14]. Insulinoma may arise either due to loss of heterozygosity (LOH) of the chromosome region 11q13 or due to presence of various mutations in the MEN-1 gene [15, 16] in accordance with the Knudson's hypothesis on cancer [17]. Most

of the insulinomas are benign and are found located anywhere in the pancreas and surgical removal is the first line of treatment. Malignant insulinomas are comparatively rare and are found in around 5–12 % of reported insulinoma cases [18] . Without curative treatment MEN1 insulinomas are found to be associated with earlier mortality in the patients[19]

In the present study, only one patient (6 %, $n = 17$; 38 years, male) had malignant insulinoma. The size of the tumor was 4.8*5.9 cm located in the head of the pancreas with multiple metastases in the liver. He was operated and died within two years of diagnosis. No MEN1 mutation was identified in this patient indicating possible presence of other important genetic events like involvement of other unidentified gene/s, chromosomal instability resulting in insulinoma development, and probably the presence of phenocopies [15, 20]. Rest of the patients had benign tumors for which they got operated and are alive without recurrence of the disease.

The MEN1 gene encodes 'menin' which is a nuclear scaffold protein that regulates gene transcription by altering chromatin remodeling. It functions as a tumor suppressor gene and interacts with several transcription factors like JUND, NFKB, SMAD3 etc. [19]. MEN1 gene mutations are well characterized with approximately 1330 mutations scattered throughout the entire gene comprises of mostly frameshift deletions or insertions, followed by nonsense, missense, splice-site mutations and either part or complete gene deletions [21].

Frameshift and nonsense mutations result in truncated and most probably inactive menin protein whereas splice site mutations result in incorrect splicing of the mRNA which leads to either exon skipping or addition of extra region to the final product.

Missense mutations of MEN1 are important as they result in change of crucial amino acids necessary for binding or interacting with various other molecules and proteins. This may further affect the functional activity of the menin protein or its expression levels. Studies have shown single amino acid change in the genes involved in oncogenic disorders to result in enhanced proteolytic degradation leading to reduced stability and loss of function of the mutant protein which is a common mechanism for inactivating tumor suppressor gene products [22, 12].

Menin has three nuclear localization signals (NLS) near the C terminus of the protein and the novel M561K mutation identified lies within the second NLS domain. This region of menin is postulated to have a role in interaction with transcription factors like Smad3 and CHES1 and cell cycle control proteins like ASK [15]. The patient with this mutation was a 65 years old woman who presented with episodes of fasting and post prandial hypoglycemia, frequency of which had increased over the last 8 years. The patient had one benign tumor measuring 1.5*1.2 cm located in the uncinate process of pancreas.

In the present study a missense mutation (Q192K) was identified at amino acid 192 in a 17-year-old male patient having symptoms of tremors, drowsiness, headache, generalized tonic clonic seizures for 13 months. A 2*2 cm insulinoma was localized in the pancreatic tail which was surgically removed. A previous study [13] has reported a nonsense mutation (Q192X) at this position. This region of menin interacts with proteins JunD responsible for transcription regulation, HDAC for epigenetic regulation, NMMHC II-A having a role in cell division and NM23A which plays a role in cell cycle control [15].

Apart from this, a silent mutation Q261Q identified had no change in the amino acid but the variation G > A is at the last nucleotide of exon 4/intron four boundary forming a part of conserved sequences required for splicing. This change might be resulting in incorrect splicing leading to an abnormal protein. Pathogenicity of the alteration was evaluated by Mutation Taster software which predicted the change to be disease causing (probability =1; indicating high security of the prediction).

An accurate splicing mechanism is required for removal of introns and forming the mature RNA which normally takes place by a large spliceosome complex that includes small nuclear ribonucleoprotein particles (snRNP) and a number of other proteins. This spliceosomal complex assembly requires the presence of conserved recognition sequences in the pre-mRNA for silencers, enhancers etc. These sequences may be present in the exons as well as introns. Alterations in any of these conserved sequences or elements may severely impair pre-mRNA splicing and gene expression. Various nonsense, missense and even silent mutations can inactivate genes by impairing the efficiency of splicing machinery thereby resulting in diseased phenotype [23].

Of the known polymorphisms identified in the present study, D418D (rs2071313) was the only one absent in the controls whereas H433H (rs540012) and A541T (rs2959656) were present in all the controls indicating that these polymorphisms may not be associated with increased tumor risk. However, the status of the polymorphism A541T is controversial as several studies report this to be a mutation associated with parathyroid tumors whereas others have reported this to be a non-pathogenic polymorphism present in pancreatic tumors [24–26].

Several reports also document intronic variations affecting mRNA splicing and leading to mild disease phenotypes with low penetrance [27, 28]. Two novel intronic variations c.445-44G → A and c.913-42G → C identified in the present study were absent in the control individuals suggesting their probable association with the disease. However, this needs further validation through more mutational and functional studies.

Conclusions

In conclusion, we report the clinical and genetic findings in 17 patients with the rare condition of sporadic insulinomas. The significance of this study is the identification of three novel exonic and two novel intronic variations. The outcome of the study considerably extends the growing list of pathogenic MEN1 mutations providing a consequential insight into phenotypic heterogeneity and in the expression of individual mutations. The new mutations identified seem to confer a role in defective binding of the menin protein to specific molecules involved in a variety of genetic and epigenetic mechanisms thereby resulting in disease pathology.

Competing interests
The authors declare that they have no competing interest.

Author contributions
VPJ was involved in the clinical diagnosis, management, literature survey and manuscript preparation. SB carried out the molecular genetic studies, literature search, data analysis and manuscript preparation. EM carried out the molecular genetic studies, literature search and data analysis. AS supervised the genetic studies, literature survey, data analysis, manuscript preparation and editing. All authors read and approved the final manuscript.

Acknowledgements
The work is supported by intramural funds by All India Institute of Medical Sciences (AIIMS), New Delhi, India. Project code No. A-12. S Birla is a recipient of senior research fellowship from the Indian Council for Medical Research.

Author details
[1]Department of Endocrinology and metabolism, All India Institute of Medical Sciences, Room No. 305, Third Floor, Biotechnology Building, New Delhi, India. [2]Department of Anatomy, All India Institute of Medical Sciences, New Delhi, India.

References
1. Abu-Zaid A, Alghuneim LA, Metawee MT, Elkabbani RO, Almana H, Amin T, et al. Sporadic insulinoma in a 10-year-old boy: a case report and literature review. JOP. 2014;15(1):53–7.

2. Jyotsna VP, Rangel N, Pal S, Seith A, Sahni P, Ammini AC. Insulinoma: Diagnosis and surgical treatment. Retrospective analysis of 31 cases. Indian J Gastroenterol. 2006;25(5):244–7.

3. Schussheim DH, Skarulis MC, Agarwal SK, Simonds WF, Burns AL, Spiegel AM, et al. Multiple endocrine neoplasia type 1: new clinical and basic findings. Trends Endocrinol Metab. 2001;12(4):173–8.

4. Pelengaris S, Khan M. Oncogenic co-operation in beta-cell tumorigenesis. Endocr Relat Cancer. 2001;8(4):307–14.

5. Davies K, Conlon KC. Neuroendocrine tumors of the pancreas. Curr Gastroenterol Rep. 2009;11(2):119–27.

6. Brandi ML, Gagel RF, Angeli A, Bilezikian JP, Beck-Peccoz P, Bordi C, et al. Guidelines for diagnosis and therapy of MEN type 1 and type 2. J Clin Endocrinol Metab. 2001;86(12):5658–71.

7. Ramkumar S, Dhingra A, Jyotsna V, Ganie MA, Das CJ, Seth A, et al. Ectopic insulin secreting neuroendocrine tumor of kidney with recurrent hypoglycemia: a diagnostic dilemma. BMC Endocr Disord. 2014;14:36.

8. Pakhetra R, Priya G, Jyotsna VP, Seith A, Ammini AC. Insulinoma: reversal of brain magnetic resonance imaging changes following resection. Neurol India. 2008;56(2):192–4.

9. Gortz B, Roth J, Speel EJ, Krähenmann A, De Krijger RR, Matias-Guiu X. Muletta- Feurer S, Rütmann K, Saremaslani P, Heitz PU, Komminoth P: MEN1 gene mutation analysis of sporadic adrenocortical lesions. Int J Cancer. 1999;80(3):373–9.

10. Chandrasekharappa SC, Guru SC, Manickam P, Olufemi SE, Collins FS, Emmert-Buck MR, et al. Positional cloning of the gene for multiple endocrine neoplasia-type 1. Science. 1997;276(5311):404–7.

11. Guru SC, Manickam P, Crabtree JS, Olufemi SE, Agarwal SK, Debelenko LV. Identification and characterization of the multiple endocrine neoplasia type 1 (MEN1) gene. J Intern Med. 1998;243(6):433–9.

12. Agarwal SK, Guru SC, Heppner C, Erdos MR, Collins RM, Park SY, et al. Menin interacts with the AP1 transcription factor JunD and represses JunD Activated transcription. Cell. 1999;96(1):143–52.

13. Jager AC, Friis-Hansen L, Hansen TV, Eskildsen PC, Sølling K, Knigge U, et al. Characteristics of the Danish families with multiple endocrine neoplasia type 1. Mol Cell Endocrinol. 2006;249(1–2):123–32.

14. Trump D, Farren B, Wooding C, Pang JT, Besser GM, Buchanan KD, et al. Clinical studies of multiple endocrine neoplasia type 1 (MEN1). QJM. 1996;89(9):653–69.

15. Thakker RV. Multiple endocrine neoplasia type 1 (MEN1) and type 4 (MEN4). Mol Cell Endocrinol. 2014;386(1–2):2–15.

16. Thakker RV, Bouloux P, Wooding C, Chotai K, Broad PM, Spurr NK, et al. Association of parathyroid tumors in multiple endocrine neoplasia type 1 with loss of alleles on chromosome 11. N Engl J Med 1989, 321(4):218–24. 15. Knudson AG: All in the (cancer) family. Nat Genet. 1993;5(2):103–4.

17. Knudson AG. All in the (cancer) family. Nat Genet. 1993;5(2):103–4.

18. Hirshberg B, Cochran C, Skarulis MC, Libutti SK, Alexander HR, Wood BJ, et al. Malignant insulinoma: spectrum of unusual clinical features. Cancer. 2005;104(2):264–72.

19. Canaff L, Vanbellinghen JF, Kaji H, Goltzman D, Hendy GN. Impaired transforming growth factor-β (TGF-β) transcriptional activity and cell proliferation control of a menin in-frame deletion mutant associated with multiple endocrine neoplasia type 1 (MEN1). J Biol Chem. 2012;287(11):8584–97.

20. Jonkers YM, Claessen SM, Perren A, Schmid S, Komminoth P, Verhofstad AA, et al. Chromosomal instability predicts metastatic disease in patients with insulinomas. Endocr Relat Cancer. 2005;12(2):435–47.

21. Lemos MC, Thakker RV. Multiple endocrine neoplasia type 1 (MEN1): analysis of 1336 mutations reported in the first decade following identification of the gene. Hum Mutat. 2008;29(1):22–32.

22. Yaguchi H, Ohkura N, Tsukada T, Yamaguchi K. Menin the multiple endocrine neoplasia type 1 gene product, exhibits GTP-hydrolyzing activity in the presenceof the tumor metastasis suppressor nm23. J Biol Chem. 2002;277(41):38197–204.

23. Cartegni L, Chew SL, Krainer AR. Listening to silence and understanding nonsense: exonic mutations that affect splicing. Nat Rev Genet. 2002;3(4):285–98.

24. Shan L, Nakamura Y, Nakamura M, Yokoi T, Tsujimoto M, Arima R, et al. Somatic mutations of multiple endocrine neoplasia type 1 gene in the sporadic endocrine tumors. Lab Invest. 1998;78(4):471–5.

25. Bazzi W, Renon M, Vercherat C, Hamze Z, Lacheretz-Bernigaud A, Wang H, et al. MEN1 missense mutations impair sensitization to apoptosis induced by wild-type menin in endocrine pancreatic tumor cells. Gastroenterology. 2008;135(5):1698–709.

26. Nozieres C, Zhang CX, Buffet A, Dupasquier S, Vargas-Poussou R, Guillaud-Bataille M, et al. Groupe français des tumeurs endocrines (GTE): p.Ala541Thr variant of MEN1 gene: a non deleterious polymorphism or a pathogenic mutation? Ann Endocrinol. 2014;75(3):133–40.

27. Carrasco CA, Gonzalez AA, Carvajal CA, Campusano C, Oestreicher E, Arteaga E, et al. Novel intronic mutation of MEN1 gene causing familial isolated primary hyperparathyroidism. J Clin Endocrinol Metab. 2004;89(8):4124–9.

28. Drori-Herishanu L, Horvath A, Nesterova M, Patronas Y, Lodish M, Bimpaki E, et al. An Intronic mutation is associated with prolactinoma in a young boy, decreased penetrance in his large family, and variable effects on MEN1 mRNA and protein. Horm Metab Res. 2009;41(8):630–4.

6

Prevalence of hypopituitarism after intracranial operations not directly associated with the pituitary gland

Steffen Kristian Fleck[1*], Henri Wallaschofski[2], Christian Rosenstengel[1], Marc Matthes[1], Thomas Kohlmann[3], Matthias Nauck[2], Henry Werner Siegfried Schroeder[1] and Christin Spielhagen[2]

Abstract

Background: Over the last few years, awareness and detection rates of hypopituitarism following traumatic brain injury (TBI) and subarachnoid hemorrhage (SAH) has steadily increased. Moreover, recent studies have found that a clinically relevant number of patients develop pituitary insufficiency after intracranial operations and radiation treatment for non-pituitary tumors. But, in a substantial portion of more than 40%, the hypopituitarism already exists before surgery. We sought to determine the frequency, pattern, and severity of endocrine disturbances using basal and advanced dynamic pituitary testing following non-pituitary intracranial procedures.

Methods: 51 patients (29 women, 22 men) with a mean age of 55 years (range of 20 to 75 years) underwent prospective evaluation of basal parameters and pituitary function testing (combined growth hormone releasing hormone (GHRH)/arginine test, insulin tolerance test (ITT), low dose adrenocorticotropic hormone (ACTH) test), performed 5 to 168 months (median 47.2 months) after intracranial operation (4 patients had additional radiation and 2 patients received additional radiation combined with chemotherapy).

Results: We discovered an overall rate of hypopituitarism with distinct magnitude in 64.7% (solitary in 45.1%, multiple in 19.6%, complete in 0%). Adrenocorticotropic hormone insufficiency was found in 51.0% (partial in 41.2%, complete in 9.8%) and growth hormone deficiency (GHD) occurred in 31.4% (partial in 25.5%, severe in 5.9%). Thyrotropic hormone deficiency was not identified. The frequency of hypogonadism was 9.1% in men. Pituitary deficits were associated with operations both in close proximity to the sella turcica and more distant regions ($p = 0.91$). Age ($p = 0.76$) and gender ($p = 0.24$) did not significantly differ across patients with versus those without hormonal deficiencies. Groups did not differ across pathology and operation type ($p = 0.07$).

Conclusion: Hypopituitarism occurs more frequently than expected in patients who have undergone neurosurgical intracranial procedures for conditions other then pituitary tumors or may already exists in a neurosurgical population before surgery. Pituitary function testing and adequate substitution may be warranted for neurosurgical patients with intracranial pathologies at least if unexplained symptoms like fatigue, weakness, altered mental activity, and decreased exercise tolerance are present.

Keywords: Hypopituitarism, Pituitary deficiency, Intracranial operation, Neurosurgery

* Correspondence: sfleck@uni-greifswald.de
[1]Department of Neurosurgery, University Medicine Greifswald,
Ferdinand-Sauerbruch-Strasse, 17475 Greifswald, Germany
Full list of author information is available at the end of the article

Background

Evaluation of endocrine function plays an essential role in pituitary tumor diagnostics. Even in experienced neurosurgical centers, high rates (ranging from 80-100%) of postoperative pituitary deficiencies have been reported. Furthermore, patients who have received radiation or chemotherapy or are suffering from childhood tumors, craniopharyngeomas, or skull base tumors carry a high risk of developing hypothalamo-hypophyseal disturbances [1,2].

Studies assessing posttraumatic hypopituitarism have only recently been published. However, earlier postmortem studies identified anterior gland necrosis in up to one third of fatal head injuries and several case reports of posttraumatic hypopituitarism exist [3,4].

Today, endocrinologists and neurosurgeons are becoming increasingly aware of the relationship between traumatic brain injury (TBI) and pituitary dysfunction [3,5-10]. However, subarachnoid hemorrhage (SAH) has also been linked with neuroendocrine dysfunction in a substantial number of patients, possibly indicating the need for endocrinology follow-up evaluations in these patients as well [11,12].

In published series, the rate of patients with hormone deficits of the hypothalamo-pituitary axis varies, ranging from 20 to 80%. These disturbances may have an important influence on health status, neurobehavioral complaints, and rehabilitation potential. Because hormonal deficiencies can develop either acutely or long after (months to years) TBI or SAH, a neuroendocrine follow-up period might be necessary to determine if hormonal replacement is necessary [5].

Schneider et al. assessed endocrine abnormalities in 68 patients who underwent surgery for non-pituitary intracranial tumors while also receiving chemotherapy or radiation and found that over 40% of all patients had hormone irregularities [13]. However, studies investigating the frequency of pituitary insufficiency after intracranial operations for non-pituitary tumors are limited [14,15] which highlight the need of more data. Therefore, we sought to prospectively determine the frequency of hypopituitarism and hypopituitarism-related factors in postoperative patients using basal parameters and advanced pituitary function tests.

Methods

Patients

This study was conducted prospectively at the Greifswald University of Medicine and was approved by the investigational and ethical review board of the University of Greifswald. Informed consent was obtained from all patients.

51 consecutive patients were eligible for enrollment having undergone a neurosurgical intracranial procedure for something other than a pituitary tumor (29 female, 22 male,

mean age 55 years, age range 20 to 75 years), (BMI mean 27.9; range of 21 to 37).

Basal hormone status and pituitary function testing was performed between 5 and 168 months (mean 47.2) after the operation. Two patients were excluded from the adrenocorticotropic function testing due to an ongoing glucocorticoid replacement therapy.

Localization of tumor/approach

The tumor or approach localization was divided into subgroups in accordance with Schneider et al. [13] (with the exception of medial and lateral sphenoid wing processes). With regard to proximity to the hypothalamic-hypophyseal region, the subgroups were characterized as, (1) central: medial sphenoid, clinoid, tuberculum sellae, intra-/supra-/parasellar, third ventricle; (2) frontal: lateral sphenoid, frontal, fronto-temporal, fronto-parietal, fronto-basal, ethmoid; (3) temporal/parietal: parieto-occipital, lateral ventricles, petrous, petroclival, acoustic nerve; and (4) occipital: occipital, cerebellar, pineal, fourth ventricle.

We additionally recorded the occurrence of hydrocephalus accompanying the operation (endoscopic third ventriculostomy (ETV), ventriculo-abdominal (VP) shunt), epilepsy, complications in the postoperative course, and radiation/chemotherapy.

Evaluation of pituitary function

All patients were tested following an overnight fast. The laboratory analytics were measured at the Institute of Clinical Chemistry and Laboratory Medicine at the University Medicine, Greifswald. The following basal measurements were performed. At 8:00 AM, we measured serum cortisol (adrenal insufficiency as indicated by < 100 nmol/l), free thyroxin (fT4), thyroid-stimulating hormone (TSH), insulin-like growth factor-I (IGF-I), follicle-stimulating hormone (FSH), luteinizing hormone (LH), and testosterone (men). Moreover, we evaluated urine and plasma sodium, osmolality, and diuresis for 24 hours. Patients underwent the following dynamic testing.

Insulin tolerance test (ITT): we performed an ITT to assess cortico- and somatotrophic secretion. In this test we measured adrenocorticotropic hormone (ACTH), cortisol, and growth hormone (GH). 0.1-0.15 IE insulin/kg body weight (BW) were intravenously administered at 0 min to induce a fall in blood glucose level to < 3 mmol/l and neuroglycopenia symptoms. ACTH, cortisol, GH, and blood glucose levels were measured at −15, 0, +30, +60, +90, and +120 minutes. In cases, where an ITT was contraindicated, a combined growth hormone releasing hormone (GHRH)/arginine test and a low dose ACTH test were performed.

Combined (GHRH)/arginine test: GHRH was given (1 μg/kg i.v. at 0 min) along with L-arginine hydrochloride 6% (i.v. infusion over 30 min from 0 to + 30 min at dosages of 0,5 g/kg, maximum 30 g). GH levels were measured at –15, 0, +30, +60, +90, and +120 minutes.

Low dose ACTH test: 1 μg ACTH (synacthen®) i.v. was injected at 0 min and cortisol was measured –15, 0 min and after 30 and 60 min.

Twenty-one patients underwent ITT, thirty patients underwent low dose ACTH test, and all patients underwent GHRH/arginine test.

Definitions of pituitary deficiencies

Pituitary deficiencies were diagnosed with respect to the clinical symptoms and result of the dynamic testing. Before study start criteria have been defined as follow:

Growth hormone deficiency (GHD): GH peak after ITT < 5 μg/l or GH peak after GHRH + Arginine test < 16 μg/l [16]. In cases where a GHRH/arginine test was performed, body mass index (BMI) dependent cut-offs were used [17]. Partial GHD was defined as patients with IGF-I levels within the age- and sex-related reference range and a pathological ITT or GHRH/arginine test. We defined severe GHD as a GH peak after ITT < 3 μg/l [18] or a GH peak following the GHRH/arginine test < 11 μg/l if BMI was < 25 [17].

Corticotrophic deficiency: was defined as baseline cortisol < 100 nmol/l [19] or cortisol < 550 nmol/l following the ITT or low dose ACTH test. Partial adrenocorticotrophic insufficiency was diagnosed if a twofold increase in baseline cortisol (above 100 nmo/l) was observed but overall cortisol levels remained lower than 550 nmol/l.

Thyrotrophic deficiency: was detected if fT4 were below the lower reference range [11,12,20] in combination with an inappropriately normal or low normal TSH. That means TSH is within the reference range and not increased as expected for primary hypothyroidism.

Hypogonadism: in men was defined as low testosterone serum concentration (< 10 nmol/l) in combination with inadequate low gonadotropins (LH, FSH) [21]. We defined hypogonadism in premenopausal women as oligo- and amenorrhea, and as low gonadotropins in postmenopausal women.

Diabetes insipidus centralis: was identified by the presence of an increased volume of dilute urine (> 6 l/24 hours) with low urine osmolality (< 300 mosmol/kg).

Statistical analysis

We performed Fisher's exact tests to assess comparisons between groups. Two-tailed p-values of <0.05 were considered significant. We conducted all analyses with SPSS 16.0 (SPSS Inc., Chicago, IL). Furthermore, we calculated 95% confidence intervals according to Altman et al. [22].

Results

We included and evaluated endocrine function in 51 patients (29 female, 22 male; mean age 54.9 years, range 20–75 years; BMI 27.9, range 21–37). Localization of

intracranial pathologies included the (1) central (n = 10), (2) frontal (n = 9), (3) temporo-parietal (n = 20), and (4) the occipital regions (n = 12).

22 patients had a meningeoma, 4 patients had an astrocytoma, 3 a vestibular schwannoma, 3 a cavernoma, 3 a brain abscess, 3 had dural arterio-venous fistula, 2 had ependymomas, 1 patient had a pinealoma, 1 an oligodendroglioma, 1 a ganglioglioma, 1 a haemangioblastoma, 1 had trigeminal nerve decompression, 1 cavum vergae, 1 patient had epilepsy surgery, 1 had an aneurysm (without SAH), 1 had an arterio-venous malformation, and finally 1 patient had a subdural hematoma. To compare pathology subgroups we categorized diagnoses as follows:

(a) meningeomas (n = 22);
(b) astrocytoma, glioblastoma, oligodendroglioma, ganglioglioma (n = 7);
(c) vestibular schwannoma, ependymoma, pinealoma (n = 7);
(d) vessel associated pathologies (9);
(e) others: subdural hematoma, cavum vergae, epileptic lesion (n = 3)
(f) brain abscess (n = 3).

Accompanying hydrocephalus occurred in five patients and a history of epileptic seizures in eight patients. Six patients underwent postoperative radiation (combined with chemotherapy in two patients). One patient developed postoperative meningitis, which resolved completely following antibiotic therapy.

As illustrated in Figure 1, a total of 35.3% of patients showed no hormonal abnormality.

Overall, we detected solitary hypopituitarism in 45.1%, multiple hypopituitarism in 19.6%, and complete insufficiency in 0% (see Figure 2).

Adrenocorticotrophic deficiency, in varying degrees, was observed in 51.0% of patients (partial 41.2%, complete 9.8%). No patient in the present study had

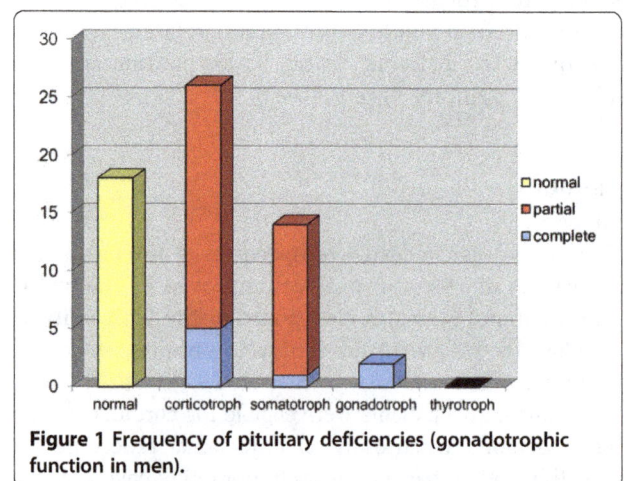

Figure 1 Frequency of pituitary deficiencies (gonadotrophic function in men).

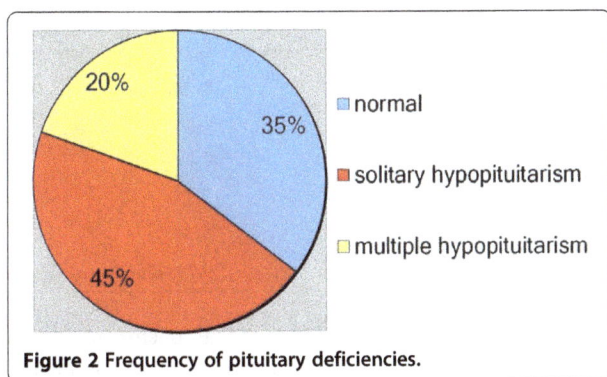

Figure 2 Frequency of pituitary deficiencies.

baseline cortisol < 100 nmol/l, therefore, we could not identify any patient to have secondary adrenal insufficiency as indicated by the basal cortisol level only. The diagnosis of adrenocorticotrophic deficiency in all patients is provided by dynamic testing. 31.4% of patients had a GHD (partial 25.5%, severe 5.9%), whereas a thyrotrophic deficiency was not observed. The prevalence of gonadotrophic deficiency was 9.1% (n = 2) in men (see Figure 1). In case of the usage of oral contraceptives or hormone replacement therapy in majority of women hypogonadism could not be exactly differentiated. Two patients developed diabetes insipidus in the early postoperative stage. Diabetes insipidus was not detected at the time of endocrine follow-up.

We observed no tendency toward a lower frequency of observed adrenal insufficiency in patients tested at longer intervals after surgery (time points 24 (p = 0.4654) and 48 months (p = 0.1441).

According to pathology localization, we classified endocrine abnormalities (complete and partial) as illustrated in Tables 1 and 2. Fischer's exact tests revealed that there was no association between endocrine abnormalities and surgical approach/pathology location (p = 0.91).

An adrenocorticotrophic deficiency (partial or complete) was observed in two of the five patients with accompanying hydrocephalus. Of these patients, a GHD was detected in one patient, but none were found to have a thyrotrophic or gonadotrophic deficiency.

Of the eight patients with a history of seizures, seven patients (87.5%) exhibited hypopituitarism along the

adrenocorticotrophic axis and 25% (two patients) along the somatotrophic axis. Thyrotrophic and gonadotrophic deficiencies were not detected in patients with epilepsy. The difference between those patients with and without epileptic seizures was significant (p = 0.018).

Six patients received radiation and/or chemotherapy. The rate of hypopituitarism (any form) did not significantly differ across patients with versus those without radiation and/or chemotherapy (p = 0.639).

No associations were found between endocrine deficiencies (binary grouping: yes/no), age (binary grouping: ≤50, >50 years; p = 0.757), gender (p = 0.236), and tumor presence (binary variable: yes/no; p = 0.761). Furthermore, pathology/operations were not associated with endocrine abnormalities (p = 0.0715; see Table 3).

Discussion

The awareness and detection rate of hypothalamo-pituitary hormone disturbances has greatly improved over the last decade, illustrating their high frequency after TBI, SAH, radiation, and neurosurgical procedures (for reasons other than pituitary tumors) [23]. Consequently, interdisciplinary expert recommendations regarding endocrine evaluation in SAH and TBI patients have been published [8,24]. The primary finding of this study is that hypopituitarism occurs more frequently than previously expected in patients who have undergone non-pituitary related intracranial procedures.

Our results are in accordance with Schneider et al. and De Marinis et al., who also found that a clinically relevant number of patients develop pituitary insufficiencies following non-pituitary operations [13,14]. However, our patient sample differs from that of Schneider et al., who evaluated 68 consecutive patients who underwent operations for non-pituitary intracranial tumors due to clinical suspicion of hormone deficiencies [13]. We detected mainly single axis disturbances (45.1%), followed by multiple axis disturbances (19.6%), and did not find any patients with total insufficiency (see Figure 2). Studies assessing endocrine disturbances in TBI and SAH patients have also primarily reported finding single axis deficiencies [12,25,26].

It has been suggested that screening for hypopituitarism (performed within 21 days after brain injury as well as 12 weeks and 12-month postoperative) is necessary [26]. We performed testing between 5 and 168 months (mean 47.2) after the procedure to evaluate possible longstanding hormonal deficiencies closer to the clinical practice. Wachter et al. [15] postulated that pituitary insufficiencies are already present before surgery but they performed the evaluation only 1 and 7 days after surgery, which might have the potential to overestimate the frequency of hypopituitarism in critical illness.

Our patients received hormone replacement therapy if hypopituitarism was diagnosed. Patients with severe GHD

Table 1 Hormonal deficiencies according to localization of tumor/approach

Region	Patients (n)	Deficiencies % (n)	Confidence interval (95%)
(A) "Central"	10	70.0% (7)	0.7 (0,40-0.89)
(B) "Frontal"	9	55.5% (5)	0.56 (0.27-0.81)
(C) "Temp.par."	20	60.0% (12)	0,60 (0.39-0.78)
(D) "Occipital"	12	66.6% (8)	0.67 (0.39-0.86)
Overall rate	51	62.7% (32)	

Table 2 Deficiencies of specific axis according to localization of tumor/approach

Region	Patients (n)	Adrenoc. deficiency % (n)	Growth hormone deficiency % (n)	Thyreotroph deficiency % (n)	Gonadotroph deficiency % (n)
A: "Central"	10	70% (7)	50% (5)	0	10% (1)
B: "Frontal"	9	44.4% (4)	22.2% (2)	0	0
C: "Temp.par."	20	50% (10)	15% (3)	0	0
D: "Occipital"	12	41.7% (5)	33.3% (4)	0	8.3% (1)
Overall rate	*51*	*50.9% (26)*	*27.4% (14)*	*0*	*9.1% (2of 2men)*

are eligible for GH replacement therapy to normalize disturbances associated with adult GHD [8]. Generally, however, neurosurgical patients are not routinely considered for endocrine evaluation following non-pituitary procedures. Furthermore, signs and symptoms of hypopituitarism are often unspecific and may be masked by what has been assumed to be a "post-traumatic" or "post-operative syndrome". The potentially life threatening condition of hypocortisolism, however, underscores the importance of screening for hypopituitarism after intracranial operations. Neurosurgeons and rehabilitation physicians should thus be aware of hypopituitarism and the screening modalities available.

It has been hypothesized that the anatomic location of the somatotrophic (in the lateral wing of the anterior lobe) and gonadotrophic cells (in the pars distalis and tuberalis), a vulnerable vascular region of the long hypophyseal portal system (passing through the sellar diaphragma), is responsible for the high rate of disturbances observed along these axes. In contrast, corticotrophic and thyrotrophic cells are located more anteromedially, in a more protected territory of the short hypophyseal portal system [2,4,9,27-29]. Apart from direct trauma, hypoperfusion of the pituitary gland may be the most common cause of postoperative disturbances [9,30,31]. Additionally, it has been postulated that a secondary hypothalamic disturbance following brain radiation in children is due to an altered neurotransmitter input from other brain centers [32].

In patients without a known history of seizures, we found a high rate (41.9%) of predominantly solitary adrenocorticotrophic deficiency using the ITT. In the eight patients with seizures, the low dose ACTH test was performed as an alternative. Of note, among these patients, we found that 87.5% had an adrenocorticotrophic deficiency. The explanation for this high rate remains unclear. False positive results must be kept in mind, although the low dose ACTH test used here has been noted to correlate highly with the ITT [33-35]. On the other hand, it might be possible that the rate of this hormonal insufficiency has been underestimated due to the absence of dynamic testing for the adrenocorticotrophic axis in other studies. Furthermore, seizure itself or accompanying seizure medication may result in hormonal disturbances. Overall, the detection of hormonal disturbances in patients with epileptic seizures differed significantly from detection in patients without a history of seizures (p = 0.0183).

Limitations of the study

We did not perform preoperative endocrine evaluations. Furthermore, by testing at a single point in time, we were unable to differentiate definitively between permanent and intermittent dysfunction.

Furthermore, the timing of postoperative testing was variable and we did not perform testing on a control group. Due to the inclusion of many different types of pathologies in small groups it is unclear to know which disease processes are strongly associated with hypopituitarism.

Conclusion

Despite the limitations described above, we found high prevalence of hypopituitarism in postoperative neurosurgery patients with non-pituitary operation procedures.

Table 3 Hormonal deficiencies according to entities

Entities	Pat. (n)	Deficiencies % (n)	Confidence interval (95%)
(A) Meningeomas	22	54% (12)	0.54 (0.35-0.73)
(B) Astrocytoma, glioma, oligodendroglioma, ganglioglioma	7	86% (6)	0.86 (0.49-0.97)
(C) Vestibular schwannoma, ependymoma, pinealoma	7	57% (4)	0.57 (0.25-0.84)
(D) Vessel associated diseases	9	88% (8)	0.88 (0.56-0.98)
(E) Subdural hematoma, epileptic lesion, Cavum vergae	3	66% (2)	0.66 (0.21-0.94)
(F) Brain abscess	3	0.00% (0)	0.00 (0.00-0.56)
Overall rate	*51*	*62.7% (32)*	

Furthermore, a recent study indicates that hypopituitarism already exists before surgery as a frequent finding. Endocrine evaluation should be part of a pre- and postoperative screening protocol, at the very least in patients suffering from unexplained and diffuse complaints. We want to appeal to perform further prospective multicenter studies with a larger number of patients and with implementation of pre-operative testing. From our point of view guidelines for example with recommendations for optimal time points of postoperative testing are required.

Abbreviations
ACTH: Adrenocorticotropic hormone; BMI: Body mass index; BW: Body weight; CI: Confidence interval; ETV: Endoscopic third ventriculostomy; fT4: Free thyroxin; FSH: Follicle-stimulating hormone; GH: Growth hormone; GHD: Growth hormone deficiency; GHRH: Growth hormone releasing hormone; IGF-I: Insulin-like growth factor-I; ITT: Insulin tolerance test (ITT-tolerance); LH: Luteinizing hormone; SAH: Subarachnoid hemorrhage; SD: Standard deviation; TBI: Traumatic brain injury; TSH: Thyroid-stimulating hormone; VP: Ventriculo-peritoneal.

Competing interests
H. Wallaschofski received travel and research grants from Pfizer and Novo Nordisk. He is a member of the German as well as the International KIMS board. C. Spielhagen received travel grants from Pfizer and Novo Nordisk. S. Fleck received a travel grant from Pfizer and Novo Nordisk.

Authors' contributions
Each author contributed to the paper according to the ICMJE guidelines for authorship. SF contributed to study conception, collecting of data, interpretation of data, and drafting the manuscript. HW contributed to study conception, analysis and interpretation of data, and revising of the manuscript. CR has been involved in data acquisition and revision of the manuscript. MM contributed to analysis and statistical interpretation, and drafting the manuscript. TM has been involved in analysis and interpretation of data, and revision of manuscript. MN contributed to analysis and interpretation of data. HS has been involved in study conception, interpretation of data. CS has been involved in study conception, acquisition and analysis of data, and drafting and revision of the manuscript. All authors have given final approval of the version to be published.

Acknowledgements
We thank Christopher O. Leonards and Sophia Lamp for the English revision of the manuscript.

Funding
This research received no specific grant from any funding agency in the public, commercial or not-for-profit sectors.

Author details
[1]Department of Neurosurgery, University Medicine Greifswald, Ferdinand-Sauerbruch-Strasse, 17475 Greifswald, Germany. [2]Institute of Clinical Chemistry and Laboratory Medicine, University Medicine Greifswald, Ferdinand-Sauerbruch-Strasse, 17475 Greifswald, Germany. [3]Institute of Community Medicine, University Medicine Greifswald, Ferdinand-Sauerbruch-Strasse, 17475 Greifswald, Germany.

References
1. Darzy KH, Shalet SM: **Radiation-induced growth hormone deficiency.** *Horm Res* 2003, **59**(Suppl 1):1–11.
2. Littley MD, Shalet SM, Beardwell CG, Ahmed SR, Applegate G, Sutton ML: **Hypopituitarism following external radiotherapy for pituitary tumours in adults.** *Q J Med* 1989, **70**:145–160.
3. Benvenga S, Campenni A, Ruggeri RM, Trimarchi F: **Clinical review 113: hypopituitarism secondary to head trauma.** *J Clin Endocrinol Metab* 2000, **85**:1353–1361.
4. Edwards OM, Clark JD: **Post-traumatic hypopituitarism: six cases and a review of the literature.** *Medicine (Baltimore)* 1986, **65**:281–290.
5. Aimaretti G, Ambrosio MR, Benvenga S, Borretta G, De Marinis L, De Menis E, Di Somma C, Faustini-Fustini M, Grottoli S, Gasco V, Gasperi M, Logoluso F, Scaroni C, Giordano G, Ghigo E: **Hypopituitarism and growth hormone deficiency (GHD) after traumatic brain injury (TBI).** *Growth Horm IGF Res* 2004, **14**(Suppl A):S114–S117.
6. Bondanelli M, De Marinis L, Ambrosio MR, Monesi M, Valle D, Zatelli MC, Fusco A, Bianchi A, Farneti M, Degli Uberti EC: **Occurrence of pituitary dysfunction following traumatic brain injury.** *J Neurotrauma* 2004, **21**:685–696.
7. Cyran E, Cyran E: **Hypophysenschädigung durch Schädelbasisfraktur.** *Dtsch Med Wochenschr* 1918, **44**:1261.
8. Ghigo E, Masel B, Aimaretti G, Leon-Carrion J, Casanueva FF, Dominguez-Morales MR, Elovic E, Perrone K, Stalla G, Thompson C, Urban R: **Consensus guidelines on screening for hypopituitarism following traumatic brain injury.** *Brain Inj* 2005, **19**:711–724.
9. Kelly DF, Gonzalo IT, Cohan P, Berman N, Swerdloff R, Wang C: **Hypopituitarism following traumatic brain injury and aneurysmal subarachnoid hemorrhage: a preliminary report.** *J Neurosurg* 2000, **93**:743–752.
10. Urban RJ, Harris P, Masel B: **Anterior hypopituitarism following traumatic brain injury.** *Brain Inj* 2005, **19**:349–358.
11. Aimaretti G, Ambrosio MR, Di Somma C, Fusco A, Cannavo S, Gasperi M, Scaroni C, De Marinis L, Benvenga S, Degli Uberti EC, Lombardi G, Mantero F, Martino E, Giordano G, Ghigo E: **Traumatic brain injury and subarachnoid haemorrhage are conditions at high risk for hypopituitarism: screening study at 3 months after the brain injury.** *Clin Endocrinol (Oxf)* 2004, **61**:320–326.
12. Kreitschmann-Andermahr I, Hoff C, Saller B, Niggemeier S, Pruemper S, Hutter BO, Rohde V, Gressner A, Matern S, Gilsbach JM: **Prevalence of pituitary deficiency in patients after aneurysmal subarachnoid hemorrhage.** *J Clin Endocrinol Metab* 2004, **89**:4986–4992.
13. Schneider HJ, Rovere S, Corneli G, Croce CG, Gasco V, Ruda R, Grottoli S, Stalla GK, Soffietti R, Ghigo E, Aimaretti G: **Endocrine dysfunction in patients operated on for non-pituitary intracranial tumors.** *Eur J Endocrinol* 2006, **155**:559–566.
14. De Marinis L, Fusco A, Bianchi A, Aimaretti G, Ambrosio MR, Scaroni C, Cannavo S, Di Somma C, Mantero F, Degli Uberti EC, Giordano G, Ghigo E: **Hypopituitarism findings in patients with primary brain tumors 1 year after neurosurgical treatment: preliminary report.** *J Endocrinol Invest* 2006, **29**:516–522.
15. Wachter D, Gondermann N, Oertel MF, Nestler U, Rohde V, Boker DK: **Pituitary insufficiency after operation of supratentorial intra- and extraaxial tumors outside of the sellar-parasellar region?** *Neurosurgical review* 2011, **34**:509–516. doi:10.1007/s10143-011-0326-5.
16. Molitch ME, Clemmons DR, Malozowski S, Merriam GR, Shalet SM, Vance ML, Stephens PA: **Evaluation and treatment of adult growth hormone deficiency: an endocrine society clinical practice guideline.** *J Clin Endocrinol Metab* 2006, **91**:1621–1634.
17. Gabellieri E, Chiovato L, Lage M, Castro AI, Casanueva FF: **Testing growth hormone deficiency in adults.** *Front Horm Res* 2010, **38**:139–144.
18. Ho KK: **Consensus guidelines for the diagnosis and treatment of adults with GH deficiency II: a statement of the GH research society in association with the European society for pediatric endocrinology, Lawson Wilkins society, European society of endocrinology, Japan endocrine society, and endocrine society of Australia.** *Eur J Endocrinol* 2007, **157**:695–700.
19. Schmidt IL, Lahner H, Mann K, Petersenn S: **Diagnosis of adrenal insufficiency: evaluation of the corticotropin-releasing hormone test and basal serum cortisol in comparison to the insulin tolerance test in patients with hypothalamic-pituitary-adrenal disease.** *J Clin Endocrinol Metab* 2003, **88**:4193–4198.
20. Volzke H, Schmidt CO, John U, Wallaschofski H, Dorr M, Nauck M: **Reference levels for serum thyroid function tests of diagnostic and prognostic significance.** *Hormone and metabolic research = Hormon- und Stoffwechselforschung = Hormones et metabolisme* 2010, **42**:809–814. doi:10.1055/s-0030-1263121.
21. Partsch CJ, Hermanussen M, Sippell WG: **Differentiation of male hypogonadotropic hypogonadism and constitutional delay of puberty by pulsatile administration of gonadotropin-releasing hormone.** *J Clin Endocrinol Metab* 1985, **60**:1196–1203.

22. Altman DMD, Bryant T, Gardner S: *Statistics with confidence: Confidence intervals and statistical guidelines (2nd ed.)*. London: British Medical Journal Books; 2000.

23. Agha A, Sherlock M, Brennan S, O'Connor SA, O'Sullivan E, Rogers B, Faul C, Rawluk D, Tormey W, Thompson CJ: **Hypothalamic-pituitary dysfunction after irradiation of nonpituitary brain tumors in adults.** *J Clin Endocrinol Metab* 2005, **90:**6355–6360.

24. Schneider HJ, Stalla GK, Buchfelder M: **Expert meeting: hypopituitarism after traumatic brain injury and subarachnoid haemorrhage.** *Acta Neurochir (Wien)* 2006, **148:**449–456.

25. Agha A, Rogers B, Sherlock M, O'Kelly P, Tormey W, Phillips J, Thompson CJ: **Anterior pituitary dysfunction in survivors of traumatic brain injury.** *J Clin Endocrinol Metab* 2004, **89:**4929–4936.

26. Aimaretti G, Ambrosio MR, Di Somma C, Gasperi M, Cannavo S, Scaroni C, Fusco A, Del Monte P, De Menis E, Faustini-Fustini M, Grimaldi F, Logoluso F, Razzore P, Rovere S, Benvenga S, Degli Uberti EC, De Marinis L, Lombardi G, Mantero F, Martino E, Giordano G, Ghigo E: **Residual pituitary function after brain injury-induced hypopituitarism: a prospective 12-month study.** *J Clin Endocrinol Metab* 2005, **90:**6085–6092.

27. Asa SKK, Melmed S: *The hypothalamic-piuitary axis*. England: Blackwell Science Cambridge; 1995.

28. Rolih CA, Ober KP: **Pituitary apoplexy.** *Endocrinol Metab Clin North Am* 1993, **22:**291–302.

29. Vance ML: **Hypopituitarism.** *N Engl J Med* 1994, **330:**1651–1662.

30. Daniel PM, Prichard MM, Treip CS: **Traumatic infarction of the anterior lobe of the pituitary gland.** *Lancet* 1959, **2:**927–931.

31. Kornblum RN, Fisher RS: **Pituitary lesions in craniocerebral injuries.** *Arch Pathol* 1969, **88:**242–248.

32. Jorgensen EV, Schwartz ID, Hvizdala E, Barbosa J, Phuphanich S, Shulman DI, Root AW, Estrada J, Hu CS, Bercu BB: **Neurotransmitter control of growth hormone secretion in children after cranial radiation therapy.** *J Pediatr Endocrinol* 1993, **6:**131–142.

33. Abdu TA, Elhadd TA, Neary R, Clayton RN: **Comparison of the low dose short synacthen test (1 microg), the conventional dose short synacthen test (250 microg), and the insulin tolerance test for assessment of the hypothalamo-pituitary-adrenal axis in patients with pituitary disease.** *J Clin Endocrinol Metab* 1999, **84:**838–843.

34. Ambrosi B, Barbetta L, Re T, Passini E, Faglia G: **The one microgram adrenocorticotropin test in the assessment of hypothalamic-pituitary-adrenal function.** *Eur J Endocrinol* 1998, **139:**575–579.

35. Stewart PM, Corrie J, Seckl JR, Edwards CR, Padfield PL: **A rational approach for assessing the hypothalamo-pituitary-adrenal axis.** *Lancet* 1988, **1:**1208–1210.

7

Natural history and outcome in chinese patients with gastroenteropancreatic neuroendocrine tumours

Doris T. Chan[1]*, Andrea O. Y. Luk[1], W. Y. So[1], Alice P. S. Kong[1], Francis C. C. Chow[1], Ronald C. W. Ma[1] and Anthony W. I. Lo[2]

Abstract

Background: There is rising incidence of gastroenteropancreatic neuroendocrine tumours (GEP- NETs) in many parts of the world, but epidemiological data from Asian populations is rare.

Methods: We conducted a retrospective study in a tertiary medical centre in Hong Kong, using updated diagnostic criteria. The presentation, clinical features, and disease outcome were reviewed for all patients with GEP-NETs confirmed histopathologically at the Prince of Wales Hospital, the Chinese University of Hong Kong, between 1996 and 2013, according to the latest 2010 World Health Organization Classification.

Results: Among 126 patients, GEP- NETs were found in pancreas (34.9 %), rectum (33.3 %), and stomach (8.7 %), and most of them were non- functional GEP- NETs (91.3 %), mostly of grade 1 (G1) (87.3 %), and about 20 % had metastases on presentation. Age under 55 years, G1 tumours and absence of metastases were significant favourable predictors for survival in univariate analysis; whereas G2/3 tumours, size ≥2 cm, and metastases were significant predictors for disease progression ($p < 0.05$). In multivariate analysis, age and metastases on presentation were significant predictors of mortality (respective hazard ratios [HR] 1.05 [95 % confidence interval {CI} 1.02-1.08] and 6.52 [95 % CI 3.22-13.2]) and disease progression (respective HRs 1.05 [95 % CI 1.02-1.07] and 4.12 [95 % CI 1.96-8.68]), while higher tumour grade also independently predicted disease progression (HR 5.17 [95 % CI 2.05-13.05]) (all $p < 0.05$).

Conclusion: Non-functional tumours with non-specific symptoms account for the vast majority of GEP-NETs in this Chinese series. Multidisciplinary approach in the management of patients with GEP-NETs may help improve the treatment efficacy and outcome.

Keywords: Neuroendocrine tumours, GEP- NETs, Carcinoids

Background

Neuroendocrine tumours (NETs) refer to tumours originating from neural and endocrine structures distributed throughout the body. They are tumours of the interface between the endocrine and the nervous systems [1]. NETs comprise a heterogeneous family with wide and complex clinical behaviours [2, 3], and they can develop at any sites, with the majority from the gastroenteropancreatic system.

Over the years, the nomenclature and classification of NETs have undergone tremendous changes. In 1907, Oberndofer first described these tumours arising from the epithelial cells in small intestine as "carcinoid", signifying their relatively indolent growth and "cancer-like" behaviour but not exactly cancers that are more aggressive [4, 5]. It was not until 2000, the term "neuroendocrine tumours" (NETs) was used officially in the WHO Classification, to replace "carcinoid", which better depicted their

* Correspondence: doris.chanting@gmail.com
[1]Department of Medicine and Therapeutics, The Chinese University of Hong Kong, Prince of Wales Hospital, Shatin, Hong Kong
Full list of author information is available at the end of the article

malignant potential. In 2010, the WHO classification added a grading system based on the proliferative activity into either G1 (equivalent to carcinoids), G2 or G3 tumours, the latter two were regarded as neuroendocrine carcinomas (NECs).

Most NETs occur in the gastrointestinal tract [6]. In the SEER database (Surveillance Epidemiology and End Results database of the National Cancer Institute) of the United States, there was substantial rise in the overall incidence of gastroenteropancreatic neuroendocrine tumours (GEP- NETs) in the past 30 years, from 1.00 case per 100,000 in the period of 1973–1977, to 3.65 cases per 100,000 in the period of 2003–2007. The statistically significant rise was persistent over the years and was observed across all GEP-NET embryologic subgroups and primary sites [5, 7]. In the SEER database and in many nation-wide cancer registries in other European countries, the increase in overall incidence of GEP-NETs was attributed to the increasing use of abdominal imaging and endoscopy, as well as the inclusion of both benign and malignant GEP-NETs in the registries.

Compared with western countries, there were only a few retrospective studies in Asian countries including Korea, China, Taiwan, India and Malaysia [8–12]. Most of the studies in Asia and the western countries have not used the most updated WHO 2010 Classification, and only very few of them provided data on the long term outcomes. This study aims to provide a detailed analysis of prognosis and outcomes among Chinese patients with GEP-NETs by describing their clinical characteristics, pathological features and clinical outcomes of these patients spanning 16 years at a tertiary endocrine centre in Hong Kong, and to identify the predictors of clinical outcomes.

Methods

Clinical information for all patients with histologically confirmed gastroenteropancreatic neuroendocrine tumours (GEP-NETs) from the Prince of Wales Hospital, Hong Kong, during the period from January 1996 to August 2013 were identified and included in this analysis. The histological diagnosis and date were retrieved from the Laboratory Information System (LIS) maintained by the Department of Anatomical and Cellular Pathology, Prince of Wales Hospital, Hong Kong. Hand-written and electronic case notes, case summaries and investigation reports of each patient were reviewed to establish patient's demographic information, details of clinical, biochemical, histopathological and endoscopic or radiological diagnosis of GEP-NETs, subsequent treatment modalities and outcomes. The date of diagnosis was defined as the date of confirmed histological diagnosis of GEP-NETs. For the diagnostic endoscopy or imaging modality, it was defined as the first investigation performed with successful detection of the tumour. Date of progression referred to the date of investigation confirming either local or metastastic progression endoscopically or radiologically. Overall survival was defined as the time from the date of diagnosis to death from all causes in deceased patients, or to the date of last follow-up otherwise. The duration for "progression-free" disease was defined as time of diagnosis to the date of death, or confirmation of regional or distant metastases.

This study was approved by the Joint Chinese University of Hong Kong – New Territories East Cluster Clinical Research Ethics Committee (Reference number: CREC 2013.031), and is in compliance with the Declaration of Helsinki.

Histological diagnosis, immunohistochemical staining and grading of tumour

The histological slides of each patient were reviewed by one pathologist. Immunohistochemical staining, Ki-67, chromogranin A and synaptophysin staining were performed for all specimens. For pancreatic NETs (pNETs), functional hormonal staining, including gastrin, somatostatin, serotonin, glucagon and insulin, was performed in all specimens. Proliferative indices, Ki-67 and mitotic rate in each specimen were reassessed again to estimate the tumour proliferative activities, and to determine the grade of the tumour according to the WHO 2010 Classification [13]. Tumours with a Ki-67 index of <2 % were classified as G1 tumours, index of 3–20 % were classified as G2, greater than 20 % as G3. Likewise, tumours with mitotic rates of <2/10 HPF were classified as G1, those of 2 to 20/10 HPF were classified as G2, greater than 20/10 HPF as G3. If the grading of Ki-67 index disaccorded with the mitotic rate, the higher one was preferred.

Statistical analysis

Data is presented as mean ± SD or median (range). Kaplan-Meier and log-rank test were used for univariate analysis of factors including gender, age, primary tumour site (pancreas versus gastro-intestinal-hepatobiliary tract), tumour size, tumour grade according to WHO 2010 classification, chromogranin A immunostaining positivity, functional status of tumour (function versus non- functional tumours), as well as presence of regional lymph node or distant metastasis on presentation. Cox proportional hazard model was used for multivariate analysis of hazard ratio. All statistical tests were two-sided with p-value <0.05 being considered as statistically significant. Statistical analysis was performed using the Statistical Package for Social Science Version 18.0 for Windows software package.

Results

Patient characteristics, clinical presentation and diagnostic trend

We identified a total of 126 patients diagnosed with GEP-NETs, 64 (50.8 %) of them were male and 62 (49.2 %) were female. The mean age of diagnosis was 56.6 ± 15.2 years old (range 21-98 years old). The most common primary sites were pancreas (34.9 %, n = 44), followed by rectum (33.3 %, $n = 42$), and stomach (8.7 %, $n = 11$). Three (2.4 %) patients had confirmed von Hippel- Lindau syndrome, and one patient had multiple endocrine neoplasia type 1 (MEN1). All of these four patients with associated familial syndromes had non-functional pNETs.

The vast majority of GEP-NETs were non- functional (91.3 %, $n = 115$). Among the 11 functional tumours, insulinoma (81.8 %, $n = 9$) accounted for the majority, while the remaining two tumours included a gastrinoma and an ACTH-secreting pancreatic tumour. As for the non-functioning GEP-NETs, most patients presented with non-specific gastrointestinal symptoms, including epigastric or abdominal pain (33.3 %, $n = 42$), gastro-intestinal bleeding (18.3 %, $n = 23$), diarrhoea or change in bowel habit (5.6 %, $n = 7$) and painless progressive jaundice (4.0 %, n = 5). Other manifestations included symptomatic anaemia (4.0 %, $n = 5$) and weight loss (2.4 %, $n = 3$), and one of them presented with pyrexia of unknown origin. About 20 % ($n = 25$) of our patients presented as incidental finding when they had abdominal imaging or endoscopies performed for other purposes such as cancer screening. The remaining four patients were identified in the regular screening of diseases associated with known familial syndromes VHL and MEN1. The distribution and presenting symptoms of patients with GEP-NETs from different sites are detailed in Table 1.

The number of GEP-NETs diagnosed in different time periods from 1996 to 2013 were presented in Table 2. This reflected a substantial increase in the number of pancreatic, rectal and stomach NETs over this time period, which can probably be attributed to the more popular use of abdominal imaging and endoscopy over the past decade. The most common diagnostic procedure was colonoscopy (31.7 %, $n = 40$), followed by oesophago-gastro-duodenoscopy (11.1 %, $n = 14$). Endoscopic ultra-sonography (7.9 %, $n = 10$) was increasingly used. On the other hand, computed tomography (CT) scan was the most common initial imaging (19.8 %, $n = 25$), followed by ultrasound (11.9 %, $n = 15$) and magnetic resonance-imaging (MRI) (2.4 %, $n = 3$). A significant proportion were identified as incidental finding during operation for other clinical indications (13.5 %, $n = 17$). The clinical diagnostic information was not available for two of the cases.

Histopathological characteristics

The median size of the tumours was 1.5 cm (range: 0.1–16.5 cm), of which 87.3 % ($n = 110$) and 98.4 % ($n = 124$) were positive for chromogranin A (CgA) and synapto-physin respectively. The majority of the tumours were G1 (87.3 %, $n = 110$). In addition, 26 patients (20.6 %) had lymph node or distant metastases on presentation and six of them had multiple metastases. The most common sites of metastases were regional lymph nodes and liver (53.8 % each). The most common tumour associated with regional or distant metastases were pancreas ($n = 8$), followed by rectum ($n = 5$), stomach ($n = 4$) and ileum ($n = 4$).

Clinical outcome

Treatment modalities

Most patients underwent curative endoscopic or surgical resections (80.2 %, $n = 101$) whereas 4.0 % ($n = 5$)

Table 1 Distribution of primary tumour sites and corresponding presenting symptoms

Primary tumour site	Patients, N (%)	Male, N	Female, N	Main clinical symptoms
GI Tract	77 (61.1 %)	43	44	
Stomach	11 (8.7 %)	6	5	Abdominal Pain, Gastrointestinal Bleeding, Anaemia
Duodenum	6 (4.8 %)	2	4	Abdominal Pain, Gastrointestinal Bleeding
Ileum	6 (4.8 %)	3	3	Abdominal Pain, Incidental Finding
Appendix	10 (7.9 %)	5	5	Abdominal Pain
Descending Colon	1 (0.8 %)	1	0	Gastrointestinal Bleeding
Sigmoid Colon	1 (0.8 %)	0	1	Abdominal Pain
Rectum	42 (33.3 %)	26	16	Gastrointestinal Bleeding, Incidental Finding
Pancreas	44 (34.9 %)	18	26	Incidental Finding, Abdominal Pain, Hypoglycaemia for Insulinoma
Hepatobiliary System	5 (4.0 %)	3	2	
Liver	4 (3.2 %)	2	2	Abdominal Pain
Cholecystoduodenal Fistula	1 (0.8 %)	1	0	Anaemia

Table 2 Distribution of GEP- NETs by site across the different periods

Site	1996–2001	2002–2007	2008–2013	Total
Pancreas	11	19	14	44
Rectum	8	17	17	42
Stomach	1	5	5	11
Appendix	3	5	2	10
Ileum	1	4	1	6
Duodenum	0	3	3	6
HBP	2	0	3	5
Colon	0	1	0	1
Sigmoid	0	0	1	1
Total number diagnosed during period	26	54	46	126

received operations as palliative measures to relieve tumour-related intestinal or biliary obstructions. Common non-chemotherapy agents administered as adjunct pre-operative medical treatment were diazoxide for insulinomas ($n = 7$) and proton-pump inhibitors ($n = 1$) for gastrinoma. Chemotherapy was used in eight patients, almost always for the purpose of palliative care ($n = 7$). The chemotherapy usually involved combination regimens with platinum-etoposide ($n = 4$), platinum with 5-fluoruracil ($n = 1$), platinum-doxorubicin ($n = 1$), irinotecan capecitabine therapy ($n = 1$) and streptozocin plus 5-fluoruracil ($n = 1$). One patient received platinum-etoposide palliative chemotherapy for recurrent metastatic liver NET and because of lack of response to transcatheter hepatic arterial chemoemobolization (TACE). Palliative radiotherapy was used in two patients with bone metastases to sacrum and right femur. Intra-arterial yttrium-90 microspheres were used in one patient with pNET with liver metastasis. Local-regional therapies such as TACE were used in six patients. Radiofrequency ablation (RFA) was used in one patient with relapse of liver metastasis. Octreotide was used in one patient as pre- operative medical treatment for benign insulinoma. Six patients who presented with metastatic diseases at the time of diagnosis received palliative care.

Mortality

One hundred and twenty three patients received long-term follow up with a median duration of 3.23 years (range 0.04–17.15 years). Three of the cases were either lost to follow-up or with their medical case notes unable to be retrieved. The 1-, 3- and 5-year-survival rates were 83.4, 76.0 and 69.3 % respectively. The majority of mortality were related to the tumour (57.9 %, $n = 22$ out of 38).

Local/ metastastic relapses

For the 101 patients who received curative surgical or endoscopic resection, 8.9 % ($n = 9$) had local ($n = 4$) or metastatic relapse ($n = 5$), all of which were secondaries to the liver. One patient had local recurrence of insulinoma in the pancreas. The remaining eight patients had their primary tumour in the pancreas ($n = 4$, 50 %), rectum ($n = 3$, 37.5 %) and descending colon ($n = 1$, 12.5 %).

Prognostic factors for survival and disease progression

Univariate analysis was performed using patients' age (55 years old as the cut-off point which corresponds to the median age in our study), gender, tumour site (gastrointestinal-biliary tract versus pancreas), tumour grade according to WHO 2010 classification (Grade 1 tumours versus Grade 2 and Grade 3 tumours), size (2 cm as cut-off point), chromogranin A immunostaining positivity, functional status, and presence of metastasis on presentation, to identify potential prognostic factors for survival and disease progression. Age younger than 55 years old ($p = 0.006$), G1 tumours ($p = 0.001$), and absence of metastasis on presentation ($p < 0.001$) were significant predictors of better survival by univariate analysis.

For disease progression, tumours grading higher than G1 ($p < 0.001$), tumours larger than or equal to 2 cm ($p = 0.031$), and presence of metastasis on presentation ($p < 0.001$) were significant predictors of disease progression (Table 3). Survival curves and disease progression-free period curves using Kaplan-Meier estimates are displayed in Figs. 1 and 2, respectively. Multivariate analysis using the Cox regression hazard model confirmed that both age and presence of metastasis on presentation were significant independent predictors of mortality and disease progression. Tumour grade was also identified as a significant independent predictor for disease progression (Table 4).

Discussion

In this large retrospective analysis of GEP-NETs in Chinese classified according to the latest WHO 2010 Classification, non-functional tumours with non-specific symptoms accounted for the vast majority disease presentation. We

Table 3 Overall survival and progression- free disease period

Factors	Overall Survival					Progression- Free Disease Period				
	Number	Mean (Yrs)	95% CI	x^2	p	Number	Mean (Yrs)	95% CI	x^2	p
All Patients	123	10.84	9.25–12.42			123	9.91	8.34-11.48		
Gender				0.122	0.727				0.919	0.338
Male	62	8.04	6.71–9.38			62	7.19	5.84–8.53		
Female	61	11.12	8.90–13.34			61	10.69	8.44–12.94		
Age				7.493	0.006				2.775	0.096
<55	56	13.56	11.68–15.44			56	11.55	9.42–13.69		
≥55	66	7.06	5.47–8.64			66	7.06	5.47–8.64		
Site				2.887	0.089				1.202	0.273
GIH	80	7.94	6.58–9.29			80	7.59	6.24–8.94		
Pancreas	43	12.53	10.14–14.93			43	10.88	8.42-13.35		
Tumour Grading										
G1	106	11.57	9.93–13.22	11.869	0.001	106	10.69	9.04–12.34	15.232	<0.001
G2 or G3	14	3.28	1.37–5.18			14	2.86	1.26–4.45		
Size				2.632	0.105				4.660	0.031
<2cm	67	12.31	10.11–14.51			67	11.82	9.63–14.01		
≥2cm	44	8.61	6.75–10.48			44	7.51	5.68–9.34		
Chromogranin A Staining				0.119	0.730				0.347	0.556
Positive	107	10.86	9.16–12.55			107	10.03	8.35–11.70		
Negative	16	7.81	4.46–11.17			16	6.93	3.71–10.14		
Functionality				2.915	0.088				2.315	0.128
Non- functional	113	8.69	7.48–9.90			113	8.04	6.83–9.24		
Functional	10	15.36	12.24–18.49			10	13.92	10.11–17.73		
Metastases on Presentation				44.760	<0.001				41.259	<0.001
Yes	26	3.39	1.83–4.94			26	3.18	1.74–4.61		
No	96	12.29	11.60–14.98			96	12.23	10.47–13.98		

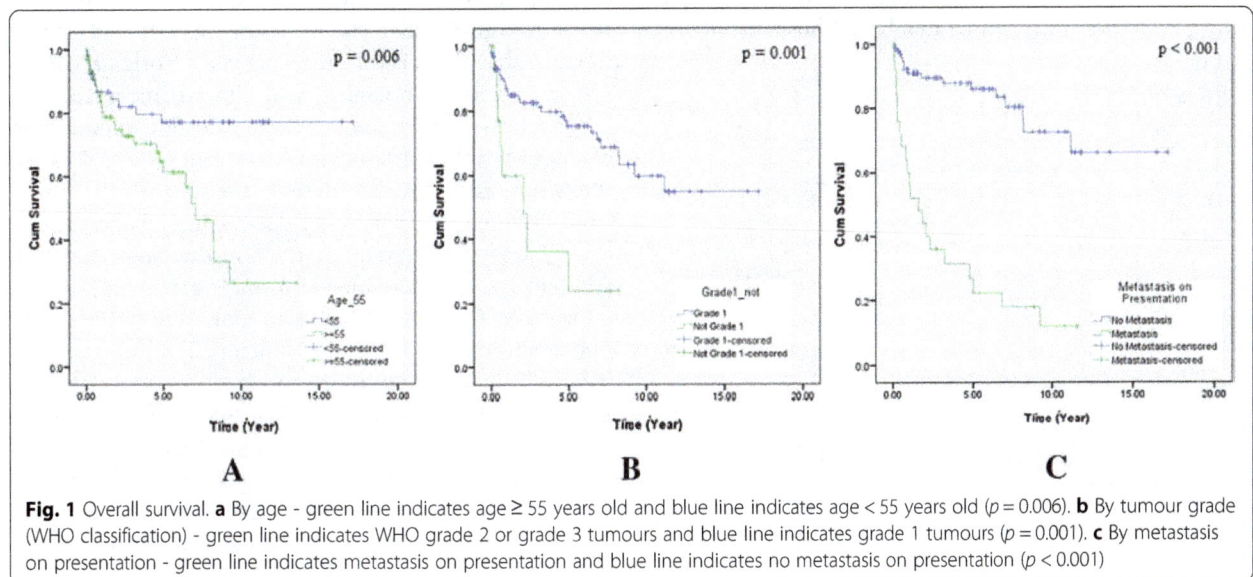

Fig. 1 Overall survival. **a** By age - green line indicates age ≥ 55 years old and blue line indicates age < 55 years old (p = 0.006). **b** By tumour grade (WHO classification) - green line indicates WHO grade 2 or grade 3 tumours and blue line indicates grade 1 tumours (p = 0.001). **c** By metastasis on presentation - green line indicates metastasis on presentation and blue line indicates no metastasis on presentation (p < 0.001)

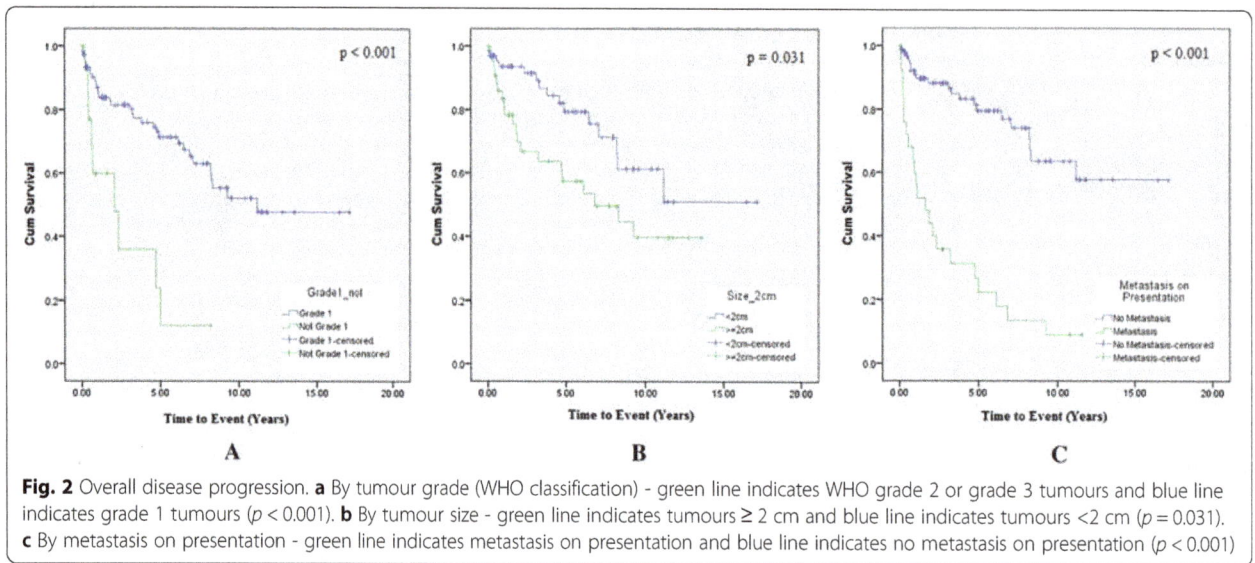

Fig. 2 Overall disease progression. **a** By tumour grade (WHO classification) - green line indicates WHO grade 2 or grade 3 tumours and blue line indicates grade 1 tumours (p < 0.001). **b** By tumour size - green line indicates tumours ≥ 2 cm and blue line indicates tumours <2 cm (p = 0.031). **c** By metastasis on presentation - green line indicates metastasis on presentation and blue line indicates no metastasis on presentation (p < 0.001)

also noted significant heterogeneity in the overall prognosis and outcome.

In older Western literature, the small intestine and the appendix were the most common sites of GEP-NETs [5, 14, 15]. Over the past two decades, with increasing availability of endoscopic imaging, rectal NETs have become more common. Among registries in Asia, rectum, pancreas and stomach were the most common primary sites [8–12]. Similarly, rectum (33.3 %) and pancreas (34.9 %) were the most frequently reported sites of GEP-NETs in this analysis, with stomach and appendix together accounting for less than 10 % each. The discrepancy between Western and Asian reports may be due to racial disparities and study design. It should be noted that most of the Western data were derived from population-based studies [5, 14–19], while data in Asia countries were often based on experiences in a single centre or "multiple-centred" studies from limited number of hospitals [8–12].

Table 4 Cox multivariate analysis for overall survival and disease progression

Variables	HR	95 % CI	p
Mortality			
Age	1.05	1.02–1.08	<0.001
Presence of Metastases on Presentation	6.52	3.22–13.19	<0.001
Disease Progression			
Age	1.05	1.02–1.07	0.001
Presence of Metastases on Presentation	4.12	1.96–8.68	<0.001
Tumour Grade	5.17	2.05–13.05	0.001

Variables included in the regression model: age (as continuous variable), tumour size (<2 cm versus ≥2 cm), tumour grade (Grade 1 versus Grade 2 and Grade 3) and status of metastases on presentation (presence of metastases versus no metastasis on presentation). Only significant variables are shown in the table
HR hazard ratio, CI confidence interval

Nevertheless, this apparent difference in the distribution of GEP-NETs between Asian series and studies reported from the US or Europe may warrant further investigation.

In some series, the Williams and Sandler classification was used [20]. This classification categorizes NETs according to their derivative origins into foregut (lung, stomach, duodenum, proximal jejunum and pancreas), midgut (distal jejunum, ileum, appendix and caecum), and hindgut (transverse and left- sided colon and rectum) [20, 21]. A nationwide epidemiological survey from Japan revealed that hindgut tumours, instead of midgut tumours, were the most common among all GEP- NETs in the Japanese population, with the midgut tumours being the least common [22]. This is in contrast to the Western population [23]. In our study, however, foregut tumours from the pancreas and the stomach accounted for more than one- thirds of all GEP- NETs when the Williams and Sandler classification was adopted. It was thought that this classification by site of origins fails to provide useful pathological and clinical information to prognosticate patients with NETs. It is also imprecise to distinguish different biologically relevant GEP- NETs entities. For example, the foregut tumours which can be from pulmonary, gastric and duodenal, or pancreatic in origin, are too different in their morphology, function and biology to be classified in a single group [24].

Over 90 % of GEP-NETs in our study were non-functional tumours. Of the functional tumours, 82 % were pNETs. The age of diagnosis of functional pNETs was almost 10 years younger than that of non-functional ones, with insulinomas being the most frequently encountered functional tumour. The younger age of presentation is due to the presence of specific symptoms by functional tumours such as recurrent unprovoked hypoglycaemic attacks in patients with insulinomas. While the majority of functional NETs resided in the pancreas, non- functional pNETs nevertheless accounted for the greater proportion. The widespread use of abdominal imaging during work-up for non-specific symptoms may have contributed to the detection of pNETs at an early stage before the development of functional manifestation. Of note, none of our patients presented with carcinoid syndrome, in contrast to the Western populations [12]. Two other single-centred studies in China and Korea also reported low rates of carcinoid syndrome [11, 12]. The reason for this ethnic disparity in the occurrence of carcinoid syndrome is not known.

In this study, regional lymph node and distant metastases occurred in 20.6 %, which is lower compared with the rates (23.0 to 53.4 %) reported by other studies [12, 23]. Most of the GEP- NETs in our review were G1 well-differentiated tumours found incidentally. The lower frequency of small intestine NETs which have greater propensity to metastasize may also account for the relatively lower rate of metastases in our data [12].

In terms of prognostic factors, smaller tumour size, lower tumour grade and absence of metastasis were associated with better survival and less likelihood of disease progression in our study, which concurred with a large retrospective cohort study in Germany [25]. In contrast to results from a single-centre study in Guangdong, China, which demonstrated positive correlation of positive functional status of GEP-NETs with survival in univariate analysis [12], functional status was not found to associate with either disease progression or survival in our analysis. Such discrepancy could be explained by the much smaller number of insulinoma, as well as the overall small proportion of functional tumours in our series.

Endoscopy, USG, CT and MRI remain the most popular diagnostic modalities of GEP-NETs in the current study. In general, the sensitivity of CT and MRI to detect GEP-NETs was estimated to be 28.6 to 94.4 %, and 84 to 95 %, respectively [26]. CT may pick up insulinomas larger than 1 cm in size but not the smaller ones. In this study, biphasic thin section helical CT was performed in all seven patients with insulinoma in whom imaging history was available. Three of them had negative CT findings and the pancreatic tumours were subsequently detected by EUS with the size of insulinomas ranging from 1.2 to 2 cm. The vast majority of NETs are slow-growing with low proliferative index, and express somatostatin receptors, especially subtype 2 (SSTR2) [26, 27]. This forms the basis of somatostatin receptor imaging (SRI) and the rationale for treatments including somatostatin analogue and peptide-receptor radionuclide therapy (PRRT) [27]. ^{111}In-DTPA-octreotide is currently the most commonly used radioactive-ligand for somatostatin receptor scintigraphy [27, 28]. The detection rate of ^{111}In-DTPA-octreotide scintigraphy is better for gastrointestinal NETs with sensitivity ranging from 80 to 100 % [28], but lower for insulinomas with sensitivity 20 to 60 % [26], as not all insulinomas express SSTR2 [29]. The only three patients with insulinoma in this study who had ^{111}In-DTPA scan performed all had negative findings, and the pancreatic lesions were detected using CT or MRI. There are no known uniform guidelines regarding imagings for GEP- NETs. In general, no single technique is 100 % sensitive and specific, multiple imaging modalities should be considered individually to detect small GEP-NETs [26].

Immunohistochemical staining for synaptophysin (Syn) and chromogranin A (CgA) is regarded as part of the standardized pathological assessment of GEP-NETs [30]. Being part of the membrane of neurosecretory hormone granules, positive staining of CgA is strongly dependent on the number of neurosecretory vesicles per cell [13]. CgA is more frequently elevated in well-differentiated tumours compared to poorly differentiated tumours. In our study, CgA was positively stained in immunohistochemical staining in 87.3 % ($n = 110$) of patients. In the remaining 16 CgA-negative patients, however, only two were poorly- differentiated neuroendocrine carcinomas. Synaptophysin (Syn) is a peptide of the small synaptic vesicles present in all neuroendocrine cells [31]. It can be demonstrated in all NETs. In our study, synaptophysin staining was positive in up to 98.4 % ($n = 124$ out of 126), consistent with the high sensitivity of Syn in diagnosis of NETs. Interestingly, immunohistochemical staining for insulin was positive in only six of the nine patients with insulinoma in this study. The negative immunoreactivity for insulin may indicate the production of precursor, or pro-insulin by tumour rather than insulin itself. Moreover, insulin molecules themselves or the antigenicity of insulin molecules may be lost during tissue processing and subsequent immunohistochemical staining.

Among the many therapeutic options for GEP-NETs, surgical treatments of both curative and debulking purposes are the mainstay treatment of choice. Most patients in this review underwent curative endoscopic or surgical resections. In patients with liver metastasis, treatment streams include surgery, loco-regional therapy, systemic medical therapy and ablative procedures such as radiofrequency ablation (RFA), and trans-arterial embolization (TAE) or chemoembolization (TACE). The six patients in our study who received RFA ($n = 1$) or TACE ($n = 5$) experienced recurrence of new metastatic liver lesions after RFA or TACE over a duration of 6 to 14 months. There have not been any randomized trials to examine the superiority of one ablative therapy over another [3].

In terms of systemic medical treatment, there has been adjuvant or neo-adjuvant therapies recommended for high grade NETs after surgery. Traditional chemotherapy is recommended for pNETs, metastatic foregut G2 NETs, and in any G3 tumours with or without liver metastases from various primary sites in the GI tract [32]. In general, well-differentiated NETs are resistant to most chemotherapeutic agents because of their slow proliferation. In our study, patients having metastatic NETs from the gut traditional chemotherapy such as platinum-based agents, all had static or progressive disease after several cycles of chemotherapy. For somatostatin analogues (SA) such as octreotide and lanreotide, they have their therapeutic values proven in functional NETs and metastatic G1 NETs in the midgut. The reported ability for SA to achieve disease stabilization is up to 50–60 % in patients with advanced or metastatic well-differentiated NETs [32, 33]. Another trial also confirmed the anti- proliferative activity of lanreotide for well-to- moderately differentiated non-functional GEP-NETs [33]. In this study, none of the patients received SA. Sunitinib and everolimus are both approved targeted therapies for well- differentiated pNETs. Only one patient of our study used sunitinib. He had von-Hippel Lindau disease and recurrent inoperable non-functional pNET. His pancreatic NET remained unchanged in size for almost three years since the commencement of sunitinib. In our locality, cost is the major constraint of using targeted therapy in metastatic pNETs. There is at present no evidence to support the efficacy of sunitinib and everolimus in treating extra- pancreatic NETs.

To the best of our knowledge, this retrospective review on GEP-NETs at a local tertiary centre is one of the first to report on the clinical presentation, pathological characteristics, investigation and treatment modalities, as well as prognostic factors of GEP-NETs in Asia. In our study, the immunohistochemical staining of chromogranin A and synaptophysin, together with the proliferative indices of Ki-67 and mitotic rate, were re-assessed by one pathologist to ensure the completeness and uniformity of the important pathological information of all specimens. In this way, the grading of the tumour according to the WHO Grade Classification 2010 was assessed accurately to facilitate the analysis of the prognostic significance of tumour grade on survival and disease progression. This approach was not possible in the previously published nation-wide registries in western countries, and was not yet adopted in the most single or multi-centre retrospective studies in Asian countries either [8–11].

There are a number of limitations in this single-centred study, with the major one being the comparatively small number of patients, as well as a small number of events especially mortality. Overall survival was adopted as endpoint rather than disease- specific survival because of this. The retrospective nature of the study also revealed the heterogeneity of disease management among different clinicians in the same tertiary centre under the lack of consensus and guidelines of the management of GEP-NETs. Individual preferences in choosing radiological or biochemical tests for disease staging in diagnosis and disease surveillance were potentially significant factors that could affect the analyses of possible prognostic factors contributing to disease- free survival and mortality. Besides, we could only evaluate the actual number of pancreatic, rectal and stomach NETs diagnosed over different time periods from 1996 to 2013 (Table 2) as it was difficult to calculate the overall incidence rate of GEP-NETs which are still overall a rare disease entity. Moreover, only GEP-NETs with confirmed histological diagnosis were included but not those with only radiological diagnosis. This might exclude patients with advanced disease and large tumour sizes, or patients with multiple metastases which was not resectable for histological diagnosis. Hence, a small number of patients with particularly poor prognosis might have been excluded from the study, leading to the reduced event rate related to the tumour. Taking this into consideration, age may be more of a predictor of overall survival rather than disease- specific survival. Given the study limitations, multidisciplinary approach for patients with GEP-NETs, which involves coordinated delivery of care by a team of specialists from related specialties [34], is expected to be the trend for treatment in the foreseeable future. Multidisciplinary practice allows a more uniform yet individualized management plan for each patient based on updated treatment guidelines and trend. From an academic and research point of view, multidisciplinary care also facilitates large- scale epidemiological research to study the disease pattern, and other opportunities for clinical trials of new treatment options in the future.

Conclusions

This single-centred retrospective review in Hong Kong provides an expedient description of the epidemiology, clinic-pathological features, management and prognostic factors of GEP-NETs in Asians. With the emergence of various diagnostic and treatment modalities, multidisciplinary care is of paramount importance to improve efficacy of treatment, and the clinical outcomes of patients with GEP- NETs. Further understanding of the molecular mechanisms may improve the treatment and prognosis of patients with GEP-NETs.

Competing interests
The authors declare that they have no competing interests.

Authors' contribution
DTC wrote the manuscript, obtained and analysed the data. AOYL obtained patient's data and helped revise the manuscript. WYS, APSK and FCCC helped revise the manuscript. RCWM was involved in the writing and revision of the manuscript. AWIL was involved in the retrieval and analyses of patients' histological slides, and in the writing and revision of the manuscript. All authors read and approved the final manuscript.

Acknowledgement

The authors thank the assistance of the staff from the Department of Anatomical and Cellular Pathology, the Chinese University of Hong Kong for providing access to the histological slides and patients' demographic databases for this study. RCWM received direct grant support for research from the Chinese University of Hong Kong (Project reference number 2041701).

Author details

[1]Department of Medicine and Therapeutics, The Chinese University of Hong Kong, Prince of Wales Hospital, Shatin, Hong Kong. [2]Department of Anatomical and Cellular Pathology, The Chinese University of Hong Kong, Prince of Wales Hospital, Shatin, Hong Kong.

References

1. Langley K. The neuroendocrine concept today. Ann N Y Acad Sci. 1994; 15(733):1–17.
2. Modlin IM, Oberg K, Chung DC, Jensen RT, de Herder WW, Thakker RV, et al. Gastroenteropancreatic neuroendocrine tumours. Lancet Oncol. 2008;9:61–72.
3. Rindi G, Wiedenmann B. Neuroendocrine neoplasms of the gut and pancreas: new insights. Nat Rev Endocrinol. 2012;8:54–64.
4. Ong SL, Garcea G, Pollard CA, Furness PN, Steward WP, Rajesh A, et al. A fuller understanding of pancreatic neuroendocrine tumours combined with aggressive management improves outcome. Pancreatology. 2009;9:583–600.
5. Yao JC, Hassan M, Phan A, Dagohoy C, Leary C, Mares JE, et al. One hundred years after "carcinoid": epidemiology of and prognostic factors for neuroendocrine tumors in 35,825 cases in the United States. J Clin Oncol. 2008;26:3063–72.
6. Fraenkel M, Kim MK, Faggiano A, Valk GD. Epidemiology of gastroenteropancreatic neuroendocrine tumours. Best Pract Res Clin Gastroenterol. 2012;26:691–703.
7. Lawrence B, Gustafsson BI, Chan A, Svejda B, Kidd M, Modlin IM. The epidemiology of gastroenteropancreatic neuroendocrine tumors. Endocrinol Metab Clin North Am. 2011;40:1–18. vii.
8. Amarapurkar DN, Juneja MP, Patel ND, Amarapurkar AD, Amarapurkar PD. A retrospective clinico-pathological analysis of neuroendocrine tumors of the gastrointestinal tract. Trop Gastroenterol. 2010;31:101–4.
9. Gunavathy M, Ghani RA, Sukor N, Kamaruddin NA. A ten-year retrospective analysis of gastroenteropancreatic-neuroendocrine tumors (GEP-NETs) in Malaysia. Med J Malaysia. 2014;69:133–7.
10. Li AF, Hsu CY, Li A, Tai LC, Liang WY, Li WY, et al. A 35-year retrospective study of carcinoid tumors in Taiwan: differences in distribution with a high probability of associated second primary malignancies. Cancer. 2008;112:274–83.
11. Lim T, Lee J, Kim JJ, Lee JK, Lee KT, Kim YH, et al. Gastroenteropancreatic neuroendocrine tumors: incidence and treatment outcome in a single institution in Korea. Asia Pac J Clin Oncol. 2011;7:293–9.
12. Wang YH, Lin Y, Xue L, Wang JH, Chen MH, Chen J. Relationship between clinical characteristics and survival of gastroenteropancreatic neuroendocrine neoplasms: A single-institution analysis (1995-2012) in South China. BMC Endocr Disord. 2012;12:30.
13. Capelli P, Fassan M, Scarpa A. Pathology - grading and staging of GEP-NETs. Best Pract Res Clin Gastroenterol. 2012;26:705–17.
14. Ellis L, Shale MJ, Coleman MP. Carcinoid tumors of the gastrointestinal tract: trends in incidence in England since 1971. Am J Gastroenterol. 2010;105: 2563–9.
15. Hemminki K, Li X. Incidence trends and risk factors of carcinoid tumors: a nationwide epidemiologic study from Sweden. Cancer. 2001;92:2204–10.
16. Newton JN, Swerdlow AJ, dos Santos Silva IM, Vessey MP, Grahame-Smith DG, Primatesta P, et al. The epidemiology of carcinoid tumours in England and Scotland. Br J Cancer. 1994;70:939–42.
17. Niederle MB, Hackl M, Kaserer K, Niederle B. Gastroenteropancreatic neuroendocrine tumours: the current incidence and staging based on the WHO and European Neuroendocrine Tumour Society classification: an analysis based on prospectively collected parameters. Endocr Relat Cancer. 2010;17:909–18.
18. Quaedvlieg PF, Visser O, Lamers CB, Janssen-Heijen ML, Taal BG. Epidemiology and survival in patients with carcinoid disease in The Netherlands. An epidemiological study with 2391 patients. Ann Oncol. 2001; 12:1295–300.
19. Westergaard T, Frisch M, Melbye M. Carcinoid tumors in Denmark 1978-1989 and the risk of subsequent cancers. A population-based study. Cancer. 1995;76:106–9.
20. Williams ED, Sandler M. The classification of carcinoid tumours. Lancet. 1963; 1:238–9.
21. Kloppel G. Tumour biology and histopathology of neuroendocrine tumours. Best Pract Res Clin Endocrinol Metab. 2007;21:15–31.
22. Ito T, Sasano H, Tanaka M, Osamura RY, Sasaki I, Kimura W, et al. Epidemiological study of gastroenteropancreatic neuroendocrine tumours in Japan. J Gastroenterol. 2010;45:234–43.
23. Rothenstein J, Cleary SP, Pond GR, Dale D, Gallinger S, Moore MJ, et al. Neuroendocrine tumors of the gastrointestinal tract: a decade of experience at the Princess Margaret Hospital. Am J Clin Oncol. 2008;31:64–70.
24. Klöppel G, Perren A, Heitz PU. The gastroenteropancreatic neuroendocrine cell system and its tumours - The WHO classification. Ann NY Acad Sci. 2004;1014:13–27.
25. Pape UF, Berndt U, Muller-Nordhorn J, Bohmig M, Roll S, Koch M, et al. Prognostic factors of long-term outcome in gastroenteropancreatic neuroendocrine tumours. Endocr Relat Cancer. 2008;15:1083–97.
26. Leung D, Schwartz L. Imaging of neuroendocrine tumors. Semin Oncol. 2013;40:109–19.
27. Sundin A. Radiological and nuclear medicine imaging of gastroenteropancreatic neuroendocrine tumours. Best Pract Res Clin Gastroenterol. 2012;26:803–18.
28. Rufini V, Calcagni ML, Baum RP. Imaging of neuroendocrine tumors. Semin Nucl Med. 2006;36:228–47.
29. Balon HR, Goldsmith SJ, Siegel BA, Silberstein EB, Krenning EP, Lang O, et al. Procedure guideline for somatostatin receptor scintigraphy with (111)In-pentetreotide. J Nucl Med. 2001;42:1134–8.
30. Modlin IM, Gustafsson BI, Moss SF, Pavel M, Tsolakis AV, Kidd M. Chromogranin A–biological function and clinical utility in neuro endocrine tumor disease. Ann Surg Oncol. 2010;17:2427–43.
31. Wiedenmann B, Franke WW, Kuhn C, Moll R, Gould VE. Synaptophysin: a marker protein for neuroendocrine cells and neoplasms. Proc Natl Acad Sci U S A. 1986;83:3500–4.
32. Pavel M, Baudin E, Couvelard A, Krenning E, Oberg K, Steinmuller T, et al. ENETS Consensus Guidelines for the management of patients with liver and other distant metastases from neuroendocrine neoplasms of foregut, ion, hindgut, and unknown primary. Neuroendocrinology. 2012;95:157–76.
33. Caplin ME, Pavel M, Cwikla JB, Phan AT, Raderer M, Sedlackova E, et al. Lanreotide in metastatic enteropancreatic neuroendocrine tumors. N Engl J Med. 2014;371:224–33.
34. Metz DC, Choi J, Strosberg J, Heaney AP, Howdend CW, Klimstra D, et al. A rationale for multidisciplinary care in treating neuroendocrine tumours. Curr Opin Endocrinol Diabetes Obes. 2012;19:306–13.

8

A rare case of anasarca caused by infiltration of the pituitary gland by diffuse large B-cell lymphoma

Ayako Kumabe[1], Tsuneaki Kenzaka[1*], Yoshioki Nishimura[1], Masaki Aikawa[2], Masaki Mori[2] and Masami Matsumura[1]

Abstract

Background: Anasarca in patients with lymphoma is a rare symptom. We report a patient with DLBCL associated with pituitary gland infiltration that was diagnosed based on significant anasarca.

Case presentation: A 72-year-old woman with a 10-year history of hypertension visited a local hospital presenting with anasarca and 15-kg weight gain in the past 3 months. we clinically diagnosed central hypothyroidism caused by pituitary gland infiltration of diffuse large B-cell lymphoma (DLBCL) (clinical stage IV in the Ann Arbor staging classification). The first course of chemotherapy improved anasarca remarkably and the patient's body weight returned to what it was 3 months before.

Conclusions: We experienced a patient with remarkable anasarca caused by DLBCL infiltration of the pituitary gland. A pituitary gland lesion with central hypothyroidism should be considered as one of the differential diagnoses of edema. This case was very valuable because we could assess it by following the time course of symptoms (edema and delayed relaxation time of the Achilles tendon reflex), laboratory data, and imaging findings (swelling anterior pituitary lobe).

Keyword: Diffuse large B-cell lymphoma, Anasarca, Edema, Hypothyroidism

Background

Correct diagnosis is occasionally difficult in some patients with lymphoma. Typical symptoms of lymphoma, called B symptoms, include fever, night sweats, and weight loss. However, atypical manifestations are observed in some patients with lymphoma. Anasarca in patients with lymphoma is a rare symptom [1].

Diffuse large B-cell lymphoma (DLBCL) reveals extranodal involvements in more than 30% of patients at diagnosis [2,3]. The gastrointestinal tract, bone marrow, pancreas, liver, intravascular system, or brain is involved in patients with DLBCL. Some reports have shown the pituitary gland with extranodal involvement in patients with lymphoma [4,5].

We report a patient with DLBCL associated with pituitary gland infiltration that was diagnosed based on significant anasarca.

* Correspondence: smile.kenzaka@jichi.ac.jp
[1]Division of General Internal Medicine, Jichi Medical University Hospital, 3311-1 Yakushiji, Shimotsuke, Tochigi 329-0498, Japan
Full list of author information is available at the end of the article

Case presentation

A 72-year-old woman with a 10-year history of hypertension visited a local hospital presenting with anasarca and 15-kg weight gain in the past 3 months. She did not have fever, appetite loss, night sweats, or dyspnea. Because of elevated liver enzymes and abdominal computed tomography (CT) abnormalities, including splenomegaly and multiple splenic tumors, she was referred to our hospital.

On admission, physical examination of the patient revealed the following: temperature, 36.3 °C; pulse rate, 84 beats per minute, regular; blood pressure, 132/74 mmHg; and respiration rate, 18 breaths per minute. Although she had remarkable anasarca, she seemed in no distress. Her height was 143.5 cm, body weight 71 kg, and body mass index 34.2. She had no jugular venous distention. Lymphadenopathy was not noted. No crackles were audible, but there were diminished breath sounds in the base of the right lung. She had remarkable nonpitting and slow pitting mixed edema of the legs. A delayed relaxation time of the Achilles tendon reflex was observed.

Laboratory test results revealed the following: white blood cell count, 7,400 cells/mm^3; hemoglobin, 11.6 g/dL; platelet count, 103,000/μL; total protein, 6.0 g/dL; albumin, 2.9 g/dL; aspartate aminotransferase, 27 IU/L; alanine aminotransferase, 20 IU/L; lactate dehydrogenase, 707 IU/L; alkaline phosphatase, 629 IU/L; total-bilirubin, 0.69 mg/dL; blood urea nitrogen, 11 mg/dL; creatinine, 0.65 mg/dL; creatinine kinase, 15 IU/L; thyroid-stimulating hormone (TSH), 0.45 μU/mL (standard value: 0.45-3.33 μU/mL); free thyroxine (FT4), 0.37 ng/dL (standard value: 0.84-1.44 ng/dL); free triiodothyronine (FT3), 0.89 pg/mL (standard value: 2.11-3.51 pg/mL); and soluble interleukin-2 receptor, 6,660 U/mL (standard value: 124–466 U/mL). Urinary protein level was 0.2 g/g creatinine. A contrast-enhanced CT of the head, neck, chest, abdomen, and pelvis revealed splenomegaly and multiple spleen tumors (Figure 1), whereas there was no lymphadenopathy. CT-guided biopsy of the spleen was performed, which showed aggregated large atypical cells. The individual cells had the chromatin-rich nuclei and relatively abundant intracytoplasmic eosinophilic inclusion bodies (Figure 2). Immunohistochemistry showed that the atypical cells were positive for CD20 and CD79a, and negative for CD3 and CD10. Histopathology and immunohistochemistry of the spleen led to the diagnosis of DLBCL.

We assessed the central hypothyroidism because of anasarca, delayed Achilles tendon reflex, and low FT4.

Head magnetic resonance imaging (MRI) revealed swelling of pituitary gland, but a normal-size of pituitary gland was confirmed in a head MRI performed 1 year before (Figure 3a, b). Luteinizing hormone (LH) and follicle-stimulating hormone (FSH) were also at low levels (LH 0.3 mIU/mL [standard value: 6.7-38.0 mIU/mL] and FSH 3.4 mIU/mL [standard value: 26.2-113.3 mIU/mL]). Cortisol level was 21.6 μg/dL [standard value: 4.0-18.3μg/dL] and ACTH was 33.4 pg/mL [standard value: 7.2-63.3 pg/mL]. Prolactin was 9.2 ng/mL[standard value: 3.12-15.39 ng/mL(menopause women)]. AVP level was not measured but there were no polyuria and hyponatremia. We diagnosed pituitary anterior lobe hormone insufficiency.

Positron emission tomography (PET) scan revealed a localized accumulation in the pituitary gland, spleen, and para-abdominal aorta lymph nodes (Figure 4). Pituitary gland biopsy was not performed; however, we clinically diagnosed central hypothyroidism caused by pituitary gland infiltration of DLBCL (clinical stage IV in the Ann Arbor staging classification).

She received 25 μg per day of levothyroxine for one week before the chemotherapy. However, the dose and duration of levothyroxine were not enough. The first course of chemotherapy for DLBCL including methotrexate, vincristine, ifosfamide, and dexamethasone, which improved anasarca remarkably and the patient's body weight returned to what it was 3 months before. Moreover, thyroid hormone, LH, and FSH levels normalized and the pituitary gland swelling improved (Figure 3c), although thyroid hormone replacement therapy was not effective before chemotherapy (Figure 5). We chose a second course of chemotherapy that comprised cyclophosphamide, hydroxydaunorubicin, vincristine, and prednisone (CHOP) because there were no atypical cells in the patient's cerebrospinal fluid. This second course of chemotherapy led to remission and the same chemotherapy regimen was repeated.

Discussion

Here, we describe a case of pituitary gland infiltration of DLBCL associated with central hypothyroidism, which caused remarkable anasarca. In this case, only a few clinical manifestation were anasarca and a delayed relaxation time of the Achilles tendon reflex, other than the typical symptoms of lymphoma (fever, night sweats, and weight loss).

Pituitary gland involvement as extranodal lymphoma is comparatively rare [4,5], and DLBCL is one of the most frequent histological types for pituitary gland involvement [2]. Infiltration of lymphoma cells to the pituitary gland lead to headache, opthalmoplegia, or hemianopia [6], and often causes diabetes insipidus [6]. Anasarca is a rare symptom in patients with lymphoma [1].

Moreover, lymphoma with pituitary gland infiltration seldom shows significant anasarca or weight gain caused

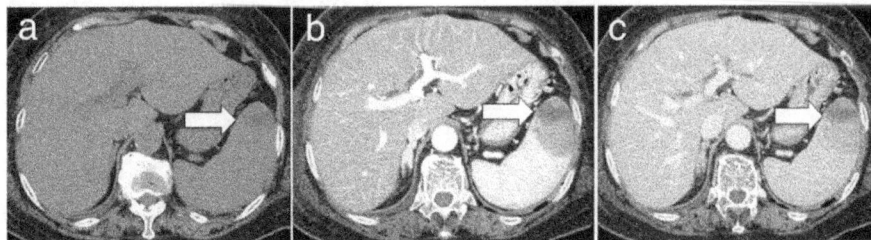

Figure 1 Contrast-enhanced abdominal computed tomography image of the abdomen. (a) Plain phase. **(b)** Arterial phase. **(c)** Equilibrium phase. Splenomegaly and multiple spleen tumors were observed. The maximal tumor size was 52 mm and the tumor had a necrotic lesion (white arrows).

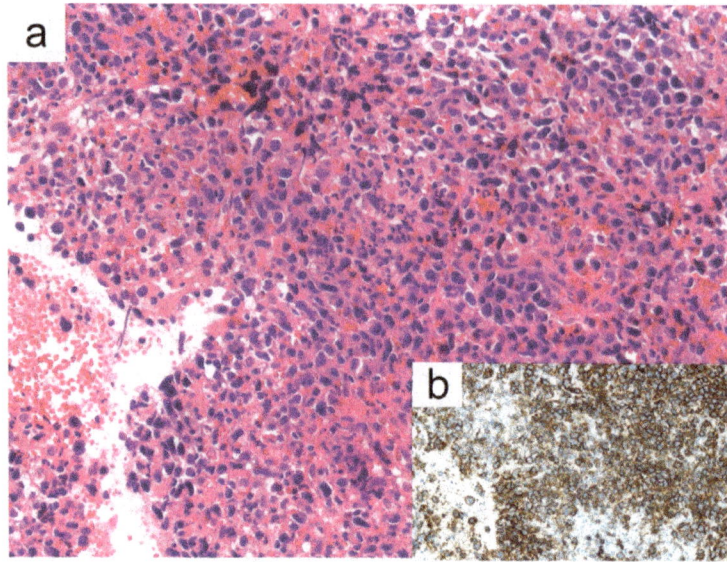

Figure 2 Histopathology finding of the spleen. (a) Hematoxylin-eosin stain. Aggregated large atypical cells were seen. The individual cells had chromatin-rich nuclei and relatively abundant intracytoplasmic eosinophilic inclusion bodies. **(b)** CD20 stain. Atypical cells were positive for CD20.

by secondary central hypothyroidism. Some patients with lymphoma who have pituitary gland involvement have no symptom, and they are incidentally detected using PET or MRI [7]. We clinically diagnosed infiltration of a malignant lymphoma in the pituitary gland based on time-dependent changes in MRI findings, thyroid hormone, LH, and FSH levels before and after chemotherapy; and PET findings.

Infiltration of DLBCL cells to the pituitary gland caused secondary central hypothyroidism, and secondary central hypothyroidism led to anasarca and weight gain in our patient. Nonpitting edema was noted, provably caused by hypothyroidism, and slow pitting edema resulting from hypoalbuminemia was observed simultaneously.

Elderly people often have several disorders at the same time; however, we believe that, in explaining manifestations, one disorder should account for every symptom. In this case, the patient had remarkable anasarca because of DLBCL involvement of the pituitary gland. This case was very valuable because we could assess the patient's abnormalities; that is to say, anasarca, weight gain, hypothyroidism, elevated lactate dehydrogenase and alkaline phosphatase, splenomegaly, and swelling of the pituitary gland caused by malignant lymphoma and its infiltration into the pituitary gland.

In this era of longevity, the prevalence of diseases increases, and we must anticipate the greater likelihood of multiple, simultaneous diagnoses [8]. Hickam's dictum and Occam's razor are well suited to this case. "A patient can have as many diagnoses as he darn well pleases" [8]. This is Hickam's dictum. However, William of Ockham stated "Among competing hypotheses, favor the simplest one" [8]. This is known as Occam's razor.

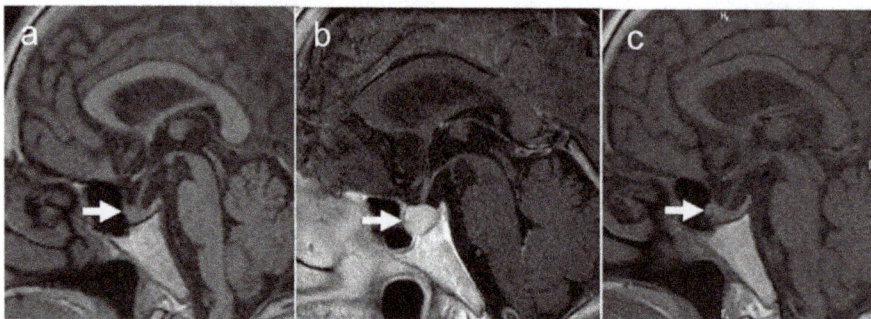

Figure 3 Head magnetic resonance imaging. White arrows indicate the pituitary gland. **(a)** One year before. Normal-sized pituitary gland. **(b)** Time of diagnosis. Pituitary gland swelling but keeping signal of posterior lobe of pituitary. **(c)** After one course of chemotherapy. Pituitary gland swelling improved.

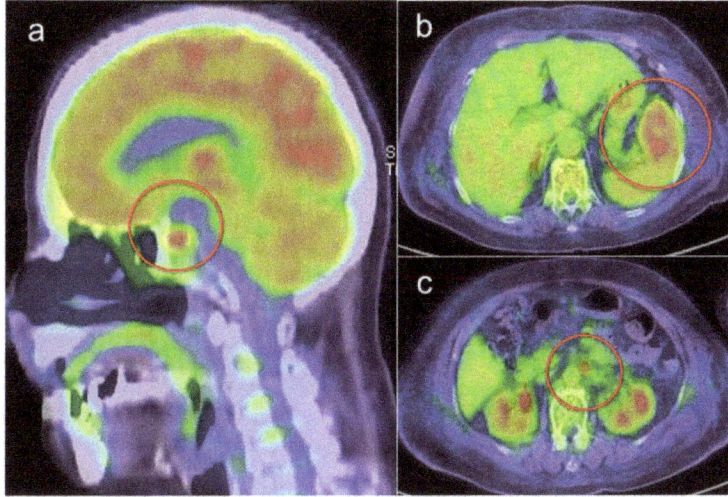

Figure 4 Positron emission tomography (PET) scan. PET scan revealed a localized accumulation in the pituitary gland **(a)**, spleen **(b)**, and para-abdominal aorta lymph nodes **(c)** (red circles).

It was easy to assess laboratory abnormalities, splenomegaly, and multiple spleen tumors that resulted from the malignant lymphoma. It was also easy to assess anasarca that was due to hypothyroidism and hypoalbuminemia. In this case, however, we reached the correct diagnosis of pituitary gland involvement from DLBCL, which manifested significant anasarca, according to Occam's razor. A pituitary gland lesion with central

hypothyroidism should be considered as one of the differential diagnoses of edema, especially nonpitting edema in some cases.

Conclusion

We experienced a patient with remarkable anasarca caused by DLBCL infiltration of the pituitary gland. A pituitary gland lesion with central hypothyroidism should be

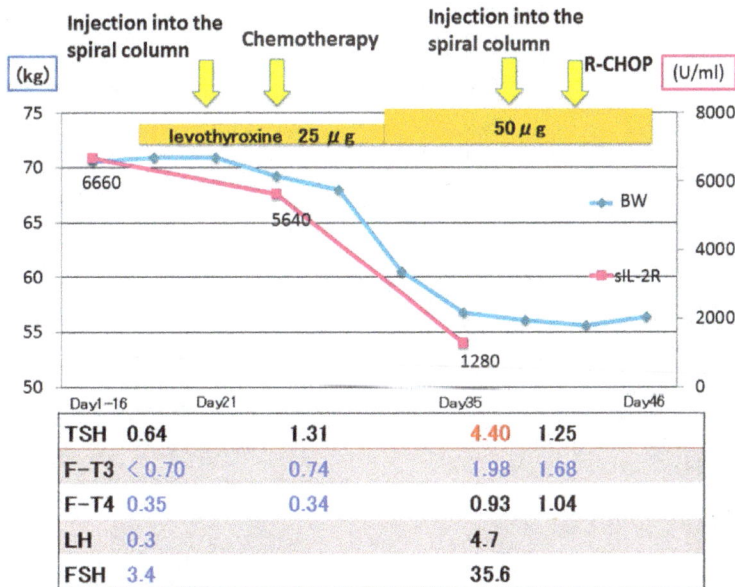

Figure 5 Clinical course. First course chemotherapy including methotrexate, vincristine, ifosfamide, and dexamethasone improved anasarca and body weight was reverted as same as 3 months before. Moreover, thyroid hormone, LH, and FSH became normal levels. Second course chemotherapy as cyclophosphamide, hydroxydaunorubicin, vincristine, and prednisone (CHOP) led to remission and the same regimen of chemotherapy was repeated.

considered as one of the differential diagnoses of edema. This case was very valuable because we could assess it by following the time course of symptoms, laboratory data, and imaging findings.

Consent

Written informed consent was obtained from the patient for publication of this Case report and any accompanying images.

A copy of the written consent is available for review by the Series Editor of this journal.

Competing interests

All authors have no financial interests to disclose and no conflict of interest to declare.

Authors' contributions

AK: Manuscript redaction. TK: Manuscript redaction, correction and relecture of the manuscript. YN, MA, and MM: Management of the case, manuscript redaction and correction. MM: Manuscript correction, redaction of the comment of the illustrations. All authors read and approved the final manuscript.

Acknowledgments

We thank Dr Yuji Sakuma (MD, PhD, Department of Integrative Pathology, Jichi Medical University) for supply of the pathological image.

Author details

[1]Division of General Internal Medicine, Jichi Medical University Hospital, 3311-1 Yakushiji, Shimotsuke, Tochigi 329-0498, Japan. [2]Department of Internal Medicine, Division of Hematology, Jichi Medical University, Shimotsuke, Japan.

References

1. Bilgili SG, Yılmaz D, Soyoral YU, Karadag AS, Bayram I. Intravascular large B-cell lymphoma presenting with anasarca-type edema and acute renal failure. Ren Fail. 2013;35:1163–6.
2. Lymphoma Study Group of Japanese Pathologists. The world health organization classification of malignant lymphomas in Japan: incidence of recently recognized entities. Pathol Int. 2000;50:696–702.
3. The Non-Hodgkin's Lymphoma Classification Project. A clinical evaluation of the International Lymphoma Study Group classification of non-Hodgkin's lymphoma. Blood. 1997;89:3909–18.
4. Yang J, Zhao N, Zhang G, Zheng W. Clinical features of patients with non-Hodgkin's lymphoma metastasizing to the pituitary glands. Oncol Lett. 2013;5:1643–8.
5. Nakashima Y, Shiratsuchi M, Abe I, Matsuda Y, Miyata N, Ohno H, et al. Pituitary and adrenal involvement in diffuse large B-cell lymphoma, with recovery of their function after chemotherapy. BMC Endocr Disord. 2013;13:45.
6. Tamer G, Kartal I, Aral F. Pituitary infiltration by non-Hodgkin lymphoma. J Med Case Rep. 2009;3:9293.
7. Akkas BE, Vural GU. The incidence of secondary central nervous system involvement in patients with non-Hodgkin's lymphoma as detected by 18 F-FDG PET/CT. Nucl Med Commun. 2013;34:50–6.
8. Hilliard AA, Weinberger SE, Tierney Jr LM, Midthun DE, Saint S. Clinical problem-solving. Occam's razor versus Saint's Triad. N Engl J Med. 2004;350:599–603.

9

Results of a prospective multicenter neuroendocrine tumor registry reporting on clinicopathologic characteristics of Greek patients

George C. Nikou[1], Kalliopi Pazaitou-Panayiotou[2], Dimitrios Dimitroulopoulos[3], Georgios Alexandrakis[4], Pavlos Papakostas[5], Michalis Vaslamatzis[6], Philippos Kaldrymidis[7], Vyron Markussis[8], Anna Koumarianou[9]* and on behalf of the "G-NET-Registry" investigators

Abstract

Background: The rare incidence of neuroendocrine neoplasms (NENs) has contributed to a paucity of large epidemiologic studies of patients with this condition. We investigated the occurrence and clinicopathologic features of NENs in Greece.

Methods: Between October 2010 and November 2012 we collected data on 246 newly diagnosed patients from a broad-based multi-institutional registry that comprises eight academic and hospital sites in Greece. The WHO 2010 pathologic classification and the 7th AJCC Staging system was applied in all cases.

Results: Of all patients 94 % had a sporadic and 6 % a multiple endocrine neoplasia tumor; 63.4 % were gastroenteropancreatic-(GEP)-NENs, 17.9 % Head & Neck NENs, 9.8 % NENs of Unknown Primary, 6.5 % Lung NENs and 2.4 % Pheochromocytomas. Gastric and pancreatic NENs were the most common primary sites. Poorly differentiated neuroendocrine carcinomas (NEC) were 9.3 %, all sporadic. Fifteen percent of patients were asymptomatic at presentation, 24 % had a first symptom of the disease related to endocrine syndrome and 61 % had symptoms related to locally advanced or metastatic disease. Metastatic disease was established in 25 % of tumors most frequently in the GEP NEN group. Findings are presented according to Ki-67 distribution. MRI had a higher diagnostic positive yield than Octreoscan. Somatostatin analogs, lanreotide and octreotide acetate, were prescribed at 38.5 & 61.5 % of NEN patients respectively and were found to be equally effective at providing symptomatic relief.

Conclusions: This is to our knowledge the first study of a Greek tumor registry and one of the few European Registries providing information regarding clinicopathologic characteristics and therapies in patients with neuroendocrine tumors of various origin sites, beyond GEP NENs.

Keywords: Neuroendocrine tumors, NET, Neuroendocrine neoplasms, NEN, Neuroendocrine carcinomas, NEC, Gastric, Enteric, Pancreatic, Head and neck, Imaging, Therapy, Registry

* Correspondence: akoumari@yahoo.com
[9]Hematology-Oncology Unit, Fourth Department of Internal Medicine,
Attikon University Hospital, Medical School, National and Kapodestrian
University of Athens, Rimini 1, 12462, Haidari, Athens, Greece
Full list of author information is available at the end of the article

Background

Neuroendocrine neoplasms (NENs) are a heterogeneous group of tumors arising from cells of the diffuse body neuroendocrine system most commonly in the gastrointestinal tract.

Since 1907, when originally described as benign tumors by Oberndorfer [1], the nomenclature and classification of NENs has changed several times, making the collection of epidemiological information and the comparison among studies published in the literature very difficult. Gastroenteropancreatic NENs (GEP NENs) were recently redefined according to the updated pathological and immunohistochemical criteria established by WHO [2]. Irrespective of the specific site of origin, GEP NENs are classified as 'well differentiated,' 'moderately differentiated' or 'poorly differentiated neuroendocrine carcinomas GEP-NEC'. Additionally the classification is based on the Ki-67 labeling index (LI) that categorizes GEP NENs into the three groups: ≤ 2, 3–20 and >20 % [2].

Despite a small number of national multicentric registry studies and an even smaller number of epidemiological studies the real incidence of NENs is unclear. This can be a reason that explains the discrepancy between the estimated incidence that differs between genders, races and among countries and continents [3, 4]. There are several explanations for this phenomenon most importantly that previous histopathologic classifications have been substituted by the most recent that encompasses more entities with malignant potential under the term neuroendocrine neoplasia [2, 5, 6].

Although there are several registries reporting on the incidence of GEP NENs [7–9] only few registries include data on NENs of other sites [10–13]. Therefore there is lack of information on the incidence and the relative frequency of many NEN subgroups including the head and neck and unknown primary (UP) that remain highly under-represented in the registries.

The primary endpoint of the study was to describe NEN subtypes in Greece and to collect information on the presenting symptoms, diagnostic evaluation, staging techniques and choice of treatment modalities, in these patients.

Methods

The neuroendocrine tumor registry in Greece

The Neuroendocrine Tumor Registry was generated by dedicated specialists involved in the diagnosis and treatment of NEN patients. The team included medical oncologists, endocrinologists and gastroenterologists from eight academic and non-academic tertiary hospitals with an established experience in the management of NEN patients. The registry was funded by IPSEN Epe, Greece. IPSEN had no influence on the setup of the database, data acquisition or data analysis and had no access to raw data. The design of the study was descriptive, multicenter and observational open-ended surveillance registry. Approval of the study was obtained from each Institutional Review Board & Ethics Committee according to the Declaration of Helsinki and Good Clinical Practice, as well as to the EU regulations [directives 95/46/EC (24/10/1995),2001/20/EC (04/04/2001) and (EC) 45/2001]. Regulatory approval was obtained from the National Organization for Medicines (EOF). All patients signed a written informed consent for participation in the study. No children were involved in this database.

Data acquisition

A dedicated database software (TMS, Athens, Greece) was built with contribution by all authors during three specifically dedicated days. The items to be included were decided upon by specialists (medical oncologists, gastroenterologists and endocrinologists) experienced in the care of patients with NEN. This prospective survey was conducted in eight Greek referral centers and recruitment of NEN patients was started after October 2010. The feasibility and utility of the database was tested in a pre-test platform and necessary modifications were performed. The resulting database consisted of data fields divided in 18 sections including demographics, symptoms, tumor characteristics, diagnostic procedures, treatments modalities and outcome. If a patient received a treatment (e.g. somatostatin analogues) for more than one continuous treatment period, then the separate treatment periods and the response to each of them were documented as separate outcomes. Possible answers were either split into "yes" or "no" or selected from a drop-down menu. All physicians were trained and were responsible for the introduction of the studied features in the registry. One trained study monitor visited each center, reviewed the patients' medical files provided by the institution and assessed the quality of data insertion to the database.

All patients were entered in the database, by trained doctors, with their initials, date of birth and date of histopathology diagnosis to exclude the possibility of more than one recordings of the same patient. Once the duplicates were removed this information was excluded. In the case of genetic syndrome data acquisition depended on its positive documentation of items. If for example multiple endocrine neoplasia (MEN) was documented either as a report of the genetic analysis or stated as diagnosis by the physician, the patient was documented as 'MEN-positive'. In the database inserted parameters included also details on the diagnostic procedures and therapies applied. Patient data were specifically checked to avoid double insertions from different centers and in that case data were merged.

Patient inclusion

Inclusion criteria were diagnosis of NEN histologically confirmed after October 2010 and a patient's signed informed consent. Patients were excluded if they had a small or large cell lung cancer histology or if they were not actively followed up. Histological classification applied was the WHO 2010 classification [2] and staging was assessed according to the 7th AJCC Staging system [14].

Statistical analysis

We performed an interim analyses after two years of patient recruitment in the registry. Continuous variables were expressed either with the use of the mean and the standard deviation or with the median and the minimum and maximum values depending on their distribution. The normality of the distribution of values was examined with the use of the Shapiro-Wilk test. Categorical variables were expressed as percentages (%). Statistical comparison between groups was performed with the use of Student's t test or with the Mann Whitney U test when the distribution of variables was normal or not, respectively. Distribution of continuous variables between more than two groups was tested with the use of ANOVA or Kruskal-Wallis test, depending on the normality or not of their distribution. Differences in categorical variables were tested with the use of the Fisher's Exact test. All statistical analyses were performed with the use of the IBM SPSS Statistics (ver. 22.0). All statistical tests were two-sided and significance was a priori determined at the $p = 0.05$ level.

Results

Patient population

During the study period, 246 eligible patients were recorded in the Greek NET Registry. Of these, 121 (49.2 %) were males. All patients were of Caucasian origin, except one of South Asian origin. The median age at diagnosis of all patients was 57 years (range 18–82).

Of all patients, 111 (45 %) were referred to the Registry Centers by a physician of a different specialty. Seventy six patients (31 %) were found incidentally during a diagnostic procedure for an apparently unrelated cause. One hundred fifty six NENs (63.4 %) were located in the gastroenteropancreatic system. The clinicopathologic characteristics are shown in Table 1. The more frequent localization in the stomach was the corpus, while it was the head for the pancreas. In the lung the typical NENs prevailed. The majority of tumors were well differentiated and with Ki-67 ≤ 2.

Of the 228 evaluable patients, 6.5 % had T4 stage (all GEP NENs), 28 % had lymph nodal infiltration (most commonly GEP NEN, bronchial and H&N) and 24 % had metastatic disease most frequently in the UP and

Table 1 Clinicopathologic characteristics of the study population

	N (%)
Primary site	
Gastrenteropancreatic	156 (63.4)
Stomach	54 (35 %)
Corpus	37 (68.5)
Antrum	11 (20.4)
Fundus	6 (11.1)
Pancreas	36 (23 %)
Head	20 (55.6)
Tail	10 (27.8)
Body	6 (16.7)
Duodenum	8 (5 %)
Jejunum	5 (3 %)
Ileum	10 (6 %)
Appendix	17 (11 %)
Colon	8 (5 %)
Rectum	18 (12 %)
Head and Neck[c]	44 (17.9)
Unknown Primary	24 (9.8)
Lung	16 (6.5)
Typical	10 (62.5)
Atypical	6 (37.5)
Pheochromocytoma	6 (2.4)
Differentiation Grade[a]	
Well	132 (58.4)
Moderate	73 (32.3)
Poor	21 (9.3)
Ki-67 [b]	
≤2 %	166 (72.8)
3–20 %	56 (24.5)
>20 %	6 (2.6)

[a]20 missing cases
[b]18 missing cases
[c]includes 41 MTC and 3 paragangliomas

GEP NEN groups. Data regarding the T stage are missing for 18 UP patients.

Multiple endocrine neoplasia was diagnosed in 14 patients (6 %), all MEN1. Mean age at diagnosis in patients with MEN1 syndrome was 48.8 ± 19 years compared to 56 ± 14 years in non-MEN patients ($p = 0.131$). Eight (57 %) had parathyroid hyperplasia, 3 (21 %) pituitary adenoma and 4 (29 %) adrenal adenomas. Neuroendocrine tumors associated with MEN1 syndrome involved 4 head and neck, 1 bronchial, 4 GEP, 2 pheochromocytomas and 3 unknown primary (UP). Clinical syndrome due to hormone secretion was present in 7 patients.

Clinical manifestations of NEN

Of all patients 38 patients (15 %) were asymptomatic, 24 % reported symptoms related to endocrine syndrome and 61 % had symptoms related to the presence of the tumoral mass. The most common clinical symptoms related to advance disease were dyspepsia (44 %), abdominal pain (38.6 %) and asthenia (35.8 %) followed by weight loss (18.3 %) and anorexia (16.7 %). Symptoms related to hormonal secretion were less reported and included mainly flushing (14.5 %), diarrhea (12 %) or both (1 %).

Regarding the symptoms according to tumor location, in gastroenteric NENs comprised abdominal pain (41 %), asthenia (41 %), weight loss (35 %), dyspepsia (35 %), and anorexia (17 %). Pancreatic NENs presented most commonly with abdominal pain (52 %), diarrhea (28 %), weight loss (28 %), dyspepsia (26 %), and asthenia (21 %). For head and neck NENs (medullary thyroid carcinomas and paragangliomas) the most common presentation was neck swelling (14 %). For adrenal NENs the most common manifestations were asthenia (25 %), weight loss (12.5 %), hyperglycemia (12.5 %), and sweating (25 %). Vein thrombosis was reported in head and neck NENs (2.5 %) but not in GEP NENs.

Diagnostic procedures

The diagnostic procedures applied according to NEN site of origin are shown in Table 2. Most commonly performed test for staging was computed tomography (CT; 82 % of patients), followed by Octreoscan (63.4 %). The procedures leading to the highest percentage of positive results (% of positive results with imaging compared to positive histopathological results) were 2-deoxy-2-(^{18}F)

fluoro-D-glucose (^{18}F-FDG) positron emission tomography (PET)-computed tomography (CT) scan and magnetic resonance.

Investigation of biochemical markers were carried out for serum chromogranin A (CgA) and for neuron specific enolase (NSE) in the serum of 60 and 43 % of patients respectively and by urinary 5-HIAA in 38 % of patients. The positive yield of these tests were 89, 28 and 33 % respectively, most commonly all three positive in NEN of UP. In patients with a suspected functioning NEN additional hormonal assessment included insulin (6.5 %), glucagon (4.1 %), gastrin (40.7 %) and VIP (3.3 %).

Histopathological characteristics

The histopathological features of all NEN patients are shown in Table 1. Specific characteristics such as vascular invasion, local infiltration and differentiation grade in relation to primary site are presented in Table 3. Local infiltration was present in 55 (38.7 %) and vascular invasion in 23 (16.7 %) of the 156 patients with GEP NENs. Ki-67 labeling index (LI) was carried out in 228 (93 %) NENs. The distribution of Ki-67 according to the primary site is shown in Table 3 and according to gender and staging in Table 4. Immunohistochemical staining for serum CgA, synaptophysin and somatostatin receptors (SSTR-2) was done in 186 (76 %), 162 (66 %) and 43 (17 %) of the entire cohort and was positive in 165 (89 %), 147 (91 %) and 31 (72 %) of the tested patients respectively.

Therapeutic interventions

Treatments applied in NEN patients are shown in Tables 4, 5 and 6.

Table 2 Diagnostic procedures used for staging, according to primary site (absolute number performed and % positive yield)

Diagnostic Procedure	Head &Neck[a]	Bronchial	GEP	Pheochromocytoma	Unknown Primary	Total
	N = 44	N = 16	N = 156	N = 6	N = 24	N = 246
(18) F-FDG PET/CT	6 (100.0)	1 (100.0)	3 (66.7)	0 (0.0)	1 (0.0)	11 (81.8)
Magnetic Resonance	12 (81.8)	4 (100.0)	52 (69.2)	3 (100.0)	14 (78.6)	85 (75.0)
Endoscopic Ultrasound	1 (0.0)	0 (0.0)	21 (81.0)	0 (0.0)	5 (60.0)	27 (74.1)
Bronchoscopy	0 (0.0)	7 (100.0)	0 (0.0)	0 (0.0)	3 (0.0)	10 (70.0)
MIBG	1 (0.0)	0 (0.0)	1 (100.0)	5 (80.0)	3 (33.3)	10 (60.0)
Enteroclysis	0 (0.0)	0 (0.0)	4 (75.0)	0 (0.0)	1 (0.0)	5 (60.0)
Computed Tomography	33 (78.8)	16 (93.8)	126 (43.2)	4 (100.0)	23 (81.8)	202 (58.5)
Abdominal Ultrasound	5 (0.0)	3 (33.3)	65 (50.8)	4 (100.0)	13 (92.3)	90 (55.6)
Gastroscopy	4 (0.0)	3 (0.0)	105 (60.0)	0 (0.0)	14 (14.3)	126 (51.6)
Octreoscan	16 (68.8)	11 (54.5)	107 (44.9)	2 (50.0)	20 (65.0)	156 (50.6)
Colonoscopy	2 (0.0)	2 (0.0)	71 (38.0)	0 (0.0)	15 (0.0)	90 (30.0)
Bone Scan	22 (18.2)	12 (25.0)	10 (22.2)	4 (25.0)	11 (18.2)	59 (20.7)
Endoscopic Capsule	0 (0.0)	0 (0.0)	10 (30.0)	0 (0.0)	6 (0.0)	16 (18.8)
x-Ray	33 (0.0)	15 (100.0)	85 (2.4)	2 (0.0)	17 (17.6)	152 (13.2)

2-deoxy-2-(^{18}F) fluoro-D-glucose: positron emission tomography/computed tomography (18F-FDG PET/CT), n: number of patients
[a]includes 41 MTC and 3 paragangliomas

Table 3 Distribution of vascular invasion, local infiltration, differentiation grading and Ki-67 LI in relation to primary site (absolute number and % of patients)

Clinicopathologic features	Head &Neck[a] N = 44	Bronchial N = 16	GEP N = 156	Pheochromocytoma N = 6	Unknown Primary N = 24	Total
Vascular invasion	13 (28.2)	5 (10.8)	23 (50.0)	2 (4.3)	3 (6.5)	46 (100.0)
Local infiltration	22 (24.4)	6 (6.6)	55 (61.1)	2 (2.2)	5 (5.5)	90 (100.0)
Differentiation grading						
G1	22 (16.6)	10 (7.5)	84 (63.6)	4 (3.0)	12 (9.0)	132 (100.0)
G2	18 (24.6)	6 (8.2)	42 (57.5)	2 (2.7)	5 (6.8)	73 (100.0)
G3	1 (4.7)	0 (0)	17 (80.9)	0 (0)	3 (14.2)	21 (100.0)
Ki-67 labelling index						
Ki-67 ≤ 2	34 (20.4)	13 (7.8)	104 (62.6)	5 (3.0)	10 (6.0)	166 (100.0)
Ki-67 3-20	3 (5.3)	3 (5.3)	39 (69.6)	1 (1.7)	10 (17.8)	56 (100.0)
Ki-67 > 20	0 (0)	0 (0)	3 (50.0)	0 (0)	3 (50.0)	6 (100.0)

[a]includes 41 MTC and 3 paragangliomas

Table 4 Distribution of Ki-67 labelling index according to gender, stage, type of treatment

Parameters	Ki-67 Labeling Index, n (%)			Total n
	≤2 (166 cases)	3–20 (56 cases)	>20 (6 cases)	
Gender				
Male	82 (74.5)	24 (21.8)	4 (3.6)	110 (100.0)
Female	84 (71.2)	32 (27.1)	2 (1.7)	118 (100.0)
Stage TNM				
T0	16 (84.2)	3 (15.8)	0 (0)	19 (100.0)
T1	68 (82.9)	14 (17.1)	0 (0)	82 (100.0)
T2	16 (64.0)	9 (36.0)	0 (0)	25 (100.0)
T3	17 (54.8)	11 (35.5)	3 (9.7)	31 (100.0)
T4	4 (28.6)	10 (71.4)	0 (0)	14 (100.0)
TX	45 (78.9)	9 (15.8)	3 (5.3)	57 (100.0)
N0	111 (78.2)	30 (21.1)	1 (0.7)	142 (100.0)
N1	39 (60.9)	20 (31.3)	5 (7.8)	64 (100.0)
NX	16 (72.7)	6 (27.3)	0 (0)	22 (100.0)
M0	97 (81.5)	22 (18.5)	0 (0)	119 (100.0)
M1	29 (52.7)	21 (38.2)	5 (9.1)	55 (100.0)
MX	40 (74.1)	13 (24.1)	1 (1.8)	54 (100.0)
Type of treatment				
Lanreotide	52 (69.3)	20 (26.6)	3 (4.1)	75 (100.0)
Octreotide	85 (71.4)	33 (27.7)	1 (0.9)	119 (100.0)
Sunitinib	5 (50.0)	5 (50.0)	0 (0)	10 (100.0)
Everolimus	3 (60.0)	2 (40.0)	0 (0)	5 (100.0)
Chemotherapy	11 (50)	9 (40.9)	2 (9.1)	22 (100.0)

Somatostatin analogs were administered in 135 patients. Lanreotide 60–120 mg and Octreotide 20–30 mg LAR was delivered for a total number of 1378 and 2473 months, respectively. Improvement of symptoms was observed in 68.2 %, stabilization in 25.9 % and deterioration in 5.8 % of the patients. There was no difference between the symptom responses observed with the two analogues ($p = 0.295$), even after controlling for the different distribution in Ki-67 LI categories in a multinomial logistic regression.

Chemotherapy was given in 22 patients and targeted therapies in 15 patients. Interferon was recorded as treatment in only 2 patients. Bevacizumab, an anti-VEGF monoclonal antibody, was delivered in 4 GEP NEN patients. Peptide Receptor Radionuclide Therapy was delivered in 17 patients and radiotherapy in 9 patients. Surgical excision was applied in 193 patients with complete excision achieved in 164 patients, all with Ki-67 < 20 % (Table 5). Local therapies in patients with liver metastases were applied on 15 occasions (Table 6).

Table 5 Primary surgery performed in NEN patients (n)

Primary Site (all Ki-67 < 20 %)	Radical Surgery (n)	Non Radical Surgery (n)	Total
Head and Neck	40	4	44
Lung	8	2	10
GEP	110	20	130
Pheochromocytoma	4	2	6
Unknown Primary	2	1	3
Type of Surgery	(n)		
Open Surgery	128		
Endoscopic/Laparoscopic Excision	65		

GEP gastroenteropancreatic, n number of patients

Table 6 Surgery and debulking procedures performed in NEN patients (n) with liver and lung metastases

	Number of patients	Primary Site (all Ki-67 < 20 %)
Patients with Liver Metastases	Total number: 49	34 GEP, 11 UP, 3 lung, 1 pheochromocyroma
Liver Metastasectomy	6	4 GEP, 1 Lung, 1 unknown primary
Chemoembolization	3	GEP
Radiofrequency Ablation	4	GEP
Other	2	GEP
Patients with Lung Metastases	Total number: 6	4 GEP, 1 lung, 1 unknown primary
Surgical Excision	1	GEP

GEP gastroenteropancreatic, *UP* unknown primary

Deaths observed

During the follow-up period of the registry and at the time of the analyses 10 deaths were documented, corresponding to 4.1 % of the registry population. The primary sites of origin of these patients were 6 gastroenteric, 2 pancreatic and 2 pheochromocytomas.

Discussion

This study presents for the first time the data of the NET registry in Greece focusing on the epidemiologic and clinico-pathologic characteristics as well as the therapeutic modalities applied in patients with all type of NENs except small and large cell lung cancer.

Greece is a European country with a reported population of 11 million in 2012 (http://countryeconomy.com/demography/population/greece). This partly explains the small number of recorded patients (246) presented in the participating centers during the first two years of this observational study. Taken into consideration that the eight centers participating in the study do not cover for the entire population definitive conclusions on the incidence of NEN tumors cannot be made.

Only few cancer NEN registries exist in the USA and Europe, mostly national. According to the SEER database (seer.cancer.gov website), that includes information on 7,262,696 cancer patients, covering for 28 % of the USA population the incidence of NENs in 2004 is 5.25/100.000 inhabitants [15]. On the other hand, data on the incidence of NENs in Europe, is limited and is usually reported by anatomic location, most commonly GEP NENs [8, 16]. Specifically, in one study including NENs of all sites, except lung, conducted by the RareCare Working Group, the overall incidence rate was 25/1,000,000 in total but it was highest when patients older than 65 years of age were considered (40 per 1,000,000) [17].

In our registry, the median age at diagnosis and the gender's ratio were in accordance to those reported in other published registries [4, 10, 12]. We found the

gastroenteropancreatic tract being the most common followed by the head and neck and UP. This is slightly different from that reported in one study from the Mediterranean area with pancreas and lung being the commonest primaries, where it was found that 63 % were GEP-NENs, 33 % thoracic-NENs including thymic, 4 % UP-NEN [10]. This difference is probably due to the fact that there was no center for lung NENs participating in our registry. With respect to the GI tract we found that gastric (35 %), pancreatic (23 %) and rectal NENs (12 %) were the commonest primary sites. An inverse frequency was found in the Italian study as the pancreatic primary (31 %) was commonest compared to gastric (10 %) [10].

The presenting symptoms of our patients were related to endocrine syndrome in 24 %, and to mass effect in 61 %, most commonly dyspepsia, similarly to our previous retrospective study [18]. Although only 15 % of patients were completely asymptomatic, the diagnosis was considered 'incidental' in 30.9 % as many patients had vague and underreported symptoms recognized after the diagnosis. In line with our study a registry from Italy reported that the first symptoms of the disease were related to tumor burden in 46 %, endocrine syndrome in 23 %, while the diagnosis was fortuity in 29 % of cases [10].

Six percent of our patients had MEN syndrome diagnosed earlier compared to patients with sporadic NENs. Multiple endocrine neoplasia associated NEN frequency was not different from that reported in an Italian (7 %), a Spanish (5 %) and a Japanese registry (4.3 %) [8, 10, 19]. As for other tumors associated with hereditary syndromes, NENs associated with MEN mandates genetic screening of the relatives, different surveillance methods and treatments for the involved patients [20, 21].

The differentiation grade and Ki-67 LI are not only obligatory requirements of the pathological classification system but represent the upmost important prognostic factors and may help tailor treatment in NEN patients [22]. Descriptions regarding the Ki-67 LI and differentiation grade are lacking in the published NEN registries and this is due not only to the frequent change in the classification system but also to the underreporting of the Ki-67 in the histological diagnosis [13]. For 93 % of our histological specimens Ki-67 LI was counted and found most commonly <2 %. With respect to the differentiation grade we could find only one similar study that reported a 52 % of well differentiated neuroendocrine tumors (NETs) and a 13 % of poorly differentiated NEC [10].

Head and neck was the second most common (20 %) primary site in our registry and included medullary tumors and paragangliomas. To our knowledge there is no information from other registries on these NENs and thus we cannot have comparable data. One possible explanation is that only in the past few years medullary tumors were included in the large family of NENs.

NENs of UP was the third most frequent subtype (9.8 %) in our registry, most commonly of Ki-67 LI > 2 % and G2/G3. A European study reported a lower incidence (4 %) and a USA study 13 % of UP [10, 15]. By definition NEN of UP site refers to a group of patients with locally advanced disease such as regional lymphadenopathy or most commonly metastatic disease [23]. It cannot be identified if these tumors arise from an occult gastrointestinal or pulmonary primary site or else from a multipotent stem cell [24]. One explanation for this high frequency of UP is the non-availability in our country of Gallium-68 PET/CT and DOPA PET/CT that have a higher sensitivity for the identification of NEN primaries such as GEPs and medullary/paragangliomas respectively [25, 26]. A recent systematic review of the studies published in the literature did not identify differences in the biology of UP NENs or in the outcome of these patients compared to NEN patients with known primary matched for grade [27].

In our study we found metastatic disease at presentation in 25 % of patients comprising 17.5 % of well, 37.5 % of moderately and 83 % of poorly differentiated neoplasms. Similar findings were reported from the SEER database as distant metastases at diagnosis comprised 21 % well, 30 % moderately and 50 % poorly differentiated tumors [15].

In our study we did not find a statistically significant difference in the distribution of histologies, primaries and staging between males and females. However, in the SEER database male patients were more likely to have metastasis at presentation, than female patients, in a statistically significant way [15]. We were able to detect in our tumors local and vascular infiltration two well-established features of malignant behavior with adverse prognostic significance [5]. As long term data of our cohort is not yet matured we cannot comment on the impact of these features on the survival of our patients.

With respect to diagnostic imaging, in our population imaging with internationally recommended techniques such as somatostatin receptor PET/CT imaging with Gallium-68 and endoscopic ultrasound (EUS) is either unavailable (^{68}Ga) or accessible in very few sites (EUS). In our study octreoscan was less sensitive compared to other procedures such as computed tomography. This is in line with an earlier study by our group showing that octreoscan compared to conventional imaging such as ultrasound and CT is less sensitive for the detection of liver metastases [28].

The most commonly applied therapy in our cohort was somatostatin analogs (SSA), octreotide 30 mg LAR and lanreotide 120 mg Autogel, both with an established role in the symptom and tumor control of patients with well and moderately differentiated NENs [29–31]. Recently, in the CLARINET trial, lanreotide 120 mg Autogel was established for its anti tumoral effect in both pancreatic and gastroenteric locally advanced or metastatic neuroendocrine tumors with Ki-67 up to 10 %. In this registry, the response was documented as improvement, stabilization or deterioration of the symptoms, without the use of the RECIST criteria, since this was out of the scope of the registry. Similarly to the previously published studies, our findings indicate an equal role of the different SSAs in the control of NEN symptoms.

Other therapies applied in our patients with Ki-67 LI < 20 % included systemic chemotherapy, with either streptozocin/5FU or temozolomide, or a targeted agent such as everolimus and sunitinib, according to previously published data [32–35]. Patients with poorly differentiated tumors or Ki-67 > 20 % were treated with systemic chemotherapy comprising cisplatin/carboplatin and etoposide doublets according to established evidence [36].

Limitations of our study include a) the fact that not all NENs diagnosed in our country between October 2010 and November 2012 were included in the present registry and b) the lack of information on survival, progressive free survival, recurrences and new metastases. As long term data of our cohort is not yet matured we cannot comment on the impact of our findings on the evolution of the disease in general and on overall survival.

Conclusions

We present for the first time the results of a Greek NET registry that includes NEN from a variety of primary sites. Our results indicate some differences in the occurrence of NENs reported from registries of other European countries and the USA. It is thus important to develop national registries for the precise description of the incidence and the handling of NENs and the possible application of the findings in prevention and pharmacoeconomics. Based on the reported occurrence of NENs and the variations in incidence observed in the literature it is important that each country develops a national registry for the recording of the incidence and clinico-pathologic characteristics of these rare tumors and to improve our understanding of the biology and survival of these tumors.

Competing interests
All authors declare no conflicts of interests.

Authors' contributions
GCN, KPP, DD, GA, PP, MV, PK, AK participated in the study design and collection of clinical data. VM assisted in the design and data management of the study. AK, KPP, DD, VM assisted in the analysis of data and the first draft of the manuscript. All authors revised the manuscript and approved its final version. The G-NET Registry investigators (TA, MP, AM, AC, SM, NA, PK, EV) contributed to data collection and revised the manuscript for important intellectual content.

Acknowledgments

The authors would like to thank Professor Philippe Ruszniewski for his invaluable comments regarding the manuscript.

Author details

[1]Neuroendocrinology Section, 1st Department of Propaedeutic Internal Medicine, Laiko University Hospital, Athens, Greece. [2]Unit of Endocrinology and Endocrine Oncology, Theagenio Cancer Hospital, Thessaloniki, Greece. [3]Gastroenterology Department, Agios Savas Cancer Hospital, Athens, Greece. [4]Gastroenterology Department, NIMTS Hospital, Athens, Greece. [5]Oncology Department, Hippokrateion Hospital, Athens, Greece. [6]Oncology Department, Evangelismos Hospital, Athens, Greece. [7]Department of Endocrinology, Metaxa Cancer Hospital, Piraeus, Greece. [8]Ipsen epe, Athens, Greece. [9]Hematology-Oncology Unit, Fourth Department of Internal Medicine, Attikon University Hospital, Medical School, National and Kapodestrian University of Athens, Rimini 1, 12462, Haidari, Athens, Greece.

References

1. Obendorfer S. Karzinoide tumoren des dünndarms. Frankf Z Pathol. 1907;1:426–32.
2. Bosman F, Carneiro F, Hruban R, Theise N. WHO Classification of Tumours of the Digestive System. Fth ed. Lyon: International Agency for Research on Cancer Press; 2010.
3. Hauso O, Gustafsson BI, Kidd M, Waldum HL, Drozdov I, Chan AK, et al. Neuroendocrine tumor epidemiology: contrasting Norway and North America. Cancer. 2008;113:2655–64.
4. Modlin IM, Oberg K, Chung DC, Jensen RT, de Herder WW, Thakker RV, et al. Gastroenteropancreatic neuroendocrine tumours. Lancet Oncol. 2008;9:61–72.
5. Klimstra DS, Modlin IR, Coppola D, Lloyd RV, Suster S. The pathologic classification of neuroendocrine tumors: a review of nomenclature, grading, and staging systems. Pancreas. 2010;39:707–12.
6. Lawrence B, Gustafsson BI, Chan A, Svejda B, Kidd M, Modlin IM. The epidemiology of gastroenteropancreatic neuroendocrine tumors. Endocrinol Metab Clin North Am. 2011;40:1–18. vii.
7. Ellis L, Shale MJ, Coleman MP. Carcinoid tumors of the gastrointestinal tract: trends in incidence in England since 1971. Am J Gastroenterol. 2010;105:2563–9.
8. Garcia-Carbonero R, Capdevila J, Crespo-Herrero G, Diaz-Perez JA, Martinez Del Prado MP, Alonso Orduna V, et al. Incidence, patterns of care and prognostic factors for outcome of gastroenteropancreatic neuroendocrine tumors (GEP-NETs): results from the National Cancer Registry of Spain (RGETNE). Ann Oncol. 2010;21:1794–803.
9. Niederle MB, Hackl M, Kaserer K, Niederle B. Gastroenteropancreatic neuroendocrine tumours: the current incidence and staging based on the WHO and European Neuroendocrine Tumour Society classification: an analysis based on prospectively collected parameters. Endocr Relat Cancer. 2010;17:909–18.
10. Faggiano A, Ferolla P, Grimaldi F, Campana D, Manzoni M, Davi MV, et al. Natural history of gastro-entero-pancreatic and thoracic neuroendocrine tumors. Data from a large prospective and retrospective Italian epidemiological study: the NET management study. J Endocrinol Invest. 2012;35:817–23.
11. Modlin IM, Lye KD, Kidd M. A 5-decade analysis of 13,715 carcinoid tumors. Cancer. 2003;97:934–59.
12. Tsai HJ, Wu CC, Tsai CR, Lin SF, Chen LT, Chang JS. The epidemiology of neuroendocrine tumors in Taiwan: a nation-wide cancer registry-based study. PLoS One. 2013;8:e62487.
13. Younes RN. Neuroendocrine tumors: a registry of 1,000 patients. Rev Assoc Med Bras. 2008;54:305–7.
14. Edge S, Byrd D, Compton C, et al. AJCC Cancer Staging Manual. 7th ed. New York: Springer; 2010.
15. Yao JC, Hassan M, Phan A, Dagohoy C, Leary C, Mares JE, et al. One hundred years after "carcinoid": epidemiology of and prognostic factors for neuroendocrine tumors in 35,825 cases in the United States. J Clin Oncol. 2008;26:3063–72.
16. Scherubl H, Streller B, Stabenow R, Herbst H, Hopfner M, Schwertner C, et al. Clinically detected gastroenteropancreatic neuroendocrine tumors are on the rise: epidemiological changes in Germany. World J Gastroenterol. 2013;19:9012–9.
17. van der Zwan JM, Trama A, Otter R, Larranaga N, Tavilla A, Marcos-Gragera R, et al. Rare neuroendocrine tumours: results of the surveillance of rare cancers in Europe project. Eur J Cancer. 2013;49:2565–78.
18. Nikou GC, Marinou K, Thomakos P, Papageorgiou D, Sanzanidis V, Nikolaou P, et al. Chromogranin a levels in diagnosis, treatment and follow-up of 42 patients with non-functioning pancreatic endocrine tumours. Pancreatology. 2008;8:510–9.
19. Ito T, Igarashi H, Nakamura K, Sasano H, Okusaka T, Takano K, Komoto I, Tanaka M, Imamura M, Jensen RT, et al. Epidemiological trends of pancreatic and gastrointestinal neuroendocrine tumors in Japan: a nationwide survey analysis. J Gastroenterol 2014;50(1):58-64.
20. Nikou GC, Toubanakis C, Nikolaou P, Giannatou E, Safioleas M, Mallas E, et al. VIPomas: an update in diagnosis and management in a series of 11 patients. Hepatogastroenterology. 2005;52:1259–65.
21. Thakker RV, Newey PJ, Walls GV, Bilezikian J, Dralle H, Ebeling PR, et al. Clinical practice guidelines for multiple endocrine neoplasia type 1 (MEN1). J Clin Endocrinol Metab. 2012;97:2990–3011.
22. Martin-Perez E, Capdevila J, Castellano D, Jimenez-Fonseca P, Salazar R, Beguiristain-Gomez A, et al. Prognostic factors and long-term outcome of pancreatic neuroendocrine neoplasms: Ki-67 index shows a greater impact on survival than disease stage. The large experience of the Spanish National Tumor Registry (RGETNE). Neuroendocrinology. 2013;98:156–68.
23. Pavlidis N, Khaled H, Gaafar R. A mini review on cancer of unknown primary site: a clinical puzzle for the oncologists. J Adv Res. 2015;6:375–82.
24. Spigel DR, Hainsworth JD, Greco FA. Neuroendocrine carcinoma of unknown primary site. Semin Oncol. 2009;36:52–9.
25. Srirajaskanthan R, Kayani I, Quigley AM, Soh J, Caplin ME, Bomanji J. The role of 68Ga-DOTATATE PET in patients with neuroendocrine tumors and negative or equivocal findings on 111In-DTPA-octreotide scintigraphy. J Nucl Med. 2010;51:875–82.
26. Timmers HJ, Chen CC, Carrasquillo JA, Whatley M, Ling A, Havekes B, et al. Comparison of 18 F-fluoro-L-DOPA, 18 F-fluoro-deoxyglucose, and 18 F-fluorodopamine PET and 123I-MIBG scintigraphy in the localization of pheochromocytoma and paraganglioma. J Clin Endocrinol Metab. 2009;94:4757–67.
27. Stoyianni A, Pentheroudakis G, Pavlidis N. Neuroendocrine carcinoma of unknown primary: a systematic review of the literature and a comparative study with other neuroendocrine tumors. Cancer Treat Rev. 2011;37:358–65.
28. Dimitroulopoulos D, Xynopoulos D, Tsamakidis K, Paraskevas E, Zisimopoulos A, Andriotis E, et al. Scintigraphic detection of carcinoid tumors with a cost effectiveness analysis. World J Gastroenterol. 2004;10:3628–33.
29. Caplin ME, Pavel M, Cwikla JB, Phan AT, Raderer M, Sedlackova E, Cadiot G, Wolin EM, Capdevila J, Wall L, Rindi G, Langley A, Martinez S, Gomez-Panzani E, Ruszniewski P, and CLARINET Investigators. Anti-tumour effects of lanreotide for pancreatic and intestinal neuroendocrine tumours: the CLARINET open-label extension study. Endocr Relat Cancer. 2016;23:191-9.
30. Rinke A, Muller HH, Schade-Brittinger C, Klose KJ, Barth P, Wied M, et al. Placebo-controlled, double-blind, prospective, randomized study on the effect of octreotide LAR in the control of tumor growth in patients with metastatic neuroendocrine midgut tumors: a report from the PROMID Study Group. J Clin Oncol. 2009;27:4656–63.
31. Ruszniewski P, Ish-Shalom S, Wymenga M, O'Toole D, Arnold R, Tomassetti P, et al. Rapid and sustained relief from the symptoms of carcinoid syndrome: results from an open 6-month study of the 28-day prolonged-release formulation of lanreotide. Neuroendocrinology. 2004;80:244–51.
32. Koumarianou A, Antoniou S, Kanakis G, Economopoulos N, Rontogianni D, Ntavatzikos A, et al. Combination treatment with metronomic temozolomide, bevacizumab and long-acting octreotide for malignant neuroendocrine tumours. Endocr Relat Cancer. 2012;19:L1–4.
33. Moertel CG, Hanley JA, Johnson LA. Streptozocin alone compared with streptozocin plus fluorouracil in the treatment of advanced islet-cell carcinoma. N Engl J Med. 1980;303:1189–94.
34. Raymond E, Dahan L, Raoul JL, Bang YJ, Borbath I, Lombard-Bohas C, et al. Sunitinib malate for the treatment of pancreatic neuroendocrine tumors. N Engl J Med. 2011;364:501–13.
35. Yao JC, Shah MH, Ito T, Bohas CL, Wolin EM, Van Cutsem E, et al. Everolimus for advanced pancreatic neuroendocrine tumors. N Engl J Med. 2011;364:514–23.
36. Koumarianou A, Chatzellis E, Boutzios G, Tsavaris N, Kaltsas G. Current concepts in the diagnosis and management of poorly differentiated gastrointestinal neuroendocrine carcinomas. Endokrynol Pol. 2013;64:60–72.

10

Chromogranin A is a reliable serum diagnostic biomarker for pancreatic neuroendocrine tumors but not for insulinomas

Xin-Wei Qiao[1†], Ling Qiu[2†], Yuan-Jia Chen[1,3*], Chang-Ting Meng[4], Zhao Sun[4], Chun-Mei Bai[4], Da-Chun Zhao[5], Tai-Ping Zhang[6], Yu-Pei Zhao[3,6], Yu-Li Song[1], Yu-Hong Wang[7], Jie Chen[7] and Chong-Mei Lu[1]

Abstract

Background: Pancreatic neuroendocrine tumors (PNETs) are a group of rare tumors. Chromogranin A (CgA) was considered as the most practical and useful serum tumor marker in PNET patients. But peripheral blood levels of CgA are not routinely tested in Chinese patients with PNETs. This study was to assess the diagnostic value of CgA in Chinese patients with PNETs especially in patients with insulinomas.

Methods: Eighty-nine patients with PNETs including 57 insulinomas and 32 non-insulinoma PNETs as well as 86 healthy participants were enrolled in this study between September 2003 and June 2013. Serum levels of CgA were measured by ELISA method. Expression of CgA protein was detected in 26 PNET tissues including 14 insulinomas by immunohistochemical staining.

Results: Serum levels of CgA in 89 PNET patients were significantly higher than that in healthy controls ($P = 7.2 \times 10^{-9}$). Serum levels of CgA in 57 patients with insulinomas (median 64.8 ng/ml, range 25–164) were slightly higher than the levels in healthy controls (median 53.4 ng/ml, range 39–94) but much lower than the levels in 32 patients with non-insulinoma PNETs (median 193 ng/ml, range 27–9021), $P = 0.001$. The serum CgA levels were reduced in 16 of 17 patients with insulinomas after tumor resection. ROC curve showed that CgA values at 60 ng/ml distinguished patients with insulinomas from healthy controls but its sensitivity and specificity were 66.7% and 73.3%, respectively. In contrast, CgA values at 74 ng/ml distinguished patients with non-insulinoma PNETs from healthy controls, and the sensitivity and specificity were 65.6% and 91.9%, respectively. Except for two insulinomas with negative staining of CgA, 12 insulinoma tissues showed positive staining of CgA.

Conclusion: CgA is a reliable serum diagnostic biomarker for PNETs but not for insulinomas.

Background

Pancreatic neuroendocrine tumors (PNETs) are a group of rare tumors. The prevalence and incidence have increased over the past 3 decades [1-5]. The clinical presentations of PNETs are very complicated due to excess of gut peptides produced by functioning PNETs while symptoms of nonfunctioning PNETs (NF) are obscure [1,3]. In addition, most of PNETs could be biologically aggressive [1,3,6]. Thus, the earlier and accurate diagnosis of PNET is important to facilitate surgical resection and/ or to initiate appropriate medical management such as molecular targeted therapy, biotherapy and other intensive care.

Chromogranin A (CgA) is a 46-kDa glycoprotein, member of the granin family, exists within all type of neurons, normal neuroendocrine cells and is expressed in NET cells [7,8]. Over the past 2 decades, many studies reported and confirmed that CgA was a reliable diagnostic biomarker for NETs including gastroentero-pancreatic NETs (GEP-NET) [1,3,5-20] and also might be a prognostic biomarker for NETs [21]. Moreover, several studies showed that

* Correspondence: yuanjchen@163.com
†Equal contributors
[1]Department of Gastroenterology, Peking Union Medical College Hospital, Peking Union Medical College, Chinese Academy of Medical Sciences, Beijing 100730, People's Republic of China
[3]Key Laboratory of Endocrinology (Ministry of Health), Department of Endocrinology, Peking Union Medical College Hospital, Peking Union Medical College, Chinese Academy of Medical Sciences, Beijing 100730, People's Republic of China
Full list of author information is available at the end of the article

peripheral blood levels of CgA were increased in endocrine-associated tumors, for example, breast cancer [22] and prostate cancer [23,24]. Recently, elevated serum/plasma levels of CgA were found in a number of non-endocrine solid tumors, such as hepatic carcinomas [25,26] and pancreatic cancer [27]. Examination of CgA levels could be used not only for diagnosis but also for prognostic evaluation in these tumors [21,23,25,27].

In recent ENETS and NANETS consensus guidelines, CgA was considered as the most practical and useful serum tumor marker in PNET patients [28,29]. Some studies suggested that testing blood CgA should be mandatory for NET diagnosis [7]. However, few attention has been paid to the insulinoma which is the most common type of functioning PNETs [7,8,14,15,17,19,21,30-32]. In addition, peripheral blood levels of CgA are not routinely tested in Chinese patients with GEP-NET. Using CgA for clinical diagnosis has not been officially approved by Sino Food Drug Administration (SFDA) because little data have been reported.

Thus, the present study is to verify the utility of CgA in diagnosis of PNETs, focusing on its diagnostic value in insulinoma. We found that serum levels of CgA were not significantly elevated in patients with insulinomas, compared to the higher levels of CgA in other PNETs. This finding was rarely reported in previous studies.

Methods
Ethics statement
This study was approved by the Scientific Ethics Committee of Peking Union Medical College Hospital and the First Affiliated Hospital of Sun Yat-sen University. Participants provided their written informed consent to participate in this study. The Scientific Ethics Committee of both hospitals approved the consent procedure.

Patients and samples collection
Eighty-nine Chinese patients with PNETs including 57 insulinomas (one with extensive hepatic metastases), and 32 non-insulinoma PNETs (8 gastrinomas, 4 glucagonomas, 1 VIPoma and 19 NF) as well as 86 healthy participants were enrolled in this study at Peking Union Medical College Hospital and the First Affiliated Hospital of Sun Yat-sen University, between September 2003 and June 2013. The diagnostic criteria for PNETs were reported previously [33-39]. Briefly, the tumors were mainly localized by computed tomography with contrast, magnetic resonance imaging, endoscopic ultrasound and somatostatin receptor scintigraphy. All patients did not suffer with inflammatory diseases (such as inflammatory bowel disease, chronic atrophic gastritis), and the renal, hepatic or cardiac insufficiency was excluded. The patients did not take proton pump inhibitors (PPIs) or histamine 2 receptor blockers as well as somatostatin analogues. The

pathological diagnosis was made by 2 experienced pathologists. We analyzed tumor grade in 54 tumors according to ENETS-WHO guideline [40] and analyzed stage in 84 patients according to the ENETS guideline [40].

Before surgery or treatment, blood samples were obtained in 89 fasted patients with PNETs. In 17 patients with insulinomas, blood samples were postoperatively collected during 3rd to 7th days after resection. The blood samples from 86 healthy participants (median age 43 years, 38 male) were collected after overnight fasting. Serum were isolated and stored in –80°C.

Detecting of serum levels of CgA
Serum levels of CgA of patients with PNETs and healthy controls were measured by ELISA method with a commercial kit (Chromoa assay; CIS Bio International, France), according to the manufacturer's protocol. Most of samples were duplicated tested, and some of samples were checked in another experiment. Ten samples were double examined in two different labs (one in Beijing and another lab in Guangzhou).

Detecting of CgA expression in tumor tissues
Expression of CgA protein was detected in 26 sections of paraffin-embedded PNETs tissues, including 14 insulinomas, 2 gastrinomas and 10 NF as well as their paired pancreatic (duodenal) tissues by immunohistochemical staining (IHC) with anti-CgA (AC-0037, clone EP38, Epitomics, Inc, Burlingame, CA) at a 1:100 dilution. The criteria of semi-quantitative grading of IHC was similar to our previous report [36,39], i.e. (–) means no positive staining in tumor cells; (±) < 20% tumor cells shown positive staining, (+) ≥20% but < 50% tumor cells shown positive staining; (++) ≥50% but < 75% tumor cells shown positive staining; (+++) ≥ 75% tumor cells shown positive staining. We defined < 20% tumor cells with staining of CgA as negative staining, i.e. (–) and (±).

Statistical analysis
To verify the diagnostic value of serum CgA, receiver operating characteristic (ROC) curves were plotted, and the area under the curve (AUC) was calculated. SPSS statistics software version 13.0 was used for statistical analysis. Mann–Whitney method was used to compare the CgA levels between each group of patients and healthy controls. Fisher exact test or Chi's test were used to analyze our data. Two-tailed test was used in all of statistic analysis. $P < 0.05$ was considered statistically significant.

Results
Clinicopathological characteristics
We studied 89 PNET patients, 73 patients underwent curative surgery and 16 patients did not undergo operation.

All tumors were well differentiated. The clinicopathological characteristics of 89 patients with PNETs and 57 patients with insulinomas were summarized in Table 1.

CgA Serum Levels in PNET Patients and ROC curves

The median values of CgA levels in 86 healthy controls, 57 patients with insulinomas and 32 patients with non-insulinoma PNETs were 53.4 ng/ml (range 39.1 – 94.1 ng/ml), 64.8 ng/ml (range 25.0 – 164.2 ng/ml) and 192.5 ng/ml (range 26.9 – 9020.7 ng/ml), respectively (Figure 1). Serum levels of CgA in 89 PNET patients were significantly higher than that in healthy controls ($P = 7.2 \times 10^{-9}$). Compared with the serum levels of CgA in the healthy controls, the CgA levels were significantly elevated in 32 patients with non-insulinoma PNETs ($P = 3.7 \times 10^{-7}$). In contrast, the levels of CgA in 57 patients with insulinomas were just slightly higher than that in healthy participants (median 64.8 ng/ml vs. 53.4 ng/ml), see Figure 1. The serum levels of CgA in patients with insulinomas (median 64.8 ng/ml) were significantly lower than that in the patients with non-insulinoma PNETs (median 192.5 ng/ml), $P = 0.001$, Figure 1.

Although the levels of CgA in patients with insulinomas were not elevated significantly, it was interesting that the serum levels of CgA were decreased in 16 of 17 patients with insulinomas after tumor resection (Figure 2A, median 64.8 ng/ml vs. 50.4 ng/ml, $P = 0.003$). The postoperative levels of CgA in patients with insulinomas were almost the same as the levels in healthy controls (Figure 2B, median 50.4 ng/ml vs. 53.4 ng/ml).

ROC curve showed that CgA values at 60.4 ng/ml distinguished patients with insulinomas from healthy controls with the sensitivity of 66.7% and specificity was 73.3%, AUC was 0.724 (Figure 3A). In contrast, CgA values at 73.9 ng/ml distinguished patients with non-insulinoma PNETs from healthy controls, with a sensitivity and specificity were 65.6% and 91.9%, respectively, AUC was 0.805 (Figure 3B). These findings suggested that the serum levels of CgA in patients with insulinomas were not obviously elevated and CgA was not a reliable diagnostic biomarker for insulinomas due to the low specificity.

Correlation of CgA levels with clinicopathological characteristics in patients with PNETs and insulinomas

We correlated the CgA levels with clinicopathological features in patients with PNETs as well as insulinomas, respectively (Table 2). We found that the serum CgA levels in 18 patients with tumor metastases were significantly higher than that in 65 patients with localized tumors (median value, 549.8 ng/ml vs. 64.3 ng/ml, respectively, $P = 4.1 \times 10^{-5}$), see Figure 4. The serum levels of CgA in PNETs patients were not significantly associated with gender, tumor size and grade but associated with age,

primary tumor location and stage, see Table 2. Furthermore, we correlated the CgA levels with clinicopathological features in patients with insulinomas. The serum levels of CgA in patients with insulinomas were not significantly associated with gender, tumor size (Figure 5A), grade and stage, but significantly associated with age (Figure 5B) and primary tumor location (Figure 5C), see Table 2.

The CgA levels in patients with localized insulinomas and in patients with localized non-insulinomas

Our data above showed that CgA levels in patients with tumor metastases were significantly higher than that in patients with localized tumors and only 1 patient with metastasic insulinoma was included in our study. We compared serum CgA levels in 56 localized insulinoma with the CgA levels in 12 patients with localized non-insulinomas. The serum levels of CgA in both groups of patients were similar, 65.2 ng/ml vs. 59.4 ng/ml, $P = 0.693$ (Figure 6). As we mentioned above, the ROC curve showed that CgA cut-off values was 60.4 ng/ml for insulinomas and 73.9 ng/ml for non-insulinomas, respectively. We noticed that only 3 of 56 patients with localized insulinomas had the CgA levels more than 120.8 ng/ml (i.e. two fold more than cut-off values for insulinoma), whereas 4 of 12 patients with localized non-insulinomas had CgA levels more than 242 ng/ml (also two fold more than cut-off values for non-insulinoma), $P = 0.015$ (Fisher exact), see Figure 6, indicating the patients with localized non-insulinomas had a more frequency of remarkable elevation of CgA than that in the patients with localized insulinomas.

The expression of CgA in PNETs tissues

Because the serum CgA levels were not elevated in patients with insulinomas, we wanted to determine whether the protein of CgA was expressed in tumor tissues or not. We observed strong or medium expression of CgA in 12 of 14 insulinomas as well as in 11 of 12 non-insulinoma PNETs, as detected by IHC (Figure 7). Two of 14 insulinomas and 1 of 12 non-insulinoma PNETs had very weak IHC staining of CgA protein. The expression of CgA in PNET tissues was not associated with serum levels of CgA in corresponding patients. These data suggested that most of insulinoma cells could synthesize a great amount of CgA protein.

Discussion

Circulating CgA levels have been confirmed to be useful diagnostic marker for NETs, with a high specificity and sensitivity [1,3,5-19,28]. In the present study, we verified the diagnostic value of serum CgA in a series of patients with non-insulinoma PNETs, in agreement with previous studies. The sensitivity and specificity were 65.6% and 91.9%, respectively, similar to the rate of 67% and 96%

Table 1 Clinicopathological characteristics of PNET patients

Clinicopathological features of patients with PNETs		Number
Gender n = 89 (%)	Male	36 (40.4)
	Female	53 (59.6)
	Male : Female	1:1.47
Age (years) at diagnosis, n = 87	Median (range)	47 (16–74)
PNET subtype n = 89 (%)	Insulinoma	57 (64.0)
	Non-insulinoma	32 (36.0)
	NF	19 (21.3)
	gastrinoma	8 (9.0)
	glucagonoma	4 (4.5)
	VIPoma	1 (1.1)
Inherited or sporadic PNETs, n = 89 (%)	Sporadic	86 (96.6)
	MEN-1 associated	3 (3.4)
Surgery or not, n = 89 (%)	Resection	73 (82.0)
	Unresection	16 (18.0)
Primary tumor location, n = 77 (%)	Pancreatic head/neck	40 (51.9)
	Pancreatic body/tail	36 (46.8)
	duodenum	1 (1.3)
Tumor size (cm) median (range) n = 82		1.6 (0.8-8)
	Insulinoma n = 56	1.5 (0.8-4)
	Non-insulinoma n = 26	4.3 (1.5-8)
Metastasis or not, n = 83 (%)	No	65 (78.3)
	Yes	18 (21.7)
Grade, n = 54 (%)	G1	37 (68.5)
	G2	15 (27.8)
	G3	2 (3.7)
Stage, n = 84 (%)	I	39 (46.4)
	II	22 (26.2)
	III	5 (6.0)
	IV	18 (21.4)

Clinicopathological features of patients with insulinomas		Number
Gender n = 57 (%)	Male	25 (43.9)
	Female	32 (56.1)
	Male : Female	1:1.28
Age (years) at diagnosis, n = 57	Median (range)	47 (16–74)
Inherited or sporadic PNETs, n = 57 (%)	Sporadic	55 (96.5)
	MEN-1 associated	2 (3.5)
Surgery or not, n = 57 (%)	Resection	54 (94.7)
	Unresection	3 (5.3)
Primary tumor location, n = 56 (%)	Pancreatic head/neck	30 (53.6)
	Pancreatic body/tail	26 (46.4)

Table 1 Clinicopathological characteristics of PNET patients (Continued)

Tumor size (cm) median (range) n = 56		1.5 (0.8-4)
Metastasis or not, n = 57 (%)	No	56 (98.2)
	Yes	1 (1.8)
Grade, n = 35 (%)	G1	31 (88.6)
	G2	4 (11.4)

when using CIS Bio kits, as Ardill and Erikkson described [12]. Similar to previous studies [9-11,14,16,41,42], we found that CgA levels in patients with gastrinomas were much higher than those in patients without gastrin-secreting PNETs.

The interesting finding in the study was that serum CgA levels were not elevated in patients with insulinomas, including one patient with extensive liver metastases (48 ng/ml). Most of previous studies on PNETs did not clarify this unusual biochemical feature of insulinoma, the most common subtype of PNETs [7,8,13-16,19,20,31] but Wouter de Herder pointed out in a review that blood levels of CgA were rarely slightly elevated in subjects with insulinomas [43] and Portela-Gomes GM et al. mentioned in a review that well-differentiated NETs expressed CgA epitopes except insulinomas [44]. A recently published guideline which was revised by the UK and Ireland Neuro-endocrine Tumor Society and the British Society of Gastroenterology addressed that CgA would not raised in benign insulinomas [45]. Moreover, Nobels et al. studied more than 200 NETs and found that serum CgA levels were rarely slightly elevated in patients with insulinomas

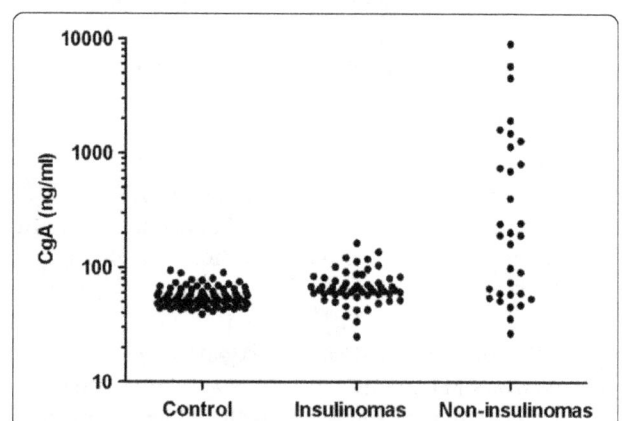

Figure 1 Serum concentrations of CgA in patients with insulinomas and non-insulinoma PNETs and in healthy controls. Individual levels were presented as dots. The results were plotted logarithmically to accommodate extreme values. The serum CgA levels were slightly elevated in 57 patients with insulinomas while the CgA levels were significantly increased in 32 patients with non-insulinoma PNETs. The serum levels of CgA in patients with insulino-mas (median 64.8 ng/ml) were significantly lower than that in the patients with non-insulinoma PNETs (median 192.5 ng/ml), $P = 0.001$.

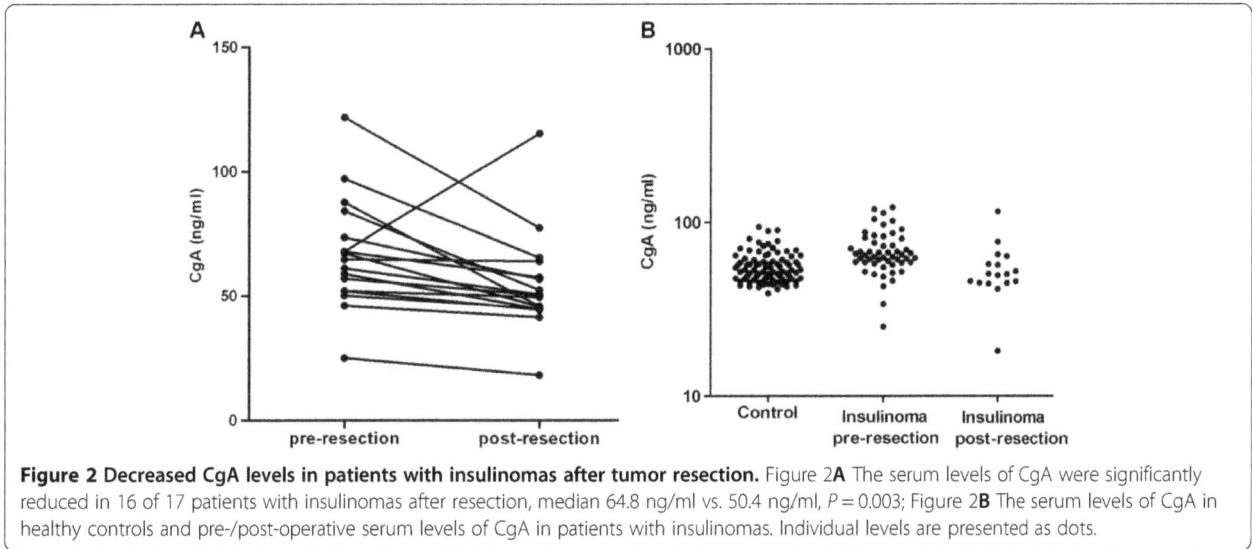

Figure 2 Decreased CgA levels in patients with insulinomas after tumor resection. Figure 2**A** The serum levels of CgA were significantly reduced in 16 of 17 patients with insulinomas after resection, median 64.8 ng/ml vs. 50.4 ng/ml, $P = 0.003$; Figure 2**B** The serum levels of CgA in healthy controls and pre-/post-operative serum levels of CgA in patients with insulinomas. Individual levels are presented as dots.

(elevated in 2 of 21 patients, range 63–236 ng/ml, upper cut-off value was 220 ng/ml) [9]. Another study showed that CgA levels were not elevated in 5 cases of insulinomas [13]. In present study, we focused on insulinomas and our findings were very similar to their data which showed only a small part of patients with insulinomas (7/57, 12%) had a slightly increased level of CgA (>100 ng/ml, the highest level: 164 ng/ml). With a relatively low specificity (73%), serum CgA was not a reliable and practicable biomarker for diagnosis of insulinoma. This finding is important. Some studies suggested that testing CgA levels should be mandatory for PNETs diagnosis [7]. Furthermore, according to recent North American Neuroendocrine Tumor Society (NANETS) and European Neuroendocrine Tumor Society (ENETS) consensus guidelines [28,29] as well as ESMO guidelines for NETs diagnosis [5], CgA was considered as a general biomarker for NETs, and CgA can be used as a marker in

patients with both Functional PNET and NF-PNET [28,29]. Insulinoma is the most common subtype of functioning PNETs [31,35,37,46]. However, whether serum levels of CgA should be tested in patients with insulinomas has not been well clarified in those guidelines for NETs diagnosis. Our data and previous reports [9,13] showed that insulinoma could be an exception for measuring serum levels of CgA for diagnostic purpose. It maybe not necessary to test CgA levels in patients with insulinomas although this issue needs to be further validated in more cases and in multiple clinical centers. In addition, using different commercial kits or assay could be useful to further validate our findings because the antibodies used in different assay were raised against the different domain or epitopes of the CgA molecular [12,15,17,47].

The underlying mechanism of low CgA levels in patients with insulinomas is not clear. Nobels et al. speculated the serum levels of CgA were only slightly elevated

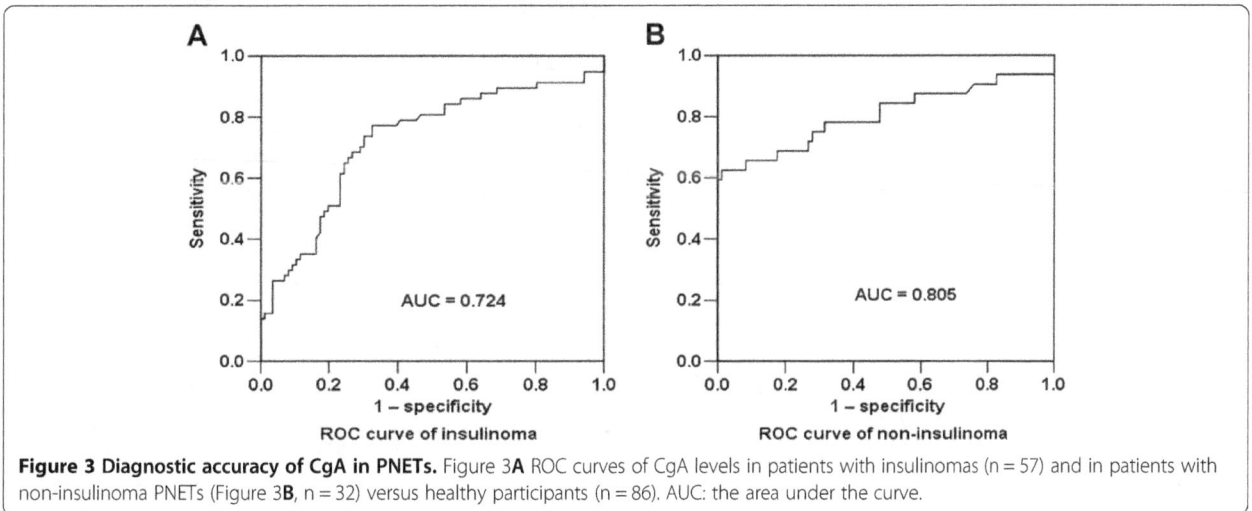

Figure 3 Diagnostic accuracy of CgA in PNETs. Figure 3**A** ROC curves of CgA levels in patients with insulinomas (n = 57) and in patients with non-insulinoma PNETs (Figure 3**B**, n = 32) versus healthy participants (n = 86). AUC: the area under the curve.

Table 2 Correlation of CgA levels with clinicopathological features in patients with PNETs and insulinomas

Clinicopathological features of patients with PNETs		CgA levels (ng/ml) median (range)	P value
Gender	Male, n = 36	67.9 (46.1-9020.7)	0.394
	Female, n = 53	67.2 (25.0-4572.3)	
Age (years)	≤48, n = 49	64.8 (25.0-5772.5)	0.039
	>48, n = 38	81.2 (26.9-9020.7)	
Primary tumor location on pancreas	Head/neck, n = 41	62.5 (25.0-5772.5)	0.019
	Body/tail, n = 36	81.9 (45.7-9020.7)	
Tumor size (cm)	n = 82, 0.8 - 8,	67.0 (25.0-9020.7)	0.545
	r = 0.068,		
Grade	G1, n = 37	67.3 (33.9-811.9)	0.103
	G2, n = 15	74.3 (26.9-1931.1)	
	G3, n = 2	323.7 (244.4-403.0)	
Stage	I, n = 39	67.2 (25.0-137.2)	0.003
	II, n = 22	61.6 (51.2-241.7)	
	III, n = 5	244.4 (26.9-811.9)	
	IV, n = 18	302.8 (45.7-9020.7)	

Clinicopathological features of patients with insulinomas		CgA levels (ng/ml) median (range)	P value
Gender	Male, n = 25	66.8 (46.1-164.2)	0.072
	Female, n = 32	62.6 (25.0-122.0)	
Age (years)	≤48, n = 32	61.4 (25.0-164.2)	0.003
	>48, n = 25	73.3 (51.2-137.2)	
Primary tumor location on pancreas	Head/neck n = 30	61.9 (25.0-122.0)	0.009
	Body/tail n = 26	68.9 (51.2-164.2)	
Tumor size (cm)	n = 56, 0.8 - 4,	64.3 (25.0-164.2)	0.942
	r = 0.01		
Grade	G1, n = 31	64.8 (33.9-164.2)	0.795
	G2, n = 4	62.5 (57.9-104.4)	
Stage	Stage I, n = 39	67.2 (25.0-137.2)	0.215
	Stage II, n = 15	61.6 (51.2-164.2)	

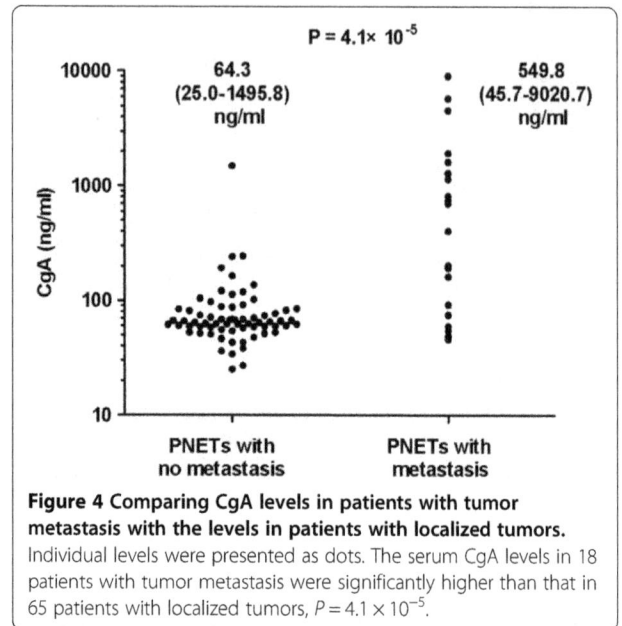

Figure 4 Comparing CgA levels in patients with tumor metastasis with the levels in patients with localized tumors. Individual levels were presented as dots. The serum CgA levels in 18 patients with tumor metastasis were significantly higher than that in 65 patients with localized tumors, $P = 4.1 \times 10^{-5}$.

in subjects with small NETs, such as insulinomas, pituitary adenomas [9]. However, there is disagreement in the literatures whether the serum CgA levels correlate with the extent of NETs or size of these tumors [7,21,32,48]. In present study, we did not observe the correlation between the tumor size and CgA levels in PNETs ($P = 0.545$) and in insulinomas alone ($P = 0.942$). Some of non-insulinoma PNETs with relatively small size still had very high serum levels of CgA, for example, CgA level was 4572 ng/ml in a gastrinoma of 1.5 cm in size, and the highest CgA level in present study was more than 9000 ng/ml in a glucagonoma of 2.5 cm in size.

Furthermore, one patient with a NF of 3.5 cm in size had a CgA level of 5772 ng/ml whereas another patient with a NF of 8 cm in size had a CgA level of 59 ng/ml.

Many previous studies [10,13,15,41,42,49] and our present data showed that CgA levels in patients with NETs metastases were much higher than that in patients with localized NETs. Thus, it may hypothesized that few metastases in insulinomas would be the reason for low serum level of CgA in insulinomas (only one metastatic insulinoma in our serial). We found CgA levels in localized insulinomas were similar to that in localized non-insulinomas, $P = 0.693$. This might imply the above hypothesis could be partly true. In fact, most of insulinomas (>90%) are benign, absent metastasis in majority of insulinomas is one of the main characteristics of this unique tumor, and in our hospital, more than 95% of insulinomas are benign [37]. However, we noticed that the rate of elevated CgA levels in patients with localized non-insulinomas was significantly higher than that in patients with localized insulinomas, $P = 0.015$. In addition, one report showed that in 9 of the 10 patients with gastrinoma, CgA values were raised, even in the absence of metastasis [41]. These data suggested that metastasis could be one of determinant factors for high levels of CgA in PNETs, but not the only one. The tumor subtype could be another important determinant for CgA serum levels. Nevertheless, more patients with metastatic insulinomas were needed to validate the low levels of CgA in insulinomas although it might be quite difficult to do so due to the limited numbers of malignant insulinomas.

It was reported that pancreastatin, a CgA-derived peptide (CgA residues 250–301) with biological activity, inhibited the releasing of insulin by islet beta cells [7,50]

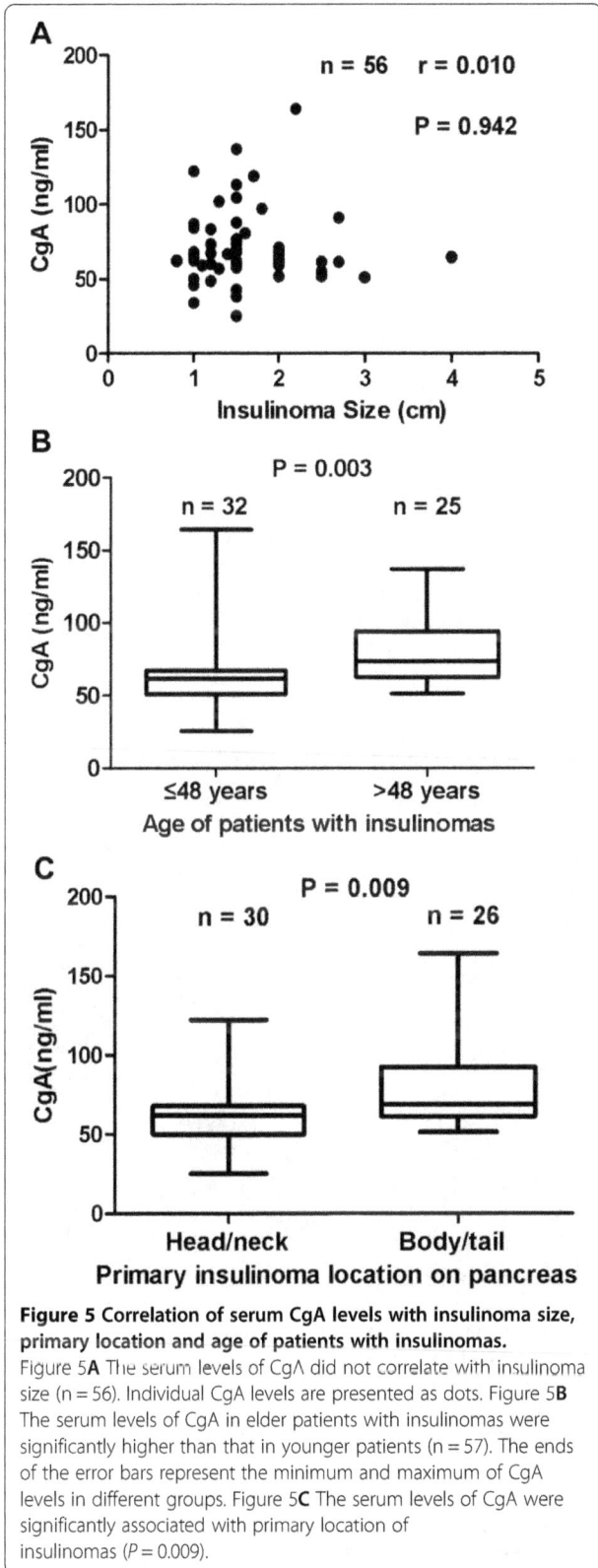

Figure 6 Comparing CgA levels in benign insulinomas with the levels in patients with localized non-insulinomas. The serum levels of CgA in 56 patinets with localized insulinomas were similar to the levels in 12 patients with localized non-insulinomas, $P = 0.693$. It can be seen that 3 of 56 patients with localized insulinomas had the CgA levels more than 120.8 ng/ml (i.e. 2 fold more than cut-off values for insulinoma), whereas 4 of 12 patients with localized non-insulinomas had CgA levels more than 242 ng/ml (2 fold more than cut-off values for non-insulinoma).

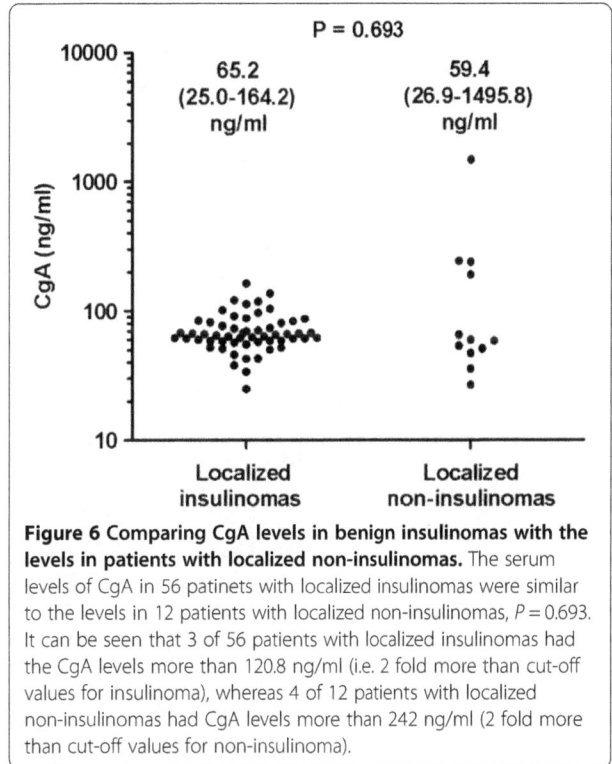

Figure 5 Correlation of serum CgA levels with insulinoma size, primary location and age of patients with insulinomas. Figure 5A The serum levels of CgA did not correlate with insulinoma size (n = 56). Individual CgA levels are presented as dots. Figure 5B The serum levels of CgA in elder patients with insulinomas were significantly higher than that in younger patients (n = 57). The ends of the error bars represent the minimum and maximum of CgA levels in different groups. Figure 5C The serum levels of CgA were significantly associated with primary location of insulinomas ($P = 0.009$).

and insulinoma cell line [51]. Gayen et al. [52] observed an inverse relationship between pancreastatin and insulin. This CgA-derived peptide might antagonize the effect of insulin via the Akt/FOXO-1 and, administration of insulin could result in low plasma levels of pancreastatin in mice (the basal pancreastatin level dropped significantly following insulin injection). In majority of insulinomas, a great deal amount of insulin is secreted by tumor cells. We speculate that high levels of insulin in patients with insulinomas might inhibit the secretion of CgA in these tumor cells. A recent study demonstrated that insulin and proinsulin were released in patients with insulinomas in response to arterial calcium stimulation, whereas CgA was not released [53].

One research suggested that CgA targeted to secretory granules in association with protein secretogranin III, a member of granin family, in pituitary and pancreatic endocrine cells [54]. If other proteins such as secretogranin III were broken down, the secretion of CgA would be disrupted. The mechanisms of hormones and peptides secretion were very complicated, it maybe concerned with molecular cellular biology and the alterations of tumor cell functions.

Other than the low blood levels of CgA in insulinomas, the biomedical behaviors of insulinomas were quite different from other PNETs. For example, its low rate of malignancy (<10%), the relatively low rate of positive Octreotide scintigraphy can be identified in benign insulinomas comparing with non-insulinoma PNETs because

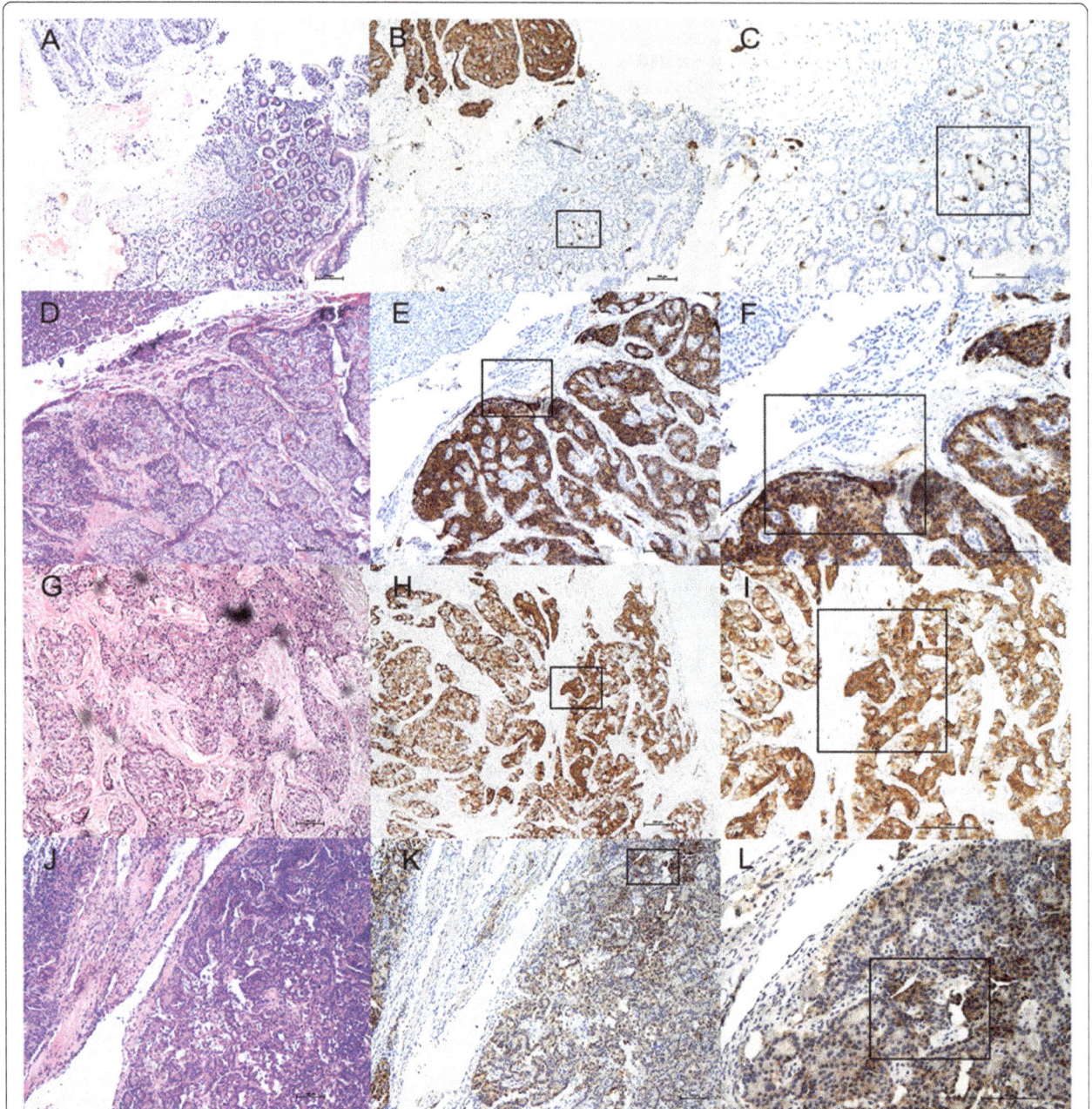

Figure 7 Representative examples of CgA expression in PNETs and their paired tissues. Left panel: HE staining; middle panel: CgA IHC, 10×; right panel: CgA IHC, 20×. Figure 7**A** shown HE staining of a gastrinoma located in duodenum, Figure 7**B** shown the strong expression of CgA protein in gastrinoma tissue and Figure 7**C** shown scattered CgA positive cells in non-tumoral duodenum tissue. Figure 7**D**, Figure 7**G** and Figure 7**J** shown HE staining of 3 different insulinomas, respectively. Figure 7**E-F**, Figure 7**H-I** and Figure 7**K-L** shown the very strong signals of CgA, strong signals of CgA and medium signals of CgA in 3 different insulinomas, respectively. In contrast, no expression of CgA can be seen in the interstitial tissues within the tumor and in the pancreatic exocrine tissues.

many insulinomas do not express somatostatin receptor subtypes [35]. All of these unusual features of insulinomas indicated that unique molecular cellular aspects and/or functions existed in insulinoma cells.

In this study, we have observed that most of insulinoma tissues (12/14) were shown strong positive staining for CgA, indicating that insulinoma cells were able to synthesize the CgA protein. This aspect of insulinoma was similar to non-insulinoma PNETs. However, only small part of the protein might be secreted into blood by the insulinoma cells because the CgA levels were not elevated and, the CgA levels were significantly reduced in 16 patients after tumor resection (from median 64.8 ng/ml to median 50.4 ng/ml, $P = 0.003$).

It is hard to explain why the serum level of CgA was postoperatively elevated in one patient who had normal liver and kidney functions. This patient did not suffer with other disease or take PPI or H2 receptor blocker. The sample was detected repeatedly and the same results were obtained.

In conclusion, our findings suggested that CgA is not a reliable biomarker for insulinomas, hence, examination of blood CgA levels could not be recommended in patients with insulinoms according to Nobels' [9] and our data. The mechanisms underlying low serum levels of CgA in insulinomas would appear to warrant further investigation.

Conclusion

The study revealed that the circulating CgA levels in patients with insulinomas were not obviously elevated, although we did validate the diagnostic value of serum CgA in a series of patients with non-insulinoma PNETs.

Competing interests
The authors declare that they have no conflict of interest.

Authors' contributions
YJC designed the study. XWQ, LQ, YJC, CTM, ZS, CMB, TPZ, YPZ, YHW and JC collected the samples and detected serum levels of CgA. XWQ, YJC, DCZ, YLS carried out the immunohistochemical staining. XWQ, LQ, CML and YJC analyzed the data and performed the statistical analysis. XWQ and YJC drafted the manuscript. All authors read and approved the final manuscript.

Acknowledgement
We thank Norvatis (China) Co. Ltd. for offering Chromogranin A ELISA kits.

Author details
[1]Department of Gastroenterology, Peking Union Medical College Hospital, Peking Union Medical College, Chinese Academy of Medical Sciences, Beijing 100730, People's Republic of China. [2]Department of Clinical Laboratory, Peking Union Medical College Hospital, Peking Union Medical College, Chinese Academy of Medical Sciences, Beijing 100730, People's Republic of China. [3]Key Laboratory of Endocrinology (Ministry of Health), Department of Endocrinology, Peking Union Medical College Hospital, Peking Union Medical College, Chinese Academy of Medical Sciences, Beijing 100730, People's Republic of China. [4]Department of Oncology, Peking Union Medical College Hospital, Peking Union Medical College, Chinese Academy of Medical Sciences, Beijing 100730, People's Republic of China. [5]Department of Pathology, Peking Union Medical College Hospital, Peking Union Medical College, Chinese Academy of Medical Sciences, Beijing 100730, People's Republic of China. [6]Department of Surgery, Peking Union Medical College Hospital, Peking Union Medical College, Chinese Academy of Medical Sciences, Beijing 100730, People's Republic of China. [7]Department of Gastroenterology, The First Affiliated Hospital of Sun Yat-sen University, Guangzhou 510000, People's Republic of China.

References
1. Rindi G, Wiedenmann B: **Neuroendocrine neoplasms of the gut and pancreas: new insights.** *Nat Rev Endocrinol* 2012, **8**(1):54–64.
2. Yao JC, Hassan M, Phan A, Dagohoy C, Leary C, Mares JE, Abdalla EK, Fleming JB, Vauthey JN, Rashid A, Evans DB: **One hundred years after "carcinoid": epidemiology of and prognostic factors for neuroendocrine tumors in 35,825 cases in the United States.** *J Clin Oncol* 2008, **26**(18):3063–3072.
3. Modlin IM, Oberg K, Chung DC, Jensen RT, de Herder WW, Thakker RV, Caplin M, Delle Fave G, Kaltsas GA, Krenning EP, Moss SF, Nilsson O, Rindi G, Salazar R, Ruszniewski P, Sundin A: **Gastroenteropancreatic neuroendocrine tumours.** *Lancet Oncol* 2008, **9**(1):61–72.
4. Lawrence B, Gustafsson BI, Chan A, Svejda B, Kidd M, Modlin IM: **The epidemiology of gastroenteropancreatic neuroendocrine tumors.** *Endocrinol Metab Clin North Am* 2011, **40**(1):1–18. vii.
5. Oberg K, Knigge U, Kwekkeboom D, Perren A, Group EGW: **Neuroendocrine gastro-entero-pancreatic tumors: ESMO clinical practice guidelines for diagnosis, treatment and follow-up.** *Ann Oncol* 2012, **23**(Suppl 7):vii124–vii130.
6. Oberg K, Eriksson B: **Endocrine tumours of the pancreas.** *Best Pract Res Clin Gastroenterol* 2005, **19**(5):753–781.
7. Modlin IM, Gustafsson BI, Moss SF, Pavel M, Tsolakis AV, Kidd M: **Chromogranin A–biological function and clinical utility in neuro endocrine tumor disease.** *Ann Surg Oncol* 2010, **17**(9):2427–2443.
8. Singh S, Law C: **Chromogranin A: a sensitive biomarker for the detection and post-treatment monitoring of gastroenteropancreatic neuroendocrine tumors.** *Expert Rev Gastroenterol Hepatol* 2012, **6**(3):313–334.
9. Nobels FR, Kwekkeboom DJ, Coopmans W, Schoenmakers CH, Lindemans J, De Herder WW, Krenning EP, Bouillon R, Lamberts SW: **Chromogranin A as serum marker for neuroendocrine neoplasia: comparison with neuron-specific enolase and the alpha-subunit of glycoprotein hormones.** *J Clin Endocrinol Metab* 1997, **82**(8):2622–2628.
10. Bashir S, Gibril F, Ojeaburu JV, Asgharian B, Entsuah LK, Ferraro G, Crafa P, Bordi C, Jensen RT: **Prospective study of the ability of histamine, serotonin or serum chromogranin A levels to identify gastric carcinoids in patients with gastrinomas.** *Aliment Pharmacol Ther* 2002, **16**(7):1367–1382.
11. Abou-Saif A, Gibril F, Ojeaburu JV, Bashir S, Entsuah LK, Asgharian B, Jensen RT: **Prospective study of the ability of serial measurements of serum chromogranin A and gastrin to detect changes in tumor burden in patients with gastrinomas.** *Cancer* 2003, **98**(2):249–261.
12. Ardill JE, Erikkson B: **The importance of the measurement of circulating markers in patients with neuroendocrine tumours of the pancreas and gut.** *Endocr Relat Cancer* 2003, **10**(4):459–462.
13. Nehar D, Lombard-Bohas C, Olivieri S, Claustrat B, Chayvialle JA, Penes MC, Sassolas G, Borson-Chazot F: **Interest of Chromogranin A for diagnosis and follow-up of endocrine tumours.** *Clin Endocrinol (Oxf)* 2004, **60**(5):644–652.
14. Campana D, Nori F, Piscitelli L, Morselli-Labate AM, Pezzilli R, Corinaldesi R, Tomassetti P: **Chromogranin A: is it a useful marker of neuroendocrine tumors?** *J Clin Oncol* 2007, **25**(15):1967–1973.
15. Zatelli MC, Torta M, Leon A, Ambrosio MR, Gion M, Tomassetti P, De Braud F, Delle Fave G, Dogliotti L, Degli Uberti EC, Italian CromaNet Working Group: **Chromogranin A as a marker of neuroendocrine neoplasia: an Italian Multicenter Study.** *Endocr Relat Cancer* 2007, **14**(2):473–482.
16. Metz DC, Jensen RT: **Gastrointestinal neuroendocrine tumors: pancreatic endocrine tumors.** *Gastroenterology* 2008, **135**(5):1469–1492.
17. Lawrence B, Gustafsson BI, Kidd M, Pavel M, Svejda B, Modlin IM: **The clinical relevance of chromogranin A as a biomarker for gastroenteropancreatic neuroendocrine tumors.** *Endocrinol Metab Clin North Am* 2011, **40**(1):111–134. viii.
18. Oberg K: **Circulating biomarkers in gastroenteropancreatic neuroendocrine tumours.** *Endocr Relat Cancer* 2011, **18**(Suppl 1):S17–S25.
19. Chou WC, Hung YS, Hsu JT, Chen JS, Lu CH, Hwang TL, Rau KM, Yeh KY, Chen TC, Sun CF: **Chromogranin A is a reliable biomarker for gastroenteropancreatic neuroendocrine tumors in an Asian population of patients.** *Neuroendocrinology* 2012, **95**(4):344–350.
20. Walter T, Chardon L, Chopin-Ialy X, Raverot V, Caffin AG, Chayvialle JA, Scoazec JY, Lombard-Bohas C: **Is the combination of chromogranin A and pancreatic polypeptide serum determinations of interest in the diagnosis and follow-up of gastro-entero-pancreatic neuroendocrine tumours?** *Eur J Cancer* 2012, **48**(12):1766–1773.
21. Arnold R, Wilke A, Rinke A, Mayer C, Kann PH, Klose KJ, Scherag A, Hahmann M, Muller HH, Barth P: **Plasma chromogranin A as marker for survival in patients with metastatic endocrine gastroenteropancreatic tumors.** *Clin Gastroenterol Hepatol* 2008, **6**(5):820–827.
22. Giovanella L, Marelli M, Ceriani L, Giardina G, Garancini S, Colombo L: **Evaluation of chromogranin A expression in serum and tissues of breast cancer patients.** *Int J Biol Markers* 2001, **16**(4):268–272.

23. Ranno S, Motta M, Rampello E, Risino C, Bennati E, Malaguarnera M: **The chromogranin-A (CgA) in prostate cancer.** *Arch Gerontol Geriatr* 2006, **43**(1):117–126.

24. Sciarra A, Di Silverio F, Autran AM, Salciccia S, Gentilucci A, Alfarone A, Gentile V: **Distribution of high chromogranin A serum levels in patients with nonmetastatic and metastatic prostate adenocarcinoma.** *Urol Int* 2009, **82**(2):147–151.

25. Malaguarnera M, Vacante M, Fichera R, Cappellani A, Cristaldi E, Motta M: **Chromogranin A (CgA) serum level as a marker of progression in hepatocellular carcinoma (HCC) of elderly patients.** *Arch Gerontol Geriatr* 2010, **51**(1):81–85.

26. Biondi A, Malaguarnera G, Vacante M, Berretta M, D'Agata V, Malaguarnera M, Basile F, Drago F, Bertino G: **Elevated serum levels of Chromogranin A in hepatocellular carcinoma.** *BMC Surg* 2012, **12**(Suppl 1):S7.

27. Malaguarnera M, Cristaldi E, Cammalleri L, Colonna V, Lipari H, Capici A, Cavallaro A, Beretta M, Alessandria I, Luca S, Motta M: **Elevated chromogranin A (CgA) serum levels in the patients with advanced pancreatic cancer.** *Arch Gerontol Geriatr* 2009, **48**(2):213–217.

28. O'Toole D, Grossman A, Gross D, Delle Fave G, Barkmanova J, O'Connor J, Pape UF, Plockinger U, Mallorca Consensus Conference p, European Neuroendocrine Tumor S: **ENETS consensus guidelines for the standards of care in neuroendocrine tumors: biochemical markers.** *Neuroendocrinology* 2009, **90**(2):194–202.

29. Vinik AI, Woltering EA, Warner RR, Caplin M, O'Dorisio TM, Wiseman GA, Coppola D, Go VL, North American Neuroendocrine Tumor S: **NANETS consensus guidelines for the diagnosis of neuroendocrine tumor.** *Pancreas* 2010, **39**(6):713–734.

30. Grant CS: **Insulinoma.** *Best Pract Res Clin Gastroenterol* 2005, **19**(5):783–798.

31. Mathur A, Gorden P, Libutti SK: **Insulinoma.** *Surg Clin North Am* 2009, **89**(5):1105–1121.

32. O'Dorisio TM, Krutzik SR, Woltering EA, Lindholm E, Joseph S, Gandolfi AE, Wang YZ, Boudreaux JP, Vinik AI, Go VL, Howe JR, Halfdanarson T, O'Dorisio MS, Mamikunian G: **Development of a highly sensitive and specific carboxy-terminal human pancreastatin assay to monitor neuroendocrine tumor behavior.** *Pancreas* 2010, **39**(5):611–616.

33. Chen YJ, Vortmeyer A, Zhuang Z, Huang S, Jensen RT: **Loss of heterozygosity of chromosome 1q in gastrinomas: occurrence and prognostic significance.** *Cancer Res* 2003, **63**(4):817–823.

34. Yang YM, Liu TH, Chen YJ, Jiang WJ, Qian JM, Lu X, Gao J, Wu SF, Sang XT, Chen J: **Chromosome 1q loss of heterozygosity frequently occurs in sporadic insulinomas and is associated with tumor malignancy.** *Int J Cancer* 2005, **117**(2):234–240.

35. de Herder WW, Niederle B, Scoazec JY, Pauwels S, Kloppel G, Falconi M, Kwekkeboom DJ, Oberg K, Eriksson B, Wiedenmann B, Rindi G, O'Toole D, Ferone D, Frascati Consensus Conference, European Neuroendocrine Tumor Society: **Well-differentiated pancreatic tumor/carcinoma: insulinoma.** *Neuroendocrinology* 2006, **84**(3):183–188.

36. Mei M, Deng D, Liu TH, Sang XT, Lu X, Xiang HD, Zhou J, Wu H, Yang Y, Chen J, Lu CM, Chen YJ: **Clinical implications of microsatellite instability and MLH1 gene inactivation in sporadic insulinomas.** *J Clin Endocrinol Metab* 2009, **94**(9):3448–3457.

37. Zhao YP, Zhan HX, Zhang TP, Cong L, Dai MH, Liao Q, Cai LX: **Surgical management of patients with insulinomas: Result of 292 cases in a single institution.** *J Surg Oncol* 2011, **103**(2):169–174.

38. Wang YH, Lin Y, Xue L, Wang JH, Chen MH, Chen J: **Relationship between clinical characteristics and survival of gastroenteropancreatic neuroendocrine neoplasms: A single-institution analysis (1995–2012) in South China.** *BMC Endocr Disord* 2012, **12**:30.

39. Liu B, Tang LH, Liu Z, Mei M, Yu R, Dhall D, Qiao XW, Zhang TP, Zhao YP, Liu TH, Xiao Y, Chen J, Xiang HD, Wu HY, Lu CM, Lv B, Zhou YR, Zhang Y, Deng DJ, Chen YJ: **Alpha-Internexin: a novel biomarker for pancreatic neuroendocrine tumor aggressiveness.** *J Clin Endocrinol Metab* 2014, **99**(5):E786–E795.

40. Rindi G, Falconi M, Klersy C, Albarello L, Boninsegna L, Buchler MW, Capella C, Caplin M, Couvelard A, Doglioni C, Delle Fave G, Fischer L, Fusai G, de Herder WW, Jann H, Komminoth P, de Krijger RR, La Rosa S, Luong TV, Pape U, Perren A, Ruszniewski P, Scarpa A, Schmitt A, Solcia E, Wiedenmann B: **TNM staging of neoplasms of the endocrine pancreas: results from a large international cohort study.** *J Natl Cancer Inst* 2012, **104**(10):764–777.

41. Tomassetti P, Migliori M, Simoni P, Casadei R, De Iasio R, Corinaldesi R, Gullo L: **Diagnostic value of plasma chromogranin A in neuroendocrine tumours.** *Eur J Gastroenterol Hepatol* 2001, **13**(1):55–58.

42. Paik WH, Ryu JK, Song BJ, Kim J, Park JK, Kim YT, Yoon YB: **Clinical usefulness of plasma chromogranin a in pancreatic neuroendocrine neoplasm.** *J Korean Med Sci* 2013, **28**(5):750–754.

43. de Herder WW: **Biochemistry of neuroendocrine tumours.** *Best Pract Res Clin Endocrinol Metab* 2007, **21**(1):33–41.

44. Portela-Gomes GM, Grimelius L, Wilander E, Stridsberg M: **Granins and granin-related peptides in neuroendocrine tumours.** *Regul Pept* 2010, **165**(1):12–20.

45. Ramage JK, Ahmed A, Ardill J, Bax N, Breen DJ, Caplin ME, Corrie P, Davar J, Davies AH, Lewington V, Meyer T, Newell-Price J, Poston G, Reed N, Rockall A, Steward W, Thakker RV, Toubanakis C, Valle J, Verbeke C, Grossman AB, Uk Ireland Neuroendocrine Tumour Society: **Guidelines for the management of gastroenteropancreatic neuroendocrine (including carcinoid) tumours (NETs).** *Gut* 2012, **61**(1):6–32.

46. Crippa S, Zerbi A, Boninsegna L, Capitanio V, Partelli S, Balzano G, Pederzoli P, Di Carlo V, Falconi M: **Surgical management of insulinomas: short- and long-term outcomes after enucleations and pancreatic resections.** *Arch Surg* 2012, **147**(3):261–266.

47. Molina R, Alvarez E, Aniel-Quiroga A, Borque M, Candas B, Leon A, Poyatos RM, Gelabert M: **Evaluation of chromogranin A determined by three different procedures in patients with benign diseases, neuroendocrine tumors and other malignancies.** *Tumour Biol* 2011, **32**(1):13–22.

48. Ito T, Igarashi H, Jensen RT: **Serum pancreastatin: the long sought universal, sensitive, specific tumor marker for neuroendocrine tumors?** *Pancreas* 2012, **41**(4):505–507.

49. Nolting S, Kuttner A, Lauseker M, Vogeser M, Haug A, Herrmann KA, Hoffmann JN, Spitzweg C, Goke B, Auernhammer CJ: **Chromogranin a as serum marker for gastroenteropancreatic neuroendocrine tumors: a single center experience and literature review.** *Cancers* 2012, **4**(1):141–155.

50. Tatemoto K, Efendic S, Mutt V, Makk G, Feistner GJ, Barchas JD: **Pancreastatin, a novel pancreatic peptide that inhibits insulin secretion.** *Nature* 1986, **324**(6096):476–478.

51. Hertelendy ZI, Patel DG, Knittel JJ: **Pancreastatin inhibits insulin secretion in RINm5F cells through obstruction of G-protein mediated, calcium-directed exocytosis.** *Cell Calcium* 1996, **19**(2):125–132.

52. Gayen JR, Saberi M, Schenk S, Biswas N, Vaingankar SM, Cheung WW, Najjar SM, O'Connor DT, Bandyopadhyay G, Mahata SK: **A novel pathway of insulin sensitivity in chromogranin A null mice: a crucial role for pancreastatin in glucose homeostasis.** *J Biol Chem* 2009, **284**(42):28498–28509.

53. Wiesli P, Uthoff H, Perren A, Pfammatter T, Zwimpfer C, Seiler H, Kindhauser R, Spinas GA, Schmid C: **Are biochemical markers of neuroendocrine tumors coreleased with insulin following local calcium stimulation in patients with insulinomas?** *Pancreas* 2011, **40**(7):995–999.

54. Hosaka M, Watanabe T, Sakai Y, Uchiyama Y, Takeuchi T: **Identification of a chromogranin A domain that mediates binding to secretogranin III and targeting to secretory granules in pituitary cells and pancreatic beta-cells.** *Mol Biol Cell* 2002, **13**(10):3388–3399.

11

Relationship between clinical characteristics and survival of gastroenteropancreatic neuroendocrine neoplasms: A single-institution analysis (1995–2012) in South China

Yu-hong Wang[1†], Yuan Lin[2†], Ling Xue[2], Jin-hui Wang[1], Min-hu Chen[1*] and Jie Chen[1*]

Abstract

Background: Gastroenteropancreatic neuroendocrine neoplasm (GEP-NEN) is the most common type of neuroendocrine tumors accounting for 65–75% of neuroendocrine neoplasms (NENs). Given the fact that there are few studies on GEP-NENs among Chinese patients, we performed a retrospective study in South China.

Methods: Totally 178 patients with GEP-NENs treated at the First Affiliated Hospital of Sun Yat-sen University between January 1995 and May 2012 were analyzed retrospectively.

Results: Pancreas was found the most common site of involvement (34.8%). 149 patients (83.7%) presented as non-functional tumors with non-specific symptoms such as abdominal pain (33.7%); carcinoid syndrome was not found in this study. Several methods are useful for localization of GEP-NENs, yielding varied detection rates from 77.8% to 98.7%. Positive rates of chromogranin A (CgA) and synaptophysin (Syn) immunhistochemically were 69.1% and 90.2%, respectively. 87 patients (51.5%) had G1 tumors, 31(18.3%) G2 tumors and 51 (30.2%) G3 tumors. Neuroendocrine tumor (NET), neuroendocrine carcinoma (NEC) and mixed adenoendocrine carcinoma (MANEC) were 69.8%, 27.2% and 3.0%, respectively. 28.1% of patients presented with distant disease. Surgery was performed in 152 (85.4%) patients, and overall 5-year survival rate was 54.5%. Functionality, G1 grading and NET classification were associated with favorable prognosis in univariate analysis. Distant metastasis contributed to unfavorable prognosis of these tumors.

Conclusions: Nonfunctional tumors with non-specific symptoms account for the majority of GEP-NENs. Diagnosis depends on pathological classification. Multidisciplinary treatments could help improve the outcome.

Keywords: Gastroenteropancreatic neuroendocrine neoplasms, Clinical pathological characteristics, Survival

Background

Neuroendocrine neoplasms, which originate from neuroendocrine cells distributed throughout the body, comprise a heterogeneous family with a wide and complex clinical behaviors [1]. The incidence of NENs ranges from 2.5 to 5 cases per 100,000 in the United States, and the gastrointestinal tract is the most commonly affected site [2,3]. According to an analysis of the National Cancer Institute's Surveillance, Epidemiology and End Results database (SEER, http://seer.cancer.gov/data/index.html), which is the largest epidemiologic series nowadays, the incidence of NENs has been rising substantially in the past 30 years.

NENs have been the subject of debate regarding optimal nomenclature, grading, staging and classification of these tumors for many years. A uniform World Health Organization (WHO) classification greatly facilitates the comparison of clinical, pathological and prognostic features and results of treatment in GEP-NENs, and so do the China Consensus Guidelines for the standards of histopathologic diagnosis as well [4,5].

* Correspondence: chenminhu@vip.163.com; chenjie7209@yahoo.com
†Equal contributors
[1]Department of Gastroenterology, The First Affiliated Hospital of Sun Yat-sen University, 58 Zhongshan II Road, Guangzhou, People's Republic of China
Full list of author information is available at the end of the article

The incidence of NENs, the treatments and survival of Caucasians have been well studied in western countries such as United States, Norway, Spain, German and the United Kingdom [2,3,6-9]. But for Asian population [10-13], especially for Chinese population, available information on these cancers is rather limited [14]. Therefore, it requires detailed data for comprehensive knowledge of NENs in China. Based on the 17-year data of our hospital, a comprehensive retrospective study was performed to examine the relationship between clinical pathological characteristic and survival of GEP-NENs. To our knowledge, it is the first study providing information on these tumors using the latest histopathologic diagnosis consensus from an Asian country.

Methods

178 patients with histologically confirmed sporadic GEP-NENs from The First Affiliated Hospital, Sun Yat-sen University (1995–2012) were enrolled in this study to collect clinical information including age, gender, locations, clinical syndromes, endoscopic and radiographic features, histopathological characteristics, metastasis patterns, treatment modalities and outcomes.

The histology of each patient was reviewed according to the WHO classification [4] and China Consensus Guidelines [5]: First, immunohistochemical staining of CgA and Syn, which are all neuroendocrine markers, were performed to recognize the histological patterns of these tumors. Specific peptide hormones (eg. insulin, glucagon and somatostatin) staining methods were not regularly used only when a functional neuroendocrine neoplasm was considered. Second, the Ki-67 index (≤2%, 3–20%, and >20% per 500–2000 tumor cells in the most active regions or hot spots, respectively) or mitotic rate (1, 2–20, and >20 mitoses per 10 high-power field in the most active regions or hot spots, respectively), which was re-stained or recounted, was used to estimate the tumor proliferative activities. Tumors with a Ki-67 index of <2% were classified as G1 tumors, index of 3–20% were classified as G2, greater than 20% as G3. Likewise, tumors with mitotic rates of <2/10 HPF were classified as G1, those of 2 to 20/10 HPF were classified as G2, greater than 20/10 HPF as G3. Once the grading of Ki-67 index disaccorded with the mitotic rate, the higher one was preferred. Thus, GEP-NENs were classified as NET (G1 and G2), NEC (G3) and MANEC (G3).

Overall survival was defined as the time from diagnosis to death or last follow-up in living patients. Survival rate was estimated according to the Kaplan–Meier product limit method, and differences between subgroups were assessed by the log-rank test with $P < 0.05$ as statistically significant. SPSS 16.0 was used for statistical analysis.

The study was approved by the ethics committee of The First Affiliated Hospital Sun Yat-sen University (with a reference number: [2012]317) and complied with the Declaration of Helsinki.

Results

Clinical features

Among the 178 Chinese patients with GEP-NENs, 108 (60.7%) were men and 70 (39.3%) were women; male-to-female ratio was 1.54. The mean age was 50.96 ± 15.01 years. The most common sites were the pancreas (62/178, 34.8%), followed by rectum (36/178, 20.2%), stomach (25/178, 14.0%), duodenum (13/178, 7.3%), metastatic NENs of unknown primary (12/178, 6.7%) and esophagus (7/178, 3.9%). Other sites included appendix, jejunum/ileum, Vater's ampulla at 12.9% (23/178). Nonfunctional tumors comprised the majority of GEP-NENs (149/178, 83.7%), whereas functional tumors accounted for the other 16.3%. A variety of gastrointestinal manifestations were caused by the effect of local compression on nearby tissues in nonfunctional tumors. The most common initial presentation was abdominal pain (60/178, 33.7%), which was not specific for the diagnosis of tumor. Other non-specific symptoms were gastrointestinal bleeding (29/178, 16.3%), jaundice (16/178, 9.0%), progressive dysphagia (9/178, 5.1%), diarrhea (8/178, 4.5%), abdominal distension (6/178, 3.4%) and so on. Incidental diagnosis occurred in 10.1% of cases which were usually asymptomatic. Insulinoma comprised 93.1% of functional tumors, which mainly occurred in pancreas, occasionally followed by the substantially rarer glucagonoma and vasoactive intestinal peptidoma (only 1 case respectively in our study). Typical symptoms included hypoglycemia, epileptic seizure and secondary diabetes mellitus, which heralded functional NENs, but carcinoid syndrome did not present in our study. The demographics and presenting symptoms of GEP-NENs are listed in Table 1.

Imaging studies

The most frequently used examination procedures included endoscopy, ultrasound, endoscopic ultrasonography (EUS), computed tomography (CT) scan, magnatic resonance imaging (MRI), and positron emission computed tomography imaging (PET-CT, using with 16 F-FDG). Endoscopy provided the highest detection rate of 98.7% (74/75). EUS was performed on 37 patients, of which a lesion was found in 34 patients, promised a detection rate of 91.9%. MRI and PET-CT, was performed in only about 10% of patients, respectively. Tumors usually appeared as polypoid prominences, ulcer type or cauliflower-like neoplasm under endoscopy; whereas on CT scan, they appeared as local space-occupying lesions which were significantly enhanced by iodinated contrast. Ultrasound and EUS usually demonstrated the tumors as rounded, homogeneous, hypoechoic, well-defined and well-vascularized masses (Table 2).

Table 1 Characteristics of study population (N = 178 patients)

Site	All patients		Men, n(%)	Women, n(%)	Clinical symptoms	Main signs
	N	%				
Pancreas	62	34.8	32(51.6)	30(48.4)	Abdominal pain, Jaundice, Hypoglycaemia	Jaundice
Rectum	36	20.2	29(80.6)	7(19.4)	Gastrointestinal bleeding, Abdominal pain, Diarrhea	Rectum mass
Somach	25	14.0	16(64.0)	9(36.0)	Abdominal pain, Gastrointestinal bleeding, Dysphagia	Abdominal tenderness
Duodenum	13	7.3	10(76.9)	3(23.1)	Abdominal pain, Jaundice, Gastrointestinal bleeding	Jaundice
Metastasis of unknown primary	12	6.7	6(50.0)	6(50.0)	Abdominal pain, Asymptomatic, Fatigue	Hepatomegaly
Esophagus	7	3.9	5(71.4)	2(28.6)	Progressive dysphagia	No signs
Appendix	6	3.4	2(33.3)	4(66.7)	Abdominal pain, Abdominal distension	Rebound pain in the Mcburney's point
Jejunum/ileum	4	2.2	3(75.0)	1(25.0)	Gastrointestinal bleeding, Small bowel obstruction	Anemia
Gallbladder	4	2.2	1(25.0)	3(75.0)	Jaundice, Asymptomatic	Jaundice
Vater's ampulla	3	1.7	3(100)	0(0)	Jaundice, Abdominal pain,	Jaundice
Peritoneum	3	1.7	0(0)	3(100)	Abdominal pain, Asymptomatic	Abdominal mass
Cecum	1	0.6	1(100)	0(0)	Abdominal pain	Abdominal mass
Choledoch	1	0.6	1(100)	0(0)	Jaundice	Jaundice
Greater omentum	1	0.6	0(0)	1(100)	Asymptomatic	No signs

Pathologic characteristics

Overall, the mean diameter of tumors was 3.95 cm (0.4–25 cm): 38.6% were smaller than 2 cm in diameter, 29.7% ranging from 2 to 4 cm, and 31.7% larger than 4 cm. Immunohistochemistry staining determined a 69.1% positive rate of CgA and a 90.2% positive rate of Syn. Ki-67 index and mitotic rate were assessed in 127 and 118 specimens to estimate the proliferative activities. Over half (51.5%) of the tumors were G1, 18.3% were at G2 and 30.2% at G3. The most common tumor type was NET (69.8%), followed by NEC (27.2%) and MANEC (3.0%). Approximately half of the assessed tumors (53/100, 53.0%) originated from gastrointestinal tract and biliary system with muscularis or serosa infiltration at diagnosis. Local infiltration and lymphatic metastasis occurred in 23.0% and 27.0% of patients respectively. Distant metastasis was a frequent event at diagnosis with an occurrence of 23.0% (41/178), which increased to 28.1% (55/178) during follow up. The liver was one of most frequently involved organs: liver metastasis occurred in 44 (80.0%) of 55 patients in the disease courses. Among the 44 patients, 29 presented with synchronous liver metastasis, whereas other 15 presented with metachronous liver metastasis during follow-up. Other locations that tumors involved were the peritoneum (12.7%, 7/55), cavitas pelvis (9.1%, 5/55), bone (7.3%, 4/55) and ovary (5.5%, 3/55). The most common site of primary tumor associated with widespread

Table 2 Characteristics of imaging studies

Imaging studies	Site	Manifestation	Case tested	Positive tests	
				n	%
Endoscopy	gastrointestinal tract		75	74	98.7
Gastroscope	esophagus, stomach, duodenum	ulcer type, bulge type, invasive type	34	34	100
Duodenoscope	duodenum	bulge type	3	3	100
Small intestinal endoscope	jejunum/ileum	small intestinal hemorrhage	2	1	50.0
Colonoscope	rectum, appendix	polypoid prominences, submucosal uplift, cauliflower-like neoplasm	36	36	100
Ultrasound	pancreas, liver, gallbladder, cho- ledoch	hypoechoic masses, well delimited and vascularized	63	49	77.8
EUS	pancreas, duodenum, stomach	hypoechoic masses	37	34	91.9
CT scan	pancreas, liver, stomach	local space-occupying lesions	123	98	91.9
MRI	pancreas, duodenum, biliary	local space-occupying lesions	20	19	95.0
PET-CT	pancreas, rectum	local space-occupying lesions	20	19	95.0

EUS, endoscopic ultrasonography; CT, computed tomography; MRI, magnatic resonance imaging; PET-CT, positron emission computed tomography imaging.

disease at diagnosis was cecum (100.0%), followed by jejunum/ileum (75.0%), gallbladder (50.0%), duodenum (38.5%), Vater's ampulla (33.3%) and stomach (28.0%) (Table 3).

Therapeutic interventions

85.4% patients underwent a surgery with curative intent (75.9%) or for palliative purpose (9.6%). Different types of endoscopic radical surgery were performed, including endoscopic mucosa resection (EMR), endoscopic sub-mucosal dissection (ESD) and endoscopic electroexcision. Local-regional therapies such as transcatheter hepatic arterial chemoembolization (TACE), radiofrequency or other ablative techniques were carried out only in 11 cases (6.2% of the population). Chemotherapy and biological therapy were performed in 31 patients, among which 15 received chemo regimen, 8 received biological therapy and 8 received both. The most common first-line chemo combinations included platinum-etoposide (6 patients, 3.4%), oxaliplatin- capecitabine (2 patients, 1.3%), oxaliplatin-TS-1 (2 patients, 1.3%) and so on. Octreotide, a somatostatin analogue, was frequently administered at a dose of 20–40 mg/month as a biological therapy, combined with chemotherapy in 1 patient (0.6%) after surgery and in 7 patients (3.9%) with unresectable tumors. 14 (7.9%) cases with progressive malignant disease were treated only with supportive care.

Table 3 Pathologic characteristics

Characteristics	Case tested	Positive tests	
		n	%
Immunohistochemistry			
CgA	149	103	69.1
Syn	143	129	90.2
Tumor grading			
G1	169	87	51.5
G2	169	31	18.3
G3	169	51	30.2
Tumor type			
NET	169	118	69.8
NEC	169	46	27.2
MANEC	169	5	3.0
Infiltration/Metastasis			
Muscularis/Serosa infiltration	100	53	53.0
Adjacent tissue/Capsule infiltration	178	41	23.0
Lymphatic metastasis	178	48	27.0
Distant metastasis			
At initial diagnosis	178	41	23.0
During follow-up	178	55	28.1

CgA, Chromogranin A; Syn, Synaptophysin;NET, neuroendocrine tumor; NEC, neuroendocrine carcinoma; MANEC, mixed adenoendocrine carcinoma.

Survival and prognostic factors

136 out of 178 patients received long-term follow up with a median duration of 8.6 years (range 0.03–13.48 years). Median survival was not obtained during the observation period. The 1-, 3- and 5-year survival rates was 74.4%, 66.7% and 54.5% respectively, and 25 patients had died at the last follow-up (14.0%). The major causes of death were tumor-related complications (84.0%), and treatment-related adverse events (12.0%); other disease contributed the other 4.0%. An analysis was performed on patients' age, gender, primary tumor site, histopathological grading, classification and condition of metastasis to identify prognostic factors for survival. Univariate analysis confirmed that functional tumors, patients were at G1 phase and classified as NET were superior to other types of NENs in survival. Distant metastasis also contributed to the prognosis of these neuroendocrine tumors. However, age, sex, primary tumor site had little impact on overall survival. The mean survival time and statistic data were provided in Table 4. Survival curves were displayed in Figure 1.

Discussion

The WHO classification system of gastroenteropancreatic neuroendocrine tumors was adopted in previous studies [3,7,8,10-12,14]. Some of these studies only focused on particular types of GEP-NENs such as well-differentiated endocrine tumors, poorly differentiated endocrine carcinomas or a single site of tumors (pancreas, colon or rectum). Our study investigated the pathologic features of GEP-NENs by using the latest histopathologic diagnosis consensus for the first time. It also analyzed any possible tumor site of digestive system including pancreas, biliary and peritoneal cavity. This study should contribute to establishing a database of the epidemiology, clinical pathological features, treatment and prognosis of GEP-NENs in China.

It is confirmed in our study that GEP-NENs comprise a heterogeneous group in relation to their primary locations. Previous researches indicated that the small intestine and appendix were the most predominant NENs locations [2,15-17]. But according to our study, pancreas is the principal site of GEP-NENs. The rectum is the most frequent sites of gastrointestinal tract, followed by the stomach and duodenum, whereas the jejunum/ileum accounts for no more than 2% tumor cases. A similar distribution of NENs was also found from a Korean study [10], which observed that rectum was the most common primary site of tumor in 470 available cases, followed by the pancreas, stomach and duodenum. Results from another three registries including SEER, National Cancer Registry for Gastroenteropancreatic Neuroendocrine Tumors (RGETNE, http://www. retegep.net) and Norwegian Registry of Cancer (NRC)

Table 4 Overall survival

Factors	Overall survival				
	Number	Mean (years)	95% CI	χ2	P
All patients	136	9.5	8.1-11.0		
Sex				2.053	0.152
Female	54	9.9	8.5-11.3		
Male	82	8.7	6.7-10.6		
Age				0.259	0.611
≤50	60	9.9	8.0-11.8		
>50	76	7.8	5.9-9.6		
Site				2.385	0.123
Gastrointestinal tract	77	6.7	5.4-8.0		
Pancreas	46	11.1	9.3-12.9		
Functional status				6.691	0.006
Functional	22	NR	NC		
Nonfunctional	114	7.7	6.1-9.2		
Tumor grading				9.087	0.011
G1	63	10.8	8.7-12.9		
G2	25	3.5	2.6-4.3		
G3	41	4.1	2.8-5.4		
Tumor type				6.634	0.010
NET	88	10.1	8.1-12.1		
NEC + MANEC	41	4.1	2.8-5.4		
Distant metastasis				23.773	0.000
Yes	44	5.0	2.7-7.3		
No	92	11.0	9.2-12.8		

CI, confidence interval; NR, not reached; NC, not computable; NET, neuroendocrine tumor; NEC, neuroendocrine carcinoma; MANEC, mixed adenoendocrine carcinoma.

significantly differed from that in our series: Rectum and jejunum/ileum were the most common sites for NENs in the SEER Program tumor registry, pancreas NENs were only the third most common NENs; The pancreas and jejunum/ileum were the most frequent positions in RGETNE; whereas the small intestine was the most frequent sites of origin, followed by the colon and rectum in NRC. These inconsistencies may be due to the racial disparities, as well as the selection bias among population based data and hospital series. So a larger patient population is required to carry on further investigation.

NENs can be classified into functional and nonfunctional tumors according to the presence or absence of symptoms associated with hormones overproduction [18]. The current study demonstrated that the majority of nonfunctional NENs usually presented with nonspecific symptoms, which may give rise to misdiagnosis of the tumors as irritable bowel syndrome or digestive adenocarcinomas. Our study also showed that insulinomas

were the most frequently encountered functional tumors in the pancreas, accounting for 93.1% of pancreatic NENs. No case, however, presented with carcinoid syndrome in this study. Interestingly, the incidence of carcinoid syndrome (10–32%) in the Western population [8,17,19-21] is significantly different from our report, with the fact that ileal tumors account for the vast majority.

Assessments of the locations and extents of GEP-NENs were crucial for management. The present study analyzed imaging methods, which is commonly used in current clinical practice, in this patient population. Conventional imaging procedures include endoscopy, ultrasound, EUS, CT scan, MRI and PET-CT, with detection rates ranging from 77.8 to 98.7%. CT scan was one of the most widely used imaging modalities (123/178) whereas endoscopy promised the highest yields of tumor detection (98.7%). The introduction of EUS provides unique advantages in evaluating the pancreatic biliary system, especially in tumors <1.0 cm in diameter and micrometastasis. The typical EUS patterns of NENs includes rounded, homogeneous, hypoechoic, well defined and vascularized masses, with the detection rate of 91.9% in our study, rather comparable to the results achieved in other series [22-24]. Small tumors and liver metastasis (i.e., tumors <0.5 cm in diameter) may be missed, resulting in underestimate of the exact disease extent. No single technique is 100% sensitive and accurate. Therefore, multiple imaging modalities should be combined to detect small, biochemically diagnosed tumors.

Despite the advances in both morphology and biology, the classification of NENs is still under debate. The lack of a uniform classification system for NENs hampers evaluation of therapy and comparison between clinical trials [25]. European Neuroendocrine Tumor Society (ENETS) and the North American Neuroendocrine Tumor Society (NANETS) have published diagnosis standard and pathology reports of NENs in 2009 and 2010 [18,26], respectively. Furthermore, the WHO revised the nomenclature and classification of GEP-NENs in 2010, version 4 [4]. In 2011, China established her own classification system for NENs [5]. Chinese Pathologic Consensus Group suggested the term "Neuroendocrine neoplasm (NEN)" instead of "Neuroendocrine Tumor (NET)" and formulated the classification criteria by the use of Ki-67 index/mitotic rate and histology. The pathologic features of NENs in our hospital were reviewed according to this diagnosis consensus in the current analysis, which to our knowledge, is the first study using the newest consensus. Overall, G1 tumors accounted for 51.5% of 169 available cases, followed by G3 (30.2%) and G2 (18.3%). The occurence of NET, NEC and MANEC were 69.8%, 27.2% and 3.0%, respectively. The availability of this uniform system for NETs greatly facilitates

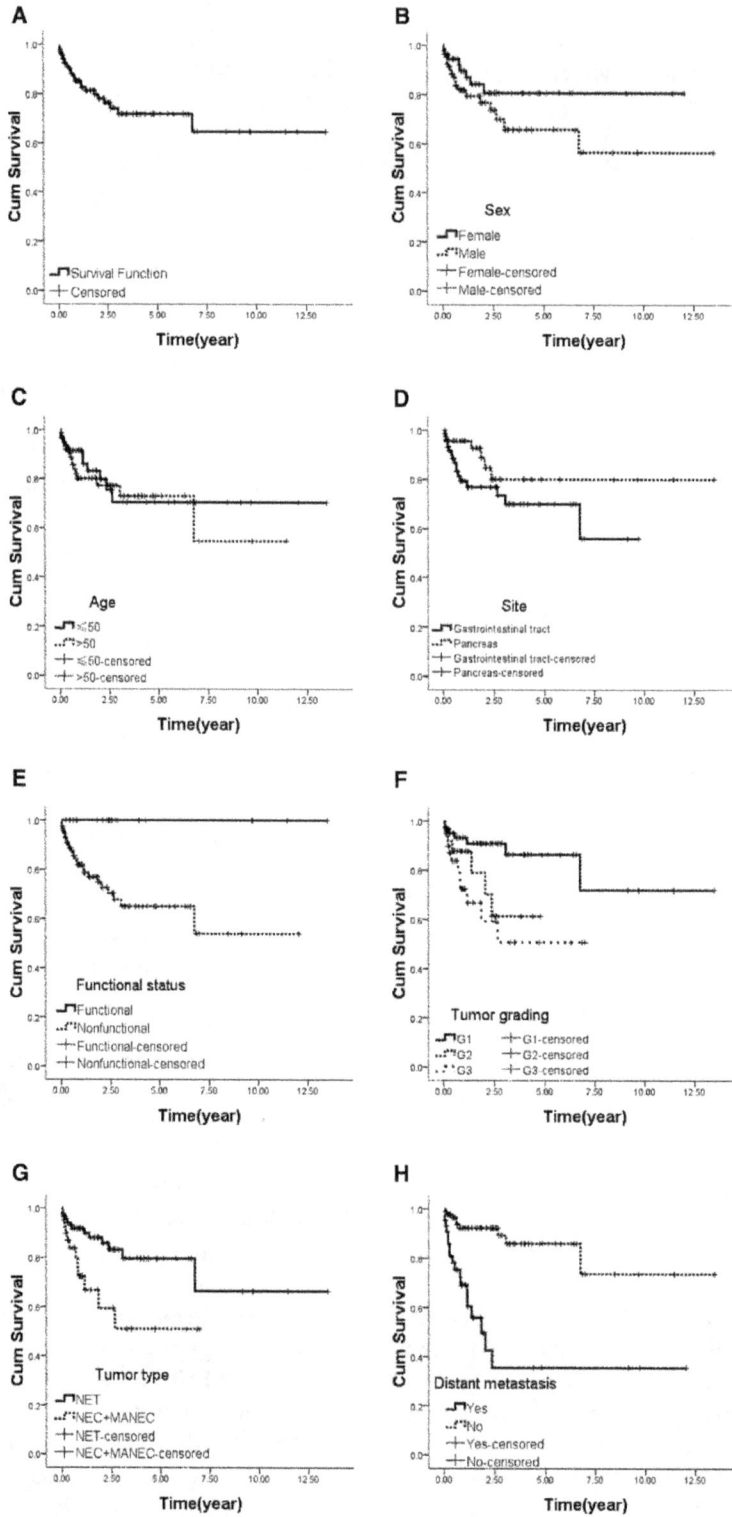

Figure 1 Overall survival (**A**) Overall survival in all patients. (**B**) Overall survival by sex. (**C**) Overall survival by age at diagnosis. (**D**) Overall survival by site of tumors. (**E**) Overall survival by functional status. (**F**) Overall survival by histological grading. (**G**) Overall survival by tumor type. (**H**) Overall survival by condition of distant metastasis.

classification of the tumors, evaluation of treatment, and comparison of clinical trials.

In our series, distant disease at initial diagnosis occurred at the rate of 23.0%, which increased to 28.1% during follow up. Liver was the most frequent site tumor involved and the distribution of distant metastasis was wider than that either in SEER or in NRC (18–22%). In RGETNE, however, a significant proportion of patients (44%) with widespread disease were reported compared with our series. The frequency of primary tumor sites associated with distant disease varied in different series: in our cohort, the most common sites was cecum (100.0%), followed by jejunum/ileum (75.0%), gallbladder (50.0%), duodenum (38.5%), Vater's ampulla (33.3%) and stomach (28.0%); in the SEER Registry, the most common site was pancreas (64%), followed by cecum/colon (44%/32%) and jejunum/ileum (30%); and in the RGETNE Registry, it was jejunum/ileum (65%), followed by colon (48%) and rectum (40%). Therefore, jejunum/ileum tumors appear to have a greater propensity for distant metastasis. However, the diversity should be taken into account.

Among the many therapeutic options for NENs, surgery is the treatment of choice. A variety of operations are available to reduce load of tumor and improve survival. The extent of surgical resection depends on the tumor size and origin and approximately 75.9% of patients have undergone a radical surgery. Radiofrequency ablation or TACE is usually adopted to treat liver involvement, accounting for 6.2% of the cases.

Besides surgery, other therapeutic options such as chemotherapy, biological therapy and targeted therapy can be used for NENs. According to the new WHO 2010 classification, well-differentiated NENs are classified as G1 and G2 neuroendocrine tumors (NETs) and poor-differentiated NENs are referred to as G3 neuroendocrine carcinomas (NECs). It has been reported that existing cytotoxic chemotherapy agents have been of limited value for the treatment of well-differentiated gastrointestinal NENs (with response rates 10% ~ 15%) [27-29], but has been the standard of care for well-differentiated metastatic pancreatic endocrine tumors (with response rates 40% ~ 70%) [30-32]. However, chemotherapy is generally considered active in poor-differentiated NENs (with response rates 50% ~ 70%) [33-35]. According to the published documents, several chemotherapeutic regimens are available, most of them are either platinum based or flurouracil based [29,34,36,37]. For the GEP-NEC, platinum-based combination regimens with etoposide or paclitaxel [33,34,36] are recommended. In our cohort, chemotherapy was performed in 23 patients. The most frequently used chemo regimen was etoposide–platinum combination. During follow-up, 3 of them died of tumor progression. It has been noticed that

biological therapy and targeted therapy promise some effect on NENs in recent years [38-43]. Somatostatin analogues are effective therapeutic option for functional neuroendocrine tumors because they reduce hormone-related symptoms [44-46]. They have also been shown to stabilize tumor growth over long periods, even to inhibit tumor growth in patients with well-differentiated metastatic neuroendocrine midgut tumors [40,47,48]. Although the treatment effect of somatostatin analogues on foregut and hindgut tumors remain to be confirmed, 16 patients including 2 patients with functional neuroendocrine tumors and 14 patients with well-differentiated metastatic GEP-NENs received long-term administration of octreotide LAR at a dose of 20–40 mg monthly in our study.

The prognosis of GEP-NENs is more favorable than that of the adenocarcinomas of the digestive system. The overall 5-year survival rate in our series was 54.5%, rather comparable to that of SEER or NRC registry [2,3,6] (50–59%), but it was lower than that in some European countries [7,9] (75–79%). The inconsistencies of survival rates may be due to the racial and geographical disparities. We also proved that prognosis differed statistically according to functional status, pathological grading and classification. As the great majority of functional tumors were insulinomas which are benign in most cases in our study, that may lead to the conclusion that functionality may be a favorable prognostic marker. The result obtained above may be caused by small sample in this series. We also confirmed that metastasis represented a worse outcome with a mean survival of 5.0 years (P = 0.000). Multivariate analysis was not done due to the small size of our series. Therefore, further evaluation in a larger patient population is required to estimate the independent prognostic factors of GEP-NENs.

A broad range of this heterogeneous tumors was reviewed in the current study, which to our knowledge, is the first report using the latest pathological diagnosis consensus of these tumors. We also confirmed that GEP-NENs may originate from any part of the digestive system, and the majority of them are nonfunctional tumors with non-specific symptoms. Endoscopy and radiographic examination play an important role in tumor detection. However, final diagnosis should be based on pathological detection. The prognosis of these tumors was more favorable compared with gastrointestinal carcinomas. Nonetheless, the outcome was extremely poor for patients with high grading tumor and distant metastasis. Further understanding of the molecular mechanisms should facilitate management of the disease. Early diagnosis is crucial for radical resection before development of local invasion or distant disease, and interdisciplinary cooperation is the direction of future.

Conclusions

Nonfunctional tumors with non-specific symptoms account for the majority of GEP-NENs. Diagnosis depends on pathological classification. Multidisciplinary treatments could help improve the outcome.

Competing interests

The authors declare that they have no competing interests.

Authors' contributions

WYH and LY contributed equally to this work; WYH and LY: Collection and/or assembly of data, Data analysis and interpretation, Manuscript writing; LY and XL: Pathological data collection and analysis; WJH: Collection of clinical data; Chen J and Chen MH: Conception and design, Financial and administrative support, manuscript editing. All authors read and approved the final manuscript.

Acknowledgments

This study was supported by the grants from National Natural Science Foundation of China (No. 30871145 and No. 81072048), the Junior Teacher Cultivation Project of Sun Yat-sen University (No. 09ykpy22), grants for major projects and emerging interdisciplinary studies of Sun Yat-sen University (No.10ykjc23) supported by the Fundamental Research Funds for the Central Universities.

Author details

[1]Department of Gastroenterology, The First Affiliated Hospital of Sun Yat-sen University, 58 Zhongshan II Road, Guangzhou, People's Republic of China. [2]Department of Pathology, The First Affiliated Hospital of Sun Yat-sen University, 58 Zhongshan II Road, Guangzhou, People's Republic of China.

References

1. Modlin IM, Oberg K, Chung DC, Jensen RT, de Herder WW, Thakker RV, Caplin M, Delle Fave G, Kaltsas GA, Krenning EP, et al: Gastroenteropancreatic neuroendocrine tumours. Lancet Oncol 2008, 9(1):61–72.
2. Modlin IM, Lye KD, Kidd M: A 5-decade analysis of 13,715 carcinoid tumors. Cancer 2003, 97(4):934–959.
3. Yao JC, Hassan M, Phan A, Dagohoy C, Leary C, Mares JE, Abdalla EK, Fleming JB, Vauthey JN, Rashid A, et al: One hundred years after "carcinoid": epidemiology of and prognostic factors for neuroendocrine tumors in 35,825 cases in the United States. J Clin Oncol 2008, 26(18):3063–3072.
4. Bosman FT, Carneiro F, Hruban RH, Theise ND: WHO classification of tumours of the digestive system. 4th edition. Lyon: International Agency for Research on Cancer; 2010.
5. Chinese Pathologic Consensus Group for Gastrointestinal and Pancreatic Neuroendocrine Neoplasm: China Consensus Guidelines for the standards of histopathologic diagnosis in Gastroenteropancreatic Neuroendocrine neoplasm. Chin J Pathol 2011, 40(4):257–262.
6. Hauso O, Gustafsson BI, Kidd M, Waldum HL, Drozdov I, Chan AK, Modlin IM: Neuroendocrine tumor epidemiology: contrasting Norway and North America. Cancer 2008, 113(10):2655–2664.
7. Garcia-Carbonero R, Capdevila J, Crespo-Herrero G, Diaz-Perez JA, Martinez Del Prado MP, Alonso Orduna V, Sevilla-Garcia I, Villabona-Artero C, Beguiristain-Gomez A, Llanos-Munoz M, et al: Incidence, patterns of care and prognostic factors for outcome of gastroenteropancreatic neuroendocrine tumors (GEP-NETs): results from the National Cancer Registry of Spain (RGETNE). Ann Oncol 2010, 21(9):1794–1803.
8. Ploeckinger U, Kloeppel G, Wiedenmann B, Lohmann R: The German NET-registry: an audit on the diagnosis and therapy of neuroendocrine tumors. Neuroendocrinology 2009, 90(4):349–363.
9. Lepage C, Rachet B, Coleman MP: Survival from malignant digestive endocrine tumors in England and Wales: a population-based study. Gastroenterology 2007, 132(3):899–904.
10. Lim T, Lee J, Kim JJ, Lee JK, Lee KT, Kim YH, Kim KW, Kim S, Sohn TS, Choi DW, et al: Gastroenteropancreatic neuroendocrine tumors: incidence and treatment outcome in a single institution in Korea. Asia Pac J Clin Oncol 2011, 7(3):293–299.
11. Li AF, Hsu CY, Li A, Tai LC, Liang WY, Li WY, Tsay SH, Chen JY: A 35-year retrospective study of carcinoid tumors in Taiwan: differences in distribution with a high probability of associated second primary malignancies. Cancer 2008, 112(2):274–283.
12. Konishi T, Watanabe T, Kishimoto J, Kotake K, Muto T, Nagawa H: Prognosis and risk factors of metastasis in colorectal carcinoids: results of a nationwide registry over 15 years. Gut 2007, 56(6):863–868.
13. Ito T, Tanaka M, Sasano H, Osamura YR, Sasaki I, Kimura W, Takano K, Obara T, Ishibashi M, Nakao K, et al: Preliminary results of a Japanese nationwide survey of neuroendocrine gastrointestinal tumors. J Gastroenterol 2007, 42(6):497–500.
14. Wang DS, Zhang DS, Qiu MZ, Wang ZQ, Luo HY, Wang FH, Li YH, Xu RH: Prognostic factors and survival in patients with neuroendocrine tumors of the pancreas. Tumour Biol 2011, 32(4):697–705.
15. Maggard MA, O'Connell JB, Ko CY: Updated population-based review of carcinoid tumors. Ann Surg 2004, 240(1):117–122.
16. Van Gompel JJ, Sippel RS, Warner TF, Chen H: Gastrointestinal carcinoid tumors: factors that predict outcome. World J Surg 2004, 28(4):387–392.
17. Onaitis MW, Kirshbom PM, Hayward TZ, Quayle FJ, Feldman JM, Seigler HF, Tyler DS: Gastrointestinal carcinoids: characterization by site of origin and hormone production. Ann Surg 2000, 232(4):549–556.
18. Klimstra DS, Modlin IR, Adsay NV, Chetty R, Deshpande V, Gonen M, Jensen RT, Kidd M, Kulke MH, Lloyd RV, et al: Pathology reporting of neuroendocrine tumors: application of the Delphic consensus process to the development of a minimum pathology data set. Am J Surg Pathol 2010, 34(3):300–313.
19. Pape UF, Bohmig M, Berndt U, Tiling N, Wiedenmann B, Plockinger U: Survival and clinical outcome of patients with neuroendocrine tumors of the gastroenteropancreatic tract in a german referral center. Ann N Y Acad Sci 2004, 1014:222–233.
20. Shebani KO, Souba WW, Finkelstein DM, Stark PC, Elgadi KM, Tanabe KK, Ott MJ: Prognosis and survival in patients with gastrointestinal tract carcinoid tumors. Ann Surg 1999, 229(6):815–821. discussion 822–813.
21. Vinik AI, Thompson N, Eckhauser F, Moattari AR: Clinical features of carcinoid syndrome and the use of somatostatin analogue in its management. Acta Oncol 1989, 28(3):389–402.
22. Anderson MA, Carpenter S, Thompson NW, Nostrant TT, Elta GH, Scheiman JM: Endoscopic ultrasound is highly accurate and directs management in patients with neuroendocrine tumors of the pancreas. Am J Gastroenterol 2000, 95(9):2271–2277.
23. Zimmer T, Scherubl H, Faiss S, Stolzel U, Riecken EO, Wiedenmann B: Endoscopic ultrasonography of neuroendocrine tumours. Digestion 2000, 62(Suppl 1):45–50.
24. Varas Lorenzo MJ, Miquel Collell JM, Maluenda Colomer MD, Boix Valverde J, Armengol Miro JR: Preoperative detection of gastrointestinal neuroendocrine tumors using endoscopic ultrasonography. Rev Esp Enferm Dig 2006, 98(11):828–883.
25. Modlin IM, Moss SF, Chung DC, Jensen RT, Snyderwine E: Priorities for improving the management of gastroenteropancreatic neuroendocrine tumors. J Natl Cancer Inst 2008, 100(18):1282–1289.
26. Kloppel G, Couvelard A, Perren A, Komminoth P, McNicol AM, Nilsson O, Scarpa A, Scoazec JY, Wiedenmann B, Papotti M, et al: ENETS Consensus Guidelines for the Standards of Care in Neuroendocrine Tumors: towards a standardized approach to the diagnosis of gastroenteropancreatic neuroendocrine tumors and their prognostic stratification. Neuroendocrinology 2009, 90(2):162–166.
27. Bukowski RM, Tangen CM, Peterson RF, Taylor SA, Rinehart JJ, Eyre HJ, Rivkin SE, Fleming TR, Macdonald JS: Phase II trial of dimethyltriazenoimidazole carboxamide in patients with metastatic carcinoid. A Southwest Oncology Group study. Cancer 1994, 73(5):1505–1508.
28. Ansell SM, Pitot HC, Burch PA, Kvols LK, Mahoney MR, Rubin J: A Phase II study of high-dose paclitaxel in patients with advanced neuroendocrine tumors. Cancer 2001, 91(8):1543–1548.
29. Sun W, Lipsitz S, Catalano P, Mailliard JA, Haller DG: Phase II/III study of doxorubicin with fluorouracil compared with streptozocin with fluorouracil or dacarbazine in the treatment of advanced carcinoid tumors: Eastern Cooperative Oncology Group Study E1281. J Clin Oncol 2005, 23(22):4897–4904.

30. Moertel CG, Hanley JA, Johnson LA: **Streptozocin alone compared with streptozocin plus fluorouracil in the treatment of advanced islet-cell carcinoma.** *N Engl J Med* 1980, **303**(21):1189–1194.

31. Moertel CG, Lefkopoulo M, Lipsitz S, Hahn RG, Klaassen D: **Streptozocin-doxorubicin, streptozocin-fluorouracil or chlorozotocin in the treatment of advanced islet-cell carcinoma.** *N Engl J Med* 1992, **326**(8):519–523.

32. Strosberg JR, Fine RL, Choi J, Nasir A, Coppola D, Chen DT, Helm J, Kvols L: **First-line chemotherapy with capecitabine and temozolomide in patients with metastatic pancreatic endocrine carcinomas.** *Cancer* 2011, **117**(2):268–275.

33. Moertel CG, Kvols LK, O'Connell MJ, Rubin J: **Treatment of neuroendocrine carcinomas with combined etoposide and cisplatin. Evidence of major therapeutic activity in the anaplastic variants of these neoplasms.** *Cancer* 1991, **68**(2):227–232.

34. Hainsworth JD, Spigel DR, Litchy S, Greco FA: **Phase II trial of paclitaxel, carboplatin, and etoposide in advanced poorly differentiated neuroendocrine carcinoma: a Minnie Pearl Cancer Research Network Study.** *J Clin Oncol* 2006, **24**(22):3548–3554.

35. Fjallskog ML, Granberg DP, Welin SL, Eriksson C, Oberg KE, Janson ET, Eriksson BK: **Treatment with cisplatin and etoposide in patients with neuroendocrine tumors.** *Cancer* 2001, **92**(5):1101–1107.

36. Mitry E, Baudin E, Ducreux M, Sabourin JC, Rufie P, Aparicio T, Lasser P, Elias D, Duvillard P, Schlumberger M, *et al*: **Treatment of poorly differentiated neuroendocrine tumours with etoposide and cisplatin.** *Br J Cancer* 1999, **81**(8):1351–1355.

37. Kouvaraki MA, Ajani JA, Hoff P, Wolff R, Evans DB, Lozano R, Yao JC: **Fluorouracil, doxorubicin, and streptozocin in the treatment of patients with locally advanced and metastatic pancreatic endocrine carcinomas.** *J Clin Oncol* 2004, **22**(23):4762–4771.

38. Yao JC, Phan AT, Chang DZ, Wolff RA, Hess K, Gupta S, Jacobs C, Mares JE, Landgraf AN, Rashid A, *et al*: **Efficacy of RAD001 (everolimus) and octreotide LAR in advanced low- to intermediate-grade neuroendocrine tumors: results of a phase II study.** *J Clin Oncol* 2008, **26**(26):4311–4318.

39. Kulke MH, Lenz HJ, Meropol NJ, Posey J, Ryan DP, Picus J, Bergsland E, Stuart K, Tye L, Huang X, *et al*: **Activity of sunitinib in patients with advanced neuroendocrine tumors.** *J Clin Oncol* 2008, **26**(20):3403–3410.

40. Rinke A, Muller HH, Schade-Brittinger C, Klose KJ, Barth P, Wied M, Mayer C, Aminossadati B, Pape UF, Blaker M, *et al*: **Placebo-controlled, double-blind, prospective, randomized study on the effect of octreotide LAR in the control of tumor growth in patients with metastatic neuroendocrine midgut tumors: a report from the PROMID Study Group.** *J Clin Oncol* 2009, **27**(28):4656–4663.

41. Yao JC, Lombard-Bohas C, Baudin E, Kvols LK, Rougier P, Ruszniewski P, Hoosen S, St Peter J, Haas T, Lebwohl D, *et al*: **Daily oral everolimus activity in patients with metastatic pancreatic neuroendocrine tumors after failure of cytotoxic chemotherapy: a phase II trial.** *J Clin Oncol* 2010, **28**(1):69–76.

42. Yao JC, Shah MH, Ito T, Bohas CL, Wolin EM, Van Cutsem E, Hobday TJ, Okusaka T, Capdevila J, de Vries EG, *et al*: **Everolimus for advanced pancreatic neuroendocrine tumors.** *N Engl J Med* 2011, **364**(6):514–523.

43. Raymond E, Dahan L, Raoul JL, Bang YJ, Borbath I, Lombard-Bohas C, Valle J, Metrakos P, Smith D, Vinik A, *et al*: **Sunitinib malate for the treatment of pancreatic neuroendocrine tumors.** *N Engl J Med* 2011, **364**(6):501–513.

44. Oberg K, Kvols L, Caplin M, Delle Fave G, de Herder W, Rindi G, Ruszniewski P, Woltering EA, Wiedenmann B: **Consensus report on the use of somatostatin analogs for the management of neuroendocrine tumors of the gastroenteropancreatic system.** *Ann Oncol* 2004, **15**(6):966–973.

45. Karashima T, Cai RZ, Schally AV: **Effects of highly potent octapeptide analogs of somatostatin on growth hormone, insulin and glucagon release.** *Life Sci* 1987, **41**(8):1011–1019.

46. Oberg K: **Future aspects of somatostatin-receptor-mediated therapy.** *Neuroendocrinology* 2004, **80**(Suppl 1):57–61.

47. Faiss S, Rath U, Mansmann U, Caird D, Clemens N, Riecken EO, Wiedenmann B: **Ultra-high-dose lanreotide treatment in patients with metastatic neuroendocrine gastroenteropancreatic tumors.** *Digestion* 1999, **60**(5):469–476.

48. Welin SV, Janson ET, Sundin A, Stridsberg M, Lavenius E, Granberg D, Skogseid B, Oberg KE, Eriksson BK: **High-dose treatment with a long-acting somatostatin analogue in patients with advanced midgut carcinoid tumours.** *Eur J Endocrinol/European Federation of Endocrine Societies* 2004, **151**(1):107–112.

12

A plausible role for actin gamma smooth muscle 2 (*ACTG2*) in small intestinal neuroendocrine tumorigenesis

Katarina Edfeldt[*], Per Hellman, Gunnar Westin and Peter Stalberg

Abstract

Background: Small intestinal neuroendocrine tumors (SI-NETs) originate from the enterochromaffin cells in the ileum and jejunum. The knowledge about genetic and epigenetic abnormalities is limited. Low mRNA expression levels of actin gamma smooth muscle 2 (*ACTG2*) have been demonstrated in metastases relative to primary SI-NETs. *ACTG2* and microRNA-145 (miR-145) are aberrantly expressed in other cancers and *ACTG2* can be induced by miR-145. The aim of this study was to investigate the role of *ACTG2* in small intestinal neuroendocrine tumorigenesis.

Methods: Protein expression was analyzed in SI-NETs ($n = 24$) and in enterochromaffin cells by immunohistochemistry. The cell line CNDT2.5 was treated with the histone methyltransferase inhibitor 3-deazaneplanocin A (DZNep), the selective EZH2 inhibitor EPZ-6438, or 5-aza-2'-deoxycytidine, a DNA hypomethylating agent. Cells were transfected with *ACTG2* expression plasmid or miR-145. Western blotting analysis, quantitative RT-PCR, colony formation- and viability assays were performed. miR-145 expression levels were measured in tumors.

Results: Eight primary tumors and two lymph node metastases displayed variable levels of positive staining. Fourteen SI-NETs and normal enterochromaffin cells stained negatively. Overexpression of *ACTG2* significantly inhibited CNDT2.5 cell growth. Treatment with DZNep or transfection with miR-145 induced *ACTG2* expression (>10-fold), but no effects were detected after treatment with EPZ-6438 or 5-aza-2'-deoxycytidine. DZNep also induced miR-145 expression. SI-NETs expressed relatively low levels of miR-145, with reduced expression in metastases compared to primary tumors.

Conclusions: *ACTG2* is expressed in a fraction of SI-NETs, can inhibit cell growth in vitro, and is positively regulated by miR-145. Theoretical therapeutic strategies based on these results are discussed.

Keywords: SI-NET, *ACTG2*, miR-145, Epigenetic regulation

Background

Small intestinal neuroendocrine tumors (SI-NETs) are small, slow growing neoplasms that originate from the enterochromaffin cells in the ileum and jejunum. These rare tumors have an incidence about 1 case per 100 000. Metastases have often already occurred at time of diagnosis and the 5-year survival rate is around 65 %. Due to excess of tumor-secreted hormones; e.g. serotonin and tachykinins, patients can suffer from the carcinoid syndrome, causing cutaneous flushing, diarrhea, carcinoid heart disease and bronchoconstriction [1, 2]. The WHO classification from 2010 divides small intestinal neuroendocrine neoplasms in three grades; G1-NETs (Ki67 < 3 %), G2-NETs (Ki67 3–20 %) and NEC (neuroendocrine carinomas, Ki67 > 20 %) [3]. SI-NETs (G1 and G2) are most often resistant to chemotherapy and radiation, and medical treatment is limited. Symptom relief can be obtained by somatostatin-analogues and interferon treatment. There is a great need of new therapeutic options that could be beneficial to the patients.

The knowledge of common genetic or epigenetic abnormalities is limited in SI-NETs. Loss of chromosome

---

* Correspondence: katarina.edfeldt@surgsci.uu.se
Department of Surgical Sciences, Uppsala University, Uppsala University Hospital, Entrance 70, 1 tr, SE-75185 Uppsala, Sweden

18 is most frequently seen, but no tumor-associated mutations have been found on chromosome 18 [4–6]. A putative role for *TCEB3C* (elongin A3), located at 18q21, as tumor suppressor gene in SI-NETs was recently suggested [7]. The mutation rate is overall low [8], and recently, exome- and genome sequencing found *CDKN1B* to be mutated in ~9 % of SI-NETs [9], implicating importance for this gene in tumorigenesis.

We have previously observed expression of actin gamma smooth muscle 2 (*ACTG2*) mRNA in a collection of primary SI-NETs, compared to undetectable expression levels in lymph node metastases [10]. Actin proteins are involved in multiple intracellular processes, including maintenance of the cytoskeleton and cell motility [11], and ACTG2 is normally found in enteric tissue. Aberrant expression has been described in several different cancer types and this can affect chemotherapy sensitivity [12–14]. Lower expression levels of *ACTG2* were detected in normal colon tissue compared to colon carcinoma [15]. High expression levels of *ACTG2* have been associated with improved disease-specific survival [16], and also with a more aggressive phenotype [17, 18]. Furthermore, microRNA-145 (miR-145) can positively regulate expression of *ACTG2* [19, 20], and overexpression of this microRNA inhibits cell proliferation, cell invasion, tumor growth and can induce apoptosis in other cancer cell types [19, 21].

The aim of this study was to investigate a possible role of *ACTG2* in small intestinal neuroendocrine tumorigenesis.

Methods

Tumor material and cell line

The patients included in the study (*n* = 28) were all diagnosed with SI-NET in the ileum and operated on at Uppsala University Hospital. This study was approved by the regional ethical review board in Uppsala (11-375/ 1.1.2011, Local ethical vetting board in Uppsala (Regionala etikprövningsnämnden i Uppsala)). Written informed consent for participation and publication of individual clinical details was obtained from all patients. All patients were above 18 years of age at time of inclusion. Fifteen tumors were classified as G1 NETs and 13 as G2 NETs. Patient characteristics are summarized in Additional file 1: Table S1. The tumors were snap frozen in liquid nitrogen and kept at –70 °C.

A SI-NET cell line, CNDT2.5, developed from a liver metastasis from a patient diagnosed with primary ileal SI-NET [22], was used in the experiments. These cells expressed neuroendocrine markers and somatostatin receptor 2 and responded to synthetic somatostatin analogue (octreotide) treatment [22, 23], although skepticism regarding the neuroendocrine authenticity of this cell line has also been raised [24]. The growth medium for CNDT2.5 was DMEM-F12 complemented with 10 % fetal bovine serum (Sigma Aldrich), 1 % vitamins, 1 % L-glutamine, 1 % sodium pyruvate, 1 % nonessential amino acids and 1 % PEST (penicillin-streptomycin), and the cells were cultured at 37 °C in 5 % CO_2.

Immunohistochemistry

Immunohistochemistry procedure is described in detail in previous research [25, 26]. Paraffin embedded tumor tissue (*n* = 24) sections (5 μm) were passed through descending alcohol concentrations and distilled water. Background staining was blocked with 3 % hydrogen peroxide and heated in citrate buffer. The tissues were treated with normal serum from goat (S-1000, Vector) and two different rabbit polyclonal anti-ACTG2 antibodies (NB100-91649 Novus Biologicals, diluted 1/200, and TA313418 Origene, diluted 1/80) and anti-chromogranin A antibodies (Ab-1, LK2H10, NeoMarkers, diluted 1/1000) were used and incubated. A biotinylated secondary antibody from goat anti-rabbit (BA-100 Vector, diluted 1/200) was added to the tissues and then treated with ABC complex. Visualization was done with DAB color reagent. Absence of primary antibody was used as a negative control. Consecutive sections from each tumor were incubated with anti-ACTG2 and anti-chromogranin A antibody. Also, consecutive sections of normal intestinal mucosa were treated with anti-ACTG2 (NB100-91649 Novus Biologicals, diluted 1/200) and anti-chromogranin A antibodies (Ab-1, LK2H10, NeoMarkers, diluted 1/1000).

Immunofluorescence

Double immunofluorescence staining was done on sections of intestinal mucosa. Paraffin-embedded sections were deparaffinized, hydrated and subjected to pretreatment (microwave heating for 10 min at 800 W, followed by 20 min at 450 W in citrate buffer, pH 6.0). The sections were blocked with normal goat serum (S-1000, Vector) for 30 min before incubation with primary antibody anti-chromogranin A (Ab-1, LK2H10, NeoMarkers, diluted 1/1000) for 90 min, followed by secondary antibody Alexa Fluor 488 goat anti-mouse for 30 min. Then, incubation with the next primary antibody anti-ACTG2 (NB100-91649 Novus Biologicals), for 90 min, was followed by the secondary antibody Alexa Fluor 594 goat anti-rabbit, for 30 min (Life Technologies). The sections were mounted with Vectashield with DAPI (Vector Laboratories Inc.) and evaluated under light microscope.

Western blotting analysis

Proteins were extracted from tumors or CNDT2.5 cells using Cytobuster™ protein extraction reagent (Novagen) supplemented with Complete mini protease inhibitor cocktail tablets (Roche Diagnostics). Analysis of ACTG2 in tumor tissue was done using a primary antibody; anti-actin gamma2 (NB100-91649). Anti-Actin antibody (sc 1616,

Santa Cruz) or coomassie blue was used as loading controls, and for verification of transfection results a mouse monoclonal anti-DDK antibody (TA50011, Origene) was used. After incubation with the appropriate secondary antibody, bands were visualized using the enhanced chemiluminescence system (GE Healthcare).

Quantitative real-time RT-PCR

For extraction and purification of RNA, RNeasy Plus Mini Kit (Qiagen) was used according to manufacturer's instructions, and for microRNA, miRNeasy Mini Kit (Qiagen) was used. Quantity was measured using NanoDrop. Reverse transcription of DNA-free RNA with random hexamer primers was performed using the "First strand cDNA Synthesis kit" according to manufacturer's instructions (Fermentas) or MicroRNA RT kit (Life Technologies) using 10 ng RNA. Successful DNase I treatment of all RNA preparations was established by PCR analysis of the MYC promoter. qRT-PCR reactions were performed on the Step I qRT-PCR system (Applied Biosystems) using TaqMan Gene Expression Master Mix and assays for *ACTG2* (Hs00242273_m1), *GAPDH* (Hs02758991_g1), hsa-miR-145 (002278) and *RNU48* (001006) (Applied Biosystems). All samples were amplified in triplicates, and non-template controls were included. Each sample's mean threshold value was corrected for the corresponding mean value for GAPDH mRNA or RNU48 miRNA, used as endogenous controls.

Drug treatment

CNDT2.5 cells were seeded onto 6 well plates and treated with different concentrations of 5-aza-dC (5-aza-2'-deoxycytidine, Sigma Chemical Co., St. Louis, MO, USA, A3656) (0.025, 0.5, 1.0, 1.25, 1.5 μM) and DZNep (3-deazaneplanocin A, 2.5, 5.0, 10.0, 12.5, 15 μM) and cell viability was accessed using WST-1 (Roche Diagnostics GmbH). Not toxic concentrations were chosen; 1 μM for 5-aza-dC and 10 μM DZNep. Freshly prepared 5-aza-dC was used in the experiments. DZNep was kindly provided by Dr. Victor Marques [27].

2×10^5 CNDT2.5 cells were seeded onto 6 well plates. After 24 h 10 μM DZNep or 1 μM 5-aza-dC was added in triplicates or 1, 2.5, or 5 μM EPZ-6438 (Selleckchem, Houston, TX, USA), a specific EZH2 inhibitor [28], was added to the wells and fresh medium and compounds were added every 24 h. The cells were harvested after 72 h, 96 h for EPZ-6438 treated cells, for RNA preparations. The DZNep treatment was repeated three times and 5-aza-dC and EPZ-6438 twice.

miR-145 analysis

CNDT2.5 cells (1×10^5) were distributed onto 6 well plates. After 24 h hsa-miR-145 or negative control miR (mirVana™miRNA mimics, Ambion) was transfected in triplicates using 20 mM miRNA and 8 μl INTERFERin siRNA transfection reagent (Polyplus Transfection). The cells were harvested and RNA prepared after 72 h. Transfections were repeated three times and successful transfection was determined by qRT-PCR using miR-145 assay. Apoptosis was measured in transfected cells using the Cell Death Detection ELISA kit (Roche Molecular Biochemicals), and as a positive control cells were incubated with 0.1 μg/ml Camptothecin (Sigma-Aldrich), a specific inhibitor of DNA topoisomerase I that induces apoptosis.

Frozen tumor sections from 24 tumors; 8 primary tumors, 9 lymph node metastases and 7 liver metastasis, were when needed macro-dissected to obtain at least 80 % tumor cells (in most cases more than 90 %) and RNA was extracted using TriZol reagent (Invitrogen), according to manufacturer's instructions. cDNA synthesis followed by qRT-PCR was performed as described above.

Proliferation and viability assays

A colony formation assay was performed and repeated three times; CNDT2.5 cells (1×10^5) were seeded onto 6 well plates and transfected with 4 μg *ACTG2*-plasmid expression vector using 8 μl Lipofectamine 2000 reagent (Life Technologies) according to manufacturer's instructions. The ACTG2 expression vector consisted of an expression-validated cDNA in pCMV6-Entry (TrueORF Gold, catalog no. RC203151. Origene Technologies, Inc., Rockville, MD, USA) and empty pcDNA3.1 was used as control. Six hours after transfection fresh medium was added complemented with 1 % PEST and 0.2 mg/ml Geneticin (G418, Sigma Aldrich). After 24 h 2000 cells were distributed onto 6 well plates and fresh medium with 0.2 mg/ml Geneticin was added every 72 h. After 8 days in selection the cells were fixed with 10 % acetic acid/10 % methanol, stained with 0.4 % crystal violet, and visible colonies were photographed and counted. Successful transfection was verified by western blotting after 24 h.

To analyze effect of *ACTG2* on viability, CNDT2.5 cells were transiently transfected and 1000 cells were seeded in a 96 well plate in triplicates. After 72 h cell viability was measured using the cell proliferation reagent WST-1 (Roche Diagnostics GmbH) according to manufacturer's instructions.

Statistical analysis

All data are presented as arithmetical mean ± standard deviation. Unpaired t test was used for statistical analysis and $p < 0.05$ was considered significant.

Results
ACTG2 protein is variably expressed in 42 % of analyzed SI-NETs

Protein expression was evaluated in 24 tumor sections from 17 patients; 16 primary tumors and 8 lymph node metastases (Additional file 1: Table S1). Fourteen tumors displayed no staining in the tumor cells (Fig. 1a) and six tumors were positive in small areas of the section (Fig. 1b). Furthermore, two tumors displayed larger areas of positive staining and two tumors were weakly positive in all of the tumor cells (Fig. 1c). No staining was detected in absence of primary antibody (Fig. 1d). In total, eight primary tumors and two lymph node metastases (10 out of 24; 42 %) displayed positive staining for ACTG2 in SI-NET cells (i.e. chromogranin-positive cells, data not shown). Connective tissue showed mostly positive staining in 19 tumors (Fig. 1a), four displayed mostly negative staining, and one tumor section lacked stromal tissue. A different anti-ACTG2 antibody was used and showed very similar results (data not shown). Western blotting analysis for ACTG2 revealed one band in the correct size range in two tumors with strong stromal staining and not in two tumors that showed negative immunohistochemical staining (Fig. 1e). No obvious relations of ACTG2 expression to clinical data were observed (not shown).

ACTG2 protein is not detected in enterochromaffin cells of the normal small intestine

In order to determine whether ACTG2 is expressed in chromogranin-positive cells of the normal intestinal mucosa (enterochromaffin cells), immunohistochemistry on consecutive tissue sections and also double immunofluorescence were performed. Thorough analysis did not reveal staining of both ACTG2 and chromogranin A in the same cell (Fig. 2). Since these enterochromaffin cells likely represent founder of SI-NET cells, our results

suggest that ACTG2 expression can be induced by unknown mechanisms in a fraction of SI-NETs.

ACTG2 expression is induced by DZNep in vitro

We next wondered whether ACTG2 expression is controlled by epigenetic mechanisms and whether it could be induced by epigenetic drugs. Treatment of the human SI-NET cell line CNDT2.5, with the global histone methyltransferase inhibitor 3-deazaneplanocin A (DZNep) but not with the DNA hypomethylating agent 5-aza-2'-deoxycytidine, induced relative ACTG2 mRNA expression approximately 20-fold (Fig. 3a, data not shown). However, this gene induction did not seem to involve the histone methyltransferase EZH2, which methylates histone 3 lysine 27 and is inhibited by DZNep, since treatment with the specific EZH2 inhibitor EPZ-6438 failed to induce ACTG2 (Fig. 3b). Thus, ACTG2 expression can be controlled directly or indirectly by mechanisms related to DZNep treatment, but other than EZH2 repression. It should be noted that positive controls for treatments with 5-aza-dC and EPZ-6438 were not included here.

Involvement of miR-145

Expression of ACTG2 is known to be positively regulated by miR-145 in other cell types, and this was also observed (~12-fold) in CNDT2.5 cells transiently transfected by miR-145 (Fig. 4a). The level of miR-145 was increased more than 1000-fold in transfected cells, as determined by quantitative RT-PCR (data not shown). Interestingly, the expression of miR-145 was induced by DZNep treatment (~11-fold) (Fig. 4b). miR-145 is known to induce apoptosis in other cell types, but this was not

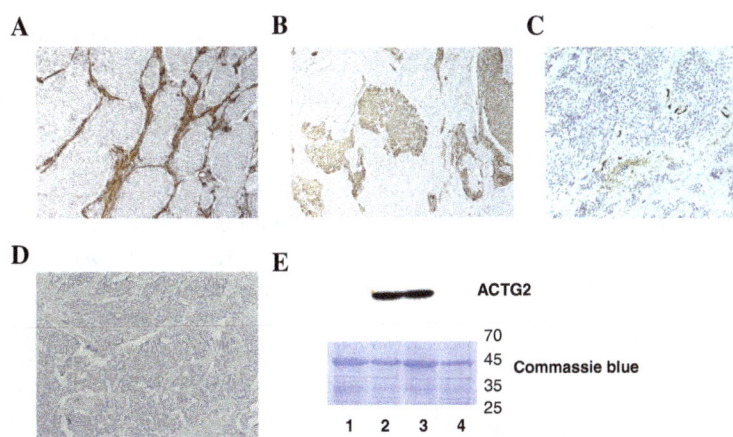

Fig. 1 Analysis of ACTG2 protein expression in SI-NETs by immunohistochemistry (**a-d**) using ACTG2 antibody (NB100-91649 Novus Biologicals) and western blotting (**e**) using another ACTG2 antibody (TA313418 Origene). **a** Negatively stained tumor cells and strong stromal staining (20x). **b** Areas with positively stained tumor cells, and negative stromal staining (20x). **c** Weak staining in all tumor cells (20x). **d** No staining in absence of primary antibody (20x). **e** Western blotting analysis showing antibody specificity and correlation to immunohistochemistry analysis. One band only was visualized in two tumors (lanes 2 and 3) displaying strong stromal staining, and no band was detected in two tumors (lanes 1 and 4) with no staining in both tumor and stromal cells. Lane 1, lymph node metastasis; lanes 2–4, primary tumors. Coomassie blue staining was used as loading control, ladder in kDa

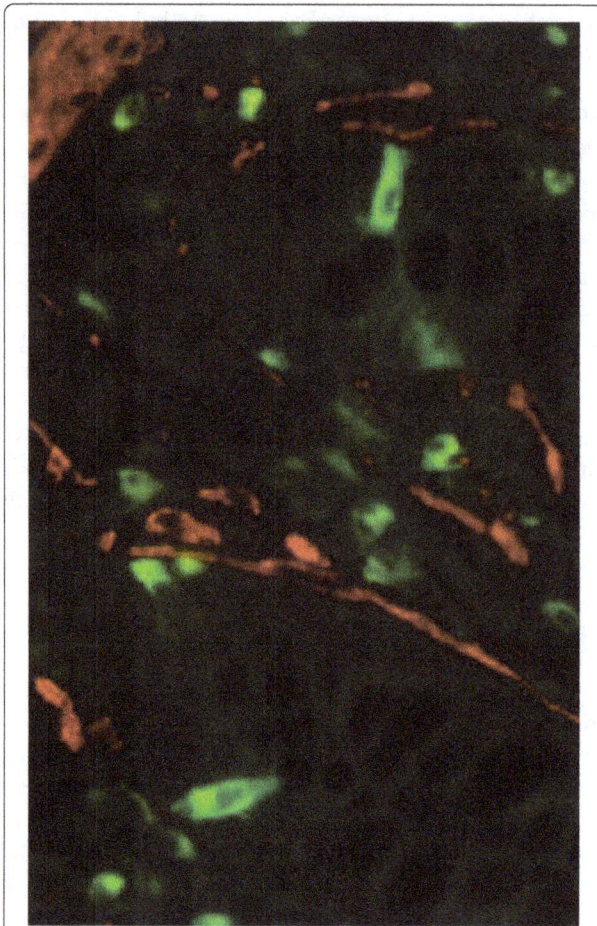

Fig. 2 Double immunofluorescence staining of intestinal mucosa. Chromogranin A is visualized as green, showing positively stained enterochromaffin cells. ACTG2 is visualized as red and no staining is detected in chromogranin A positive cells (yellow)

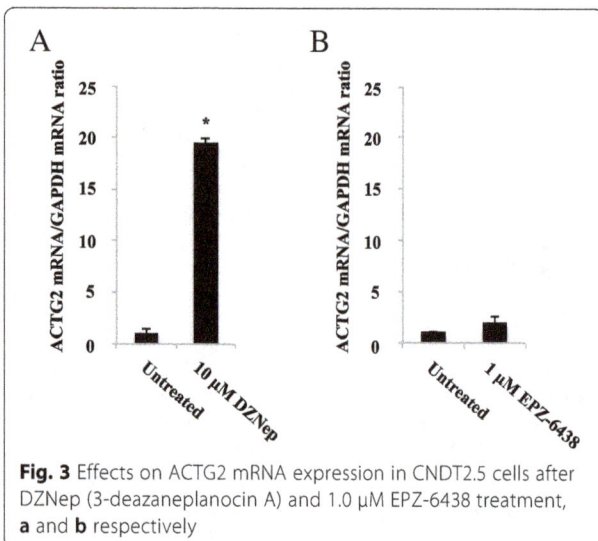

Fig. 3 Effects on ACTG2 mRNA expression in CNDT2.5 cells after DZNep (3-deazaneplanocin A) and 1.0 µM EPZ-6438 treatment, **a** and **b** respectively

observed here (Fig. 4c). Relative miR-145 expression was then determined in 24 SI-NETs; with a mean threshold cycle (Ct)-value of 32.4 and somewhat higher expression in 5 primary tumors compared to metastases and CNDT2.5 cells. miR-145 was significantly less expressed in liver metastases compared to primary tumors (Fig. 5a). There was a tendency towards decreased expression in lymph node metastases compared to primary tumors ($p = 0.09$). This needs to be examined in a larger cohort, although in line with these results, previously published experiments have shown significantly reduced expression of *ACTG2* mRNA in lymph node metastases compared to primary tumors (Fig. 5b) [10].

Growth inhibition by *ACTG2* in vitro

To investigate whether *ACTG2* could control SI-NET cell growth, a colony formation assay was performed on CNDT2.5 cells stably transfected with an *ACTG2* expression plasmid or empty vector. A significantly reduced ability to form colonies (by 32 %) compared to control cells was observed (Fig. 6a and b). This finding was supported by the reduced viability (Fig. 6c and d), supporting a growth inhibitory effect of *ACTG2* in vitro.

Discussion

ACTG2 is often aberrantly expressed in multiple cancers [15, 17, 18], and low levels have been associated with worse disease-specific survival [16]. Previously, low mRNA expression levels of *ACTG2* were demonstrated in metastases relatively to primary SI-NETs [10]. To investigate a possible role and function of *ACTG2* in SI-NET tumorigenesis this finding was first confirmed by immunohistochemistry, demonstrating absence of protein expression in the majority of investigated SI-NETs. Interestingly, eight primary tumors and two lymph node metastases displayed positive staining for ACTG2 in tumor cells, albeit at variable level and appearance. We could not detect ACTG2 expression in the enterochromaffin cells of the normal intestinal mucosa, suggesting that expression of *ACTG2* can be induced at some point during tumor progression representing a dedifferentiated phenotype, rather than being normally expressed in this cell type. Induction of *ACTG2* at some point during primary tumor growth may have beneficial effects as *ACTG2* showed growth inhibitory effects, at least in vitro. Expression of *ACTG2* was detected in stromal cells and whether ACTG2 can display growth effects here remains to be investigated.

This study demonstrated that expression of *ACTG2* can be induced by DZNep treatment or miR-145 transfection of the human SI-NET cell line CNDT2.5. Treatment with DZNep also induced expression of miR-145, indicating a possibility that induction of *ACTG2* by DZNep may be due to the effects on miR-145 expression. DZNep is a

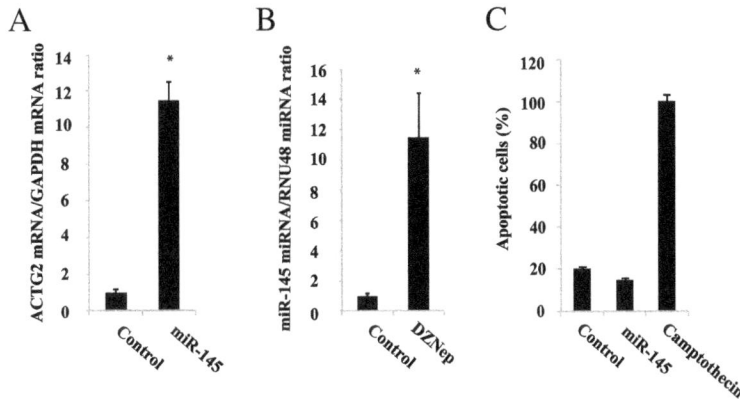

Fig. 4 a Effects on ACTG2 mRNA expression in CNDT2.5 cells after miR-145 transfection. **b** Effects on miR-145 expression after DZNep treatment. **c** Quantitative determination of cytoplasmic histone-associated-DNA-fragments (mono- and oligonucleosomes) after miR-145 transfection. Camptothecin at 0.1 μg/ml was used as positive control

potential drug in cancer treatment [29]. DZNep can inhibit the histone methyltransferase EZH2, which is the catalytic subunit of polycomb repressive complex 2 and is responsible for methylation of lysine 27 on histone 3, a repressive mark [30]. A role of EZH2 was however excluded here since EPZ-6438, a newly developed specific drug inhibiting EZH2 enzymatic activity [28], was not able to induce *ACTG2* expression. MiR-145 is often deregulated in cancer cells [31, 32] and is known to induce *ACTG2* expression in breast cancer [19]. Here, it is demonstrated that this occurs also in SI-NET cells; overexpression of miR-145 increased expression of *ACTG2* in vitro. There was a decrease of miR-145 expression in metastasis compared to primary tumors, as observed for *ACTG2* [10].

Low levels of *ACTG2* are correlated to chemotherapy resistance [12, 14] and inducing this gene in SI-NETs would, not only have a growth inhibitory effect, but also potentially make the tumors more sensitive to treatment. SI-NETs are difficult to cure due to their resistance to chemotherapy and radiation, and new treatment strategies are warranted. MicroRNAs are involved in gene regulation and cancer development, and thus, have a potential role as therapeutic targets. miR-145 has been suggested to be a candidate for RNA medicine in colon tumors with a reduced expression [33]. miR-145 have multiple gene targets, and seems to be able to act as both a tumor suppressor and an oncogene depending on tumor type. Ruebel et al. [34] detected a difference in expression levels

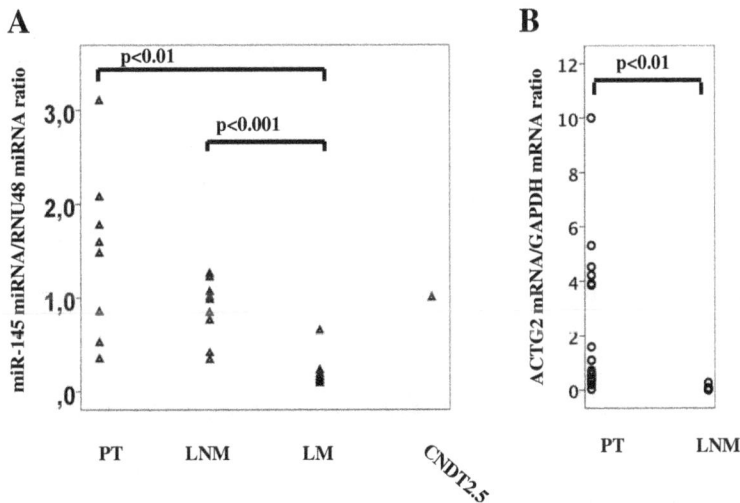

Fig. 5 a miR-145 expression levels in 24 SI-NETs, and in CNDT2.5. A significant (*p* < 0.01) difference between primary tumors and liver metastases, and also between lymph node and liver metastasis (*p* < 0.001) was observed. A tendency towards decreased expression in lymph node metastases compared to primary tumors was detected (*p* = 0.09). **b** *ACTG2* mRNA expression levels in 18 PT and 16 LNM. A significant (*p* < 0.01) difference between primary tumors and lymph node metastases was observed. PT, primary tumor. LNM, lymph node metastasis. LM, liver metastasis

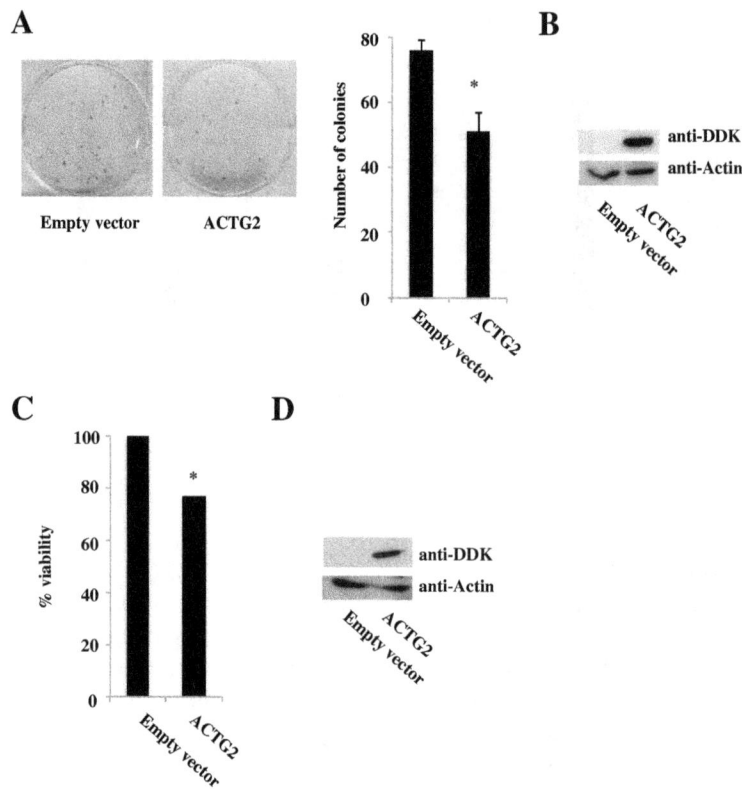

Fig. 6 a Colony formation assay in CNDT2.5 cells stably transfected with a plasmid expressing ACTG2 or with empty expression vector. **b** Western blotting demonstrating successful transfection of the DDK epitope fused to ACTG2. **c** Viability assay using WST-1 after transient overexpression of ACTG2. **d** Western blotting demonstrating successful transfection of the DDK epitope fused to ACTG2

of miR-145 between primary SI-NETs and metastases, and here we confirmed a decrease in expression by tumor progression. These results suggest that miR-145 may be a tumor suppressor and may be important for the ability to metastasize. Inducing or introducing miR-145 may be a potential new therapeutic strategy in SI-NETs.

Conclusions
Involvement of *ACTG2* in small intestinal neuroendocrine tumorigenensis has not been investigated previously. Here, we demonstrate that ACTG2 protein expression can be detected in a fraction of SI-NETs and absent in others, and that it is regulated by miR-145. Overexpression of *ACTG2* inhibited cell growth and reduced cell viability in vitro. Further investigation is needed to determine if introducing miR-145 in SI-NETs could have therapeutic advantages.

Competing interest
The authors declare that they have no competing interests.

Authors' contributions
KE carried out the molecular, cell line and IHC studies and drafted the

manuscript. PH has been involved in revising the manuscript critically for important intellectual content. GW has made substantial contributions to conception and design and interpretation of data. He has been involved in revising the manuscript critically for important intellectual content and has given the final approval of the version to be published. PS has been involved in, design and interpretation of data, and revising the manuscript critically for important intellectual content and has given the final approval of the version to be published. All authors have read and approved the final manuscript.

Acknowledgements
The authors are grateful to B Bondeson and E Persson for skillful technical assistance. The authors thank Dr. Lee Ellis for making the CNDT2.5 cell line available to them.

Funding
This study was supported Medical Research Council.

References
1. Dierdorf SF. Carcinoid tumor and carcinoid syndrome. Curr Opin Anaesthesiol. 2003;16:343–7.
2. Norlen O, Stalberg P, Oberg K, Eriksson J, Hedberg J, Hessman O, et al. Long-term results of surgery for small intestinal neuroendocrine tumors at a tertiary referral center. World J Surg. 2012;36:1419–31.
3. Bosman FT, Carneiro F, Hruban RH, Theise ND. WHO classification of tumours of the digestive system. 2010; (Ed):417.

4. Cunningham JL, Diaz de Stahl T, Sjoblom T, Westin G, Dumanski JP, Janson ET. Common pathogenetic mechanism involving human chromosome 18 in familial and sporadic ileal carcinoid tumors. Genes Chromosomes Cancer. 2011;50:82–94.

5. Kulke MH, Freed E, Chiang DY, Philips J, Zahrieh D, Glickman JN, et al. High-resolution analysis of genetic alterations in small bowel carcinoid tumors reveals areas of recurrent amplification and loss. Genes Chromosomes Cancer. 2008;47:591–603.

6. Lollgen RM, Hessman O, Szabo E, Westin G, Akerstrom G. Chromosome 18 deletions are common events in classical midgut carcinoid tumors. Int J Cancer. 2001;92:812–5.

7. Edfeldt K, Ahmad T, Akerstrom G, Janson ET, Hellman P, Stalberg P, et al. TCEB3C a putative tumor suppressor gene of small intestinal neuroendocrine tumors. Endocr Relat Cancer. 2014;21:2,275–284.

8. Banck MS, Kanwar R, Kulkarni AA, Boora GK, Metge F, Kipp BR, et al. The genomic landscape of small intestine neuroendocrine tumors. J Clin Invest. 2013;123:2502–8.

9. Francis JM, Kiezun A, Ramos AH, Serra S, Pedamallu CS, Qian ZR, et al. Somatic mutation of CDKN1B in small intestine neuroendocrine tumors. Nat Genet. 2013;45(12):1483–6.

10. Edfeldt K, Bjorklund P, Akerstrom G, Westin G, Hellman P, Stalberg P. Different gene expression profiles in metastasizing midgut carcinoid tumors. Endocr Relat Cancer. 2011;18:479–89.

11. Pollard TD, Cooper JA. Actin, a central player in cell shape and movement. Science. 2009;326:1208–12.

12. Lu X, Pan J, Li S, Shen S, Chi P, Lin H, et al. Establishment of a predictive genetic model for estimating chemotherapy sensitivity of colorectal cancer with synchronous liver metastasis. Cancer Biother Radiopharm. 2009;28:552–8.

13. Watson MB, Lind MJ, Smith L, Drew PJ, Cawkwell L. Expression microarray analysis reveals genes associated with in vitro resistance to cisplatin in a cell line model. Acta Oncology. 2007;46:651–8.

14. Xu CZ, Xie J, Jin B, Chen XW, Sun ZF, Wang BX, et al. Gene and microRNA expression reveals sensitivity to paclitaxel in laryngeal cancer cell line. Int J Clin Exp Pathol. 2013;6:1351–61.

15. Drew JE, Farquharson AJ, Mayer CD, Vase HF, Coates PJ, Steele RJ, et al. Predictive gene signatures: molecular markers distinguishing colon adenomatous polyp and carcinoma. PLoS One. 2014;9(11):e113071.

16. Beck AH, Lee CH, Witten DM, Gleason BC, Edris B, Espinosa I, et al. Discovery of molecular subtypes in leiomyosarcoma through integrative molecular profiling. Oncogene. 2010;29:845–54.

17. Lauvrak SU, Munthe E, Kresse SH, Stratford EW, Namlos HM, Meza-Zepeda LA, et al. Functional characterisation of osteosarcoma cell lines and identification of mRNAs and miRNAs associated with aggressive cancer phenotypes. Br J Cancer. 2013;109(8):2228–36.

18. Lin ZY, Chuang WL. Genes responsible for the characteristics of primary cultured invasive phenotype hepatocellular carcinoma cells. Biomed Pharmacother. 2012;66:454–8.

19. Adammek M, Greve B, Kassens N, Schneider C, Bruggmann K, Schuring AN, et al. MicroRNA miR-145 inhibits proliferation, invasiveness, and stem cell phenotype of an in vitro endometriosis model by targeting multiple cytoskeletal elements and pluripotency factors. Fertil Steril. 2013;99(5):1346–55.

20. Gotte M, Mohr C, Koo CY, Stock C, Vaske AK, Viola M. miR-145-dependent targeting of junctional adhesion molecule A and modulation of fascin expression are associated with reduced breast cancer cell motility and invasiveness. Oncogene. 2010;29:6569–80.

21. Akao Y, Nakagawa Y, Naoe T. MicroRNAs 143 and 145 are possible common onco-microRNAs in human cancers. Oncol Rep. 2006;16:845–50.

22. Van Buren 2nd G, Rashid A, Yang AD, Abdalla EK, Gray MJ, Liu W, et al. The development and characterization of a human midgut carcinoid cell line. Clin Cancer Res. 2007;13:4704–12.

23. Li SC, Martijn C, Cui T, Essaghir A, Luque RM, Demoulin JB, et al. The somatostatin analogue octreotide inhibits growth of small intestinal neuroendocrine tumour cells. PLoS One. 2012;7, e48411.

24. Ellis LM, Samuel S, Sceusi E. Varying opinoins on the authenticity of a human midgut carcinoid cell line - letter. Clin Cancer Res. 2010;16:5365–6.

25. Björklund P, Åkerström G, Westin G. Accumulation of nonphosphorylated ß-catenin and c-myc in primary and uremic secondary hyperparathyroid tumors. J Clin Endocrinol Metab. 2007;92:338–44.

26. Segersten U, Correa P, Hewison M, Hellman P, Dralle H, Carling T, Åkerström G, Westin G. 25-hydroxyvitamin D(3)-1alpha-hydroxylase expression in normal and pathological parathyroid glands. J Clin Endocrinol Metab. 2002; 87:2967–72.

27. Svedlund J, Koskinen Edblom S, Marquez VE, Åkerström G, Björklund P, Westin G. Hypermethylated in cancer 1 (HIC1), a tumor suppressor gene epigenetically deregulated in hyperparathyroid tumors by histone H3 lysine modification. J Clin Endocrinol Metab. 2012;97:E1307–15.

28. Knutson SK, Warholic NM, Wigle TJ, Klaus CR, Allain CJ, Raimondi A, et al. Durable tumor regression in genetically altered malignant rhabdoid tumors by inhibition of methyltransferase EZH2. Proc Natl Acad Sci U S A. 2013;110:7922–7.

29. Miranda TB, Cortez CC, Yoo CB, Liang G, Abe M, Kelly TK. DZNep is a global histone methylation inhibitor that reactivates developmental genes not silenced by DNA methylation. Mol Cancer Ther. 2009;8:1579–88.

30. Margueron R, Reinberg D. The Polycomb complex PRC2 and its mark in life. Nature. 2011;469:343–9.

31. Akao Y, Nakagawa Y, Naoe T. MicroRNA-143 and −145 in colon cancer. DNA Cell Biol. 2007;26:311–20.

32. Tazawa H, Kagawa S, Fujiwara T. MicroRNAs as potential target gene in cancer gene therapy of gastrointestinal tumors. Expert Opin Biol Ther. 2011; 11:145–55.

33. Kitade Y, Akao Y. MicroRNAs and their therapeutic potential for human diseases: microRNAs, miR-143 and −145, function as anti-oncomirs and the application of chemically modified miR-143 as an anti-cancer drug. J Pharmacol Sci. 2010;114:276–80.

34. Ruebel K, Leontovich A, Stilling G, Zhang S, Righi A, Jin L, et al. MicroRNA expression in ileal carcinoid tumors: downregulation of microRNA-133a with tumor progression. Mod Pathol. 2010;23:367–75.

13

Evolution in functionality of a metastatic pancreatic neuroendocrine tumour (pNET) causing Cushing's syndrome: treatment response with chemotherapy

Surya Panicker Rajeev[1], Steffan McDougall[1], Monica Terlizzo[2], Daniel Palmer[3], Christina Daousi[1,4] and Daniel J Cuthbertson[1,4*]

Abstract

Background: We report the case of a patient who had a non-functional metastatic pancreatic neuroendocrine tumour (pNET), which changed in functionality during the course of the disease. This case demonstrates the effectiveness of conventional cytotoxic chemotherapy in the management of select group of patients with this rare, challenging condition.

Case presentation: Our patient was a 34 year old man under oncology follow up, diagnosed with a non-functional metastatic pancreatic neuroendocrine tumour treated with a Whipple's procedure two years ago. Despite treatment with somatostatin analogues and sunitinib, a tyrosine kinase inhibitor, he had demonstrated radiological progression of his metastatic disease. He now presented with a short history of Cushing's syndrome. A presumptive diagnosis of a rapidly progressive, metastatic, functional pNET with ectopic ACTH production was made, confirmed biochemically and with liver biopsy. The proliferative index, Ki-67 of 20% of the liver biopsy prompted us to treat him with conventional cytotoxic chemotherapy using streptozocin, 5-fluorouracil and doxorubicin. Prior to its administration clinical and biochemical control of the hypercortisolemic state was achieved with metyrapone. However the clinical, biochemical and radiological response to chemotherapy was so dramatic obviating the need for metyrapone therapy.

Conclusions: Non-functional pNETs may evolve in their clinical and biologic behaviour producing functional hormonal syndromes. Chemotherapy may be an effective therapeutic modality in such circumstances.

Keywords: Pancreatic neuroendocrine tumour, Cushing's syndrome, Chemotherapy

Background

ACTH secretion in functional pNETS is rare and it is even more rare for non-functional pNETs to evolve into ACTH secreting functional tumours with only very few cases reported in literature. We describe such an interesting and rare case of evolution in functionality of a non-functional pNET. Apart from control of hypercortisolaemic state, preventing disease progression can be a real challenge despite various therapeutic modalities being increasingly used in the last decade. We report the case of a young patient who had a non-functional pNET,

which later started secreting ACTH, highlighting the importance of being very vigilant during the follow up of such patients. Despite novel chemotherapeutic options and PRRT (Peptide Receptor Radionuclide Therapy), conventional chemotherapeutic agents still have a very important role and should be tried if the above agents fail to control disease state as demonstrated by our case.

Case presentation

We report the case of a 34-year-old man who presented with a one-month history of lethargy, generalised upper and lower limb weakness and significant weight gain. He had been recently diagnosed with type 2 diabetes mellitus and initiated on pre-mixed insulin injections 30 units twice daily (HbA1c 85 mmol/mol).

* Correspondence: daniel.cuthbertson@liverpool.ac.uk
[1]Department of Obesity and Endocrinology, University Hospital Aintree, Liverpool L9 7AL, UK
[4]Department of Obesity and Endocrinology, Institute of Ageing and Chronic Disease, University of Liverpool, Liverpool L69 3BX, UK
Full list of author information is available at the end of the article

He had been diagnosed with a pancreatic neuroendocrine tumour (pNET) two years previously, having presented with jaundice and abdominal pain. An abdominal CT had demonstrated tumour in the head of the pancreas with loco-regional metastases (peripancreatic lymph nodes and nine hepatic metastatic lesions varying in size from 7–18 mm) for which he underwent a Whipple's procedure with resection of lymph nodes and an intra-operative liver biopsy. Measurement of a full fasting gut hormone profile showed elevated chromogranin A but was otherwise normal, consistent with a non-functional tumour. Immunohistochemistry of the pancreatic specimen was positive for chromogranin and synaptophysin with a Ki-67 index of 2% confirming the diagnosis of a Grade 2 pNET (ACTH staining not performed); the liver biopsy appearances were similar morphologically. A careful family history of endocrine tumours or endocrine disorders had been unremarkable.

On follow up imaging he had developed further liver metastases, so was commenced on a long-acting somatostatin analogue (Lanreotide), for its anti-proliferative potential, and a tyrosine kinase inhibitor (Sunitinib) was thereafter added upon evidence of further radiological progression.

Two years subsequently, he presented with cushingoid features with a moon face, easy bruising, abdominal striae, centripetal fat distribution and marked proximal myopathy. Blood pressure was normal. Biochemical investigations revealed serum potassium concentration of 2.5 mmol/l, glucose 17 mmol/l and significantly elevated random serum cortisol of 2003 nmol/L and serum ACTH concentration 50 pmol/L (normal range 2–11 pmol/L). Basal pituitary biochemistry and gadolinium enhanced MRI imaging was otherwise unremarkable. MRI scan of the liver revealed solid and cystic metastatic deposits ranging between 7.8-9.2 cm in segments 6, 7 and 8 indicating further progression despite sunitinib.[111]In-labeled octreotide scanning demonstrated somatostatin receptor positive disease in five of his liver metastatic deposits but not in any other sites (Figure 1).

A diagnosis of a rapidly progressive, functional, metastatic pNET with ectopic ACTH production causing Cushing's syndrome was made, with an assumption that the tumour had evolved in its functionality from its previous non-functional status. Treatment options discussed at the supra-regional multidisciplinary team meeting (ENETS Centre of Excellence) considered metyrapone, bilateral adrenalectomy, peptide receptor radionuclide therapy (PRRT) or cytotoxic chemotherapy. Mutational analysis of the gene for multiple endocrine neoplasia type 1 (MEN 1) was negative.

A repeat liver biopsy was performed to provide an accurate histological grade of the liver metastases, on the premise that primary NETs, and their synchronous/

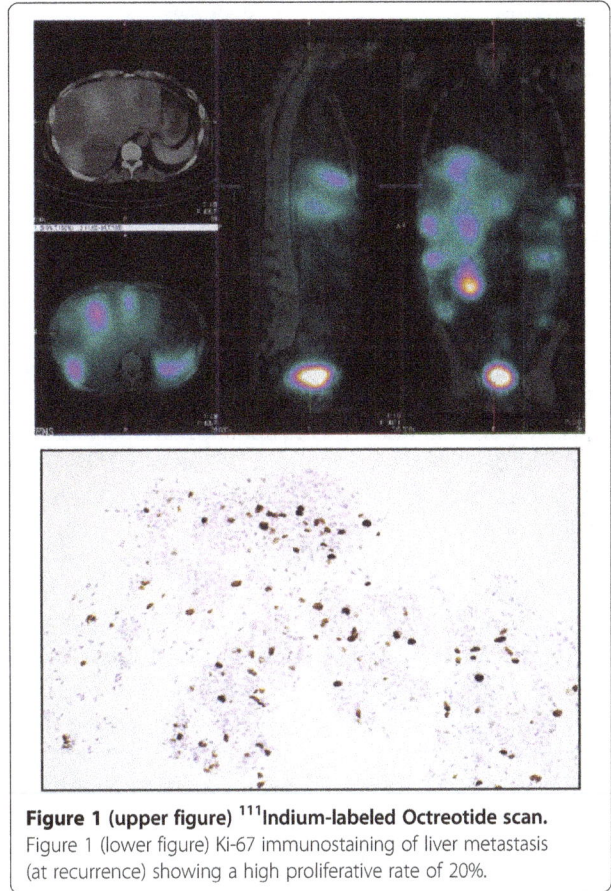

Figure 1 (upper figure) [111]Indium-labeled Octreotide scan.
Figure 1 (lower figure) Ki-67 immunostaining of liver metastasis (at recurrence) showing a high proliferative rate of 20%.

metachronous metastases, frequently differ in grade and proliferative index (Ki-67). Immunohistochemistry was strongly positive for chromogranin and synaptophysin with a Ki-67 index of 20% (ACTH staining not performed) (Figure 1). The treatment decision based on this result was to administer conventional cytotoxic chemotherapy with streptozocin, 5-fluorouracil and doxorubicin, with metyrapone given pre-chemotherapy to control the hypercortisolaemic state. Incremental doses of metyrapone (up to 1 g qds) effected a dramatic clinical response (with resolution of his symptoms and reduction of his insulin dosage) and an equally dramatic biochemical response (normalisation of serum potassium and lowering of mean cortisol concentrations on cortisol day curves) prior to his chemotherapy.

Three months after starting his chemotherapy, he had managed to completely discontinue his metyrapone with excellent mean cortisol concentrations on his cortisol day curve of 315 nmol/L (Figure 2 graph), with serum ACTH concentration of 11pmol/l. He discontinued all insulin injections with excellent glycaemic control (HbA1c 53 mmol/mol) and cross-sectional imaging (abdominal CT) showing a dramatic reduction in the size of the hepatic metastases with more necrotic/cystic contents than previously. He remains clinically stable three months later.

Discussion

pNETs are rare with a reported incidence of 1-2/100,000. They may be functional tumours, with an associated clinical syndrome, or non-functional, which despite not producing any hormone-specific symptoms, frequently either secrete other peptides (such as pancreatic polypeptide, chromogranin A, neuron specific enolase) or may stain positively on immunohistochemistry for certain hormones.

The most common functional pancreatic NET syndromes relate to insulinoma and gastrinoma. ACTH secretion occurs only rarely, presenting with features of Cushing's syndrome, but more than 95% are malignant with an average age at diagnosis of 50–55 years and an equal sex distribution [1]. Functional pNETs account for 4-16% of patients with ectopic ACTH secretion [1]. The diagnostic approach is similar to that in suspected Cushing's syndrome, first to confirm excess cortisol production and then to localise the tumour source.

Even more rarely, initially non-functional pNETs have been reported to evolve into functional tumours. In a series of 353 patients described by Wynick et al., 24 patients demonstrated de novo evidence of secretion of a second hormone during the course of the disease (median delay of 19 months and 92% reflecting liver metastases) [2]. Several reports have highlighted clinical cases of ectopic ACTH/Cushing's syndrome, where secondary deposits stained strongly positive for ACTH despite a primary tumour being negative on ACTH staining [3]. In our case, ACTH staining was not deemed necessary with biochemical confirmation, considering the high cost involved and availability of ACTH staining in only a single United Kingdom centre. However, as above, our patient presented after 24 months of the initial diagnosis of non-functional pNET with hepatic metastatic disease and de novo Cushing's syndrome, highlighting evolution in tumour functionality should be considered during follow up of patients with pNETs.

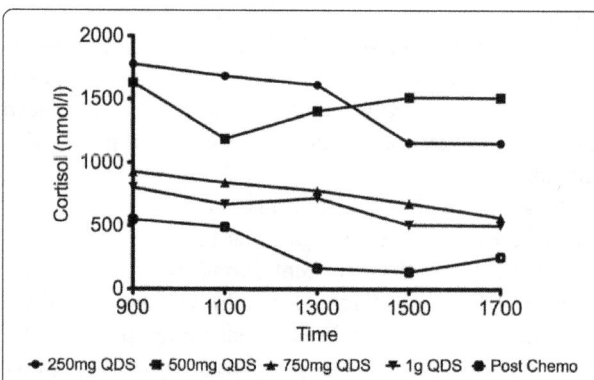

Figure 2 Cortisol day curves demonstrating cortisol concentrations on incremental doses of metyrapone, up to 1 g qds prior to chemotherapy, and effects of chemotherapy with patient having discontinued metyrapone.

Treatment aims are twofold involving biochemical control of hypercortisolaemia and preventing disease progression. Adrenal blocking agents like metyrapone, or bilateral adrenalectomy in patients who fail to respond to metyrapone therapy, may be used to address hypercortisolaemia. Medical treatment of the neuroendocrine tumour may involve long acting somatostatin analogues (SSA) or occasionally alpha interferon may be effective. Surgery is recommended even in the presence of metastatic disease, including localized liver metastases, if potentially resectable, and symptomatic control of the hormone excess state through cytoreductive surgery or radiofrequency ablation. However, our patient had large, multiple liver metastatic deposits and hence surgery was not deemed to be an option.

In patients with advanced, surgically non-resectable, progressive pNETs, everolimus [4] and sunitinib [5] are novel chemotherapeutic options and PRRT (Peptide Receptor Radionuclide Therapy) may also have a role. Ki-67 index is important in deciding treatment options and triage patients into the most appropriate treatment arm. Conventional chemotherapy with streptozocin, 5- fluorouarcil and doxorubicin still has a place as in the management of some patients with more aggressive tumours. Our patient failed to respond to SSAs and sunitinib, but had an excellent treatment response to conventional chemotherapy.

Conclusions

This clinical case offers several important learning points. Firstly, there should be vigilance to the possibility of an evolution or change of functionality of pNETs, during tumour progression, particularly in non-functional pNETs considering their pluripotency with awareness of the various clinical syndromes that may arise. Secondly, repeat histological examination of metastatic deposits may indicate different biological behaviour of the tumour and this may modify the treatment regime. In the case described, we observed the evolution towards Cushing's syndrome from a non-functional tumour, with repeat histological findings modifying our treatment approach and facilitating effective treatment with chemotherapy. The different proliferative potential may represent inherent heterogeneity within the tumour or across different anatomical sites but may reflect evolution in the histology towards a higher grade.

Consent

Written informed consent was obtained from the patient for publication of this Case report and any accompanying images. A copy of the written consent is available for review by the Editor of this journal.

Abbreviations
pNET: Pancreatic neuroendocrine tumour; PRRT: Peptide receptor radionuclide therapy; MEN: Multiple endocrine neoplasia; SSA: Somatostatin analogues; ACTH: Adrenocorticotrophic hormone.

Competing interests
The authors declare that they have no competing interest.

Authors' contributions
SPR drafted the initial manuscript, which was revised by DJC and CD. SM was involved in the management of our patient and helped in preparing the manuscript. MT performed the immunohistochemistry. DHP was involved in the oncological management and helped in the revision of the script. All authors have read and approved the final manuscript.

Author details
[1]Department of Obesity and Endocrinology, University Hospital Aintree, Liverpool L9 7AL, UK. [2]Department of Pathology, University Hospital Aintree, Liverpool L9 7AL, UK. [3]Department of Molecular and Clinical Cancer Medicine, Institute of Translational Medicine, University of Liverpool, Liverpool L69 3BX, UK. [4]Department of Obesity and Endocrinology, Institute of Ageing and Chronic Disease, University of Liverpool, Liverpool L69 3BX, UK.

References
1. Jensen RT, Cadiot G, Brandi ML, de Herder WW, Kaltsas G, Komminoth P, Scoazec J-Y, Salazar R, Sauvanet A, Kianmanesh R: *ENETS Consensus Guidelines for the Management of Patients with Digestive Neuroendocrine Neoplasms: Functional Pancreatic Endocrine Tumor Syndromes*; 2012:98–119.
2. Wynick D, Williams SJ, Bloom SR: **Symptomatic secondary hormone syndromes in patients with established malignant pancreatic endocrine tumors.** *N Engl J Med* 1988, **319**:605–607.
3. Miehle K, Tannapfel A, Lamesch P, Borte G, Schenker E, Kluge R, Ott RA, Wiechmann V, Koch M, Kassahun W, Passchke R, Koch CM: **Pancreatic neuroendocrine tumor with ectopic adrenocorticotropin production upon second recurrence.** *J Clin Endocrinol Metab* 2004, **89**:3731–3736.
4. Yao JC, Shah MH, Ito T, Bohas CL, Wolin EM, van Cutsem E, Hobday TJ, Okusaka T, Capdevila J, de Vries EGE, Tomassetti P, Pavel ME, Hoosen S, Haas T, Lincy J, Lebwohl D, Oberg K: **Everolimus for advanced pancreatic neuroendocrine tumors.** *N Engl J Med* 2011, **364**:514–523.
5. Raymond E, Dahan L, Raoul J-L, Bang Y-J, Borbath I, Lombard-Bohas C, Valle J, Metrakos P, Smith D, Vinik A, Chen JS, Horsch D, Hammel P, Wiedenmann B, Van Custem E, Patyna S, Lu DR, Blanckmeister C, Chao R, Ruszniewski P: **Sunitinib malate for the treatment of pancreatic neuroendocrine tumors.** *N Engl J Med* 2011, **364**:501–513.

Genetic analyses of bone morphogenetic protein 2, 4 and 7 in congenital combined pituitary hormone deficiency

Jana Breitfeld[1,2†], Susanne Martens[1,2†], Jürgen Klammt[3], Marina Schlicke[3], Roland Pfäffle[3], Kerstin Krause[1], Kerstin Weidle[1], Dorit Schleinitz[1], Michael Stumvoll[1], Dagmar Führer[4], Peter Kovacs[1,2] and Anke Tönjes[1,2*]

Abstract

Background: The complex process of development of the pituitary gland is regulated by a number of signalling molecules and transcription factors. Mutations in these factors have been identified in rare cases of congenital hypopituitarism but for most subjects with combined pituitary hormone deficiency (CPHD) genetic causes are unknown. Bone morphogenetic proteins (BMPs) affect induction and growth of the pituitary primordium and thus represent plausible candidates for mutational screening of patients with CPHD.

Methods: We sequenced *BMP2, 4* and *7* in 19 subjects with CPHD. For validation purposes, novel genetic variants were genotyped in 1046 healthy subjects. Additionally, potential functional relevance for most promising variants has been assessed by phylogenetic analyses and prediction of effects on protein structure.

Results: Sequencing revealed two novel variants and confirmed 30 previously known polymorphisms and mutations in *BMP2, 4* and *7*. Although phylogenetic analyses indicated that these variants map within strongly conserved gene regions, there was no direct support for their impact on protein structure when applying predictive bioinformatics tools.

Conclusions: A mutation in the *BMP4* coding region resulting in an amino acid exchange (p.Arg300Pro) appeared most interesting among the identified variants. Further functional analyses are required to ultimately map the relevance of these novel variants in CPHD.

Keywords: Combined pituitary hormone deficiency, Bone morphogenetic proteins, BMP2, BMP4, BMP7

Background

The development of the pituitary gland is a highly complex process, involving many signalling molecules and transcription factors [1-3]. During embryogenesis cells from the oral ectoderm form the adenohypophysis, while the posterior part develops from neural tissue. With the help of animal models it has been shown that transcription factors like HesX1, Prop1, Pou1F1, Lhx3, Lhx4, Pitx1, Pitx2, Otx2, Sox2 and Sox3 play a crucial role in the development of the pituitary gland [4-6]. Several mutations in genes encoding these transcription factors

have been reported in combined pituitary hormone deficiency (CPHD). However, for most of the patients the genetic cause of hypoplasia or at least functional insufficiency of the pituitary gland remains to be discovered.

Bone morphogenetic proteins (BMP) 2, 4 and 7 have a crucial role during the embryonic development of the pituitary gland [7]. In early development Bmp4 contributes to the formation of the rudimentary Rathke's pouch in the mouse (reviewed in [4]). Later BMP 2, 4 and 7 secreted by surrounding tissues contribute to the polarisation of the pouch [7,8]. The development of the pituitary gland is completed within the first trimester of pregnancy in humans [9].

The BMPs are members of the transforming growth factor (TGF)-ß family and bind to type 1 and 2 serine-threonine kinase receptors (BMPR1A and BMPR2). Among different isoforms, three type 1 receptors (BMPR1A/ALK3,

* Correspondence: Anke.Toenjes@medizin.uni-leipzig.de
†Equal contributors
[1]Department of Medicine, University of Leipzig, Liebigstrasse 20, Leipzig 04103, Germany
[2]IFB Adiposity Diseases, University of Leipzig, Philipp-Rosenthal-Str. 27, Leipzig 04103, Germany
Full list of author information is available at the end of the article

BMPR1B/ALK6, and ACVR1A/ALK2) and three type 2 receptors (BMPR2, ACTR2A, and ACTR2B) mediate most of the effects of BMPs [10-14]. *Bmp2* null mice die between embryonic day E.7.5 and E.10.5, suffering from cardiac defects [15]. Selective inhibition of *Bmp4* in mouse embryos results in a loss of nearly all pituitary cell lines except a few corticotrophs [8]. *Bmp4* knock-out mice are characterized by pituitary aplasia, suffer from severe facial, kidney and skeletal abnormalities, and die early in embryogenesis [16]. Severe eye defects and skeletal and renal anomalies are found also in *Bmp7* null mice [17], which die shortly after birth [18]. However, systematic search for mutations in *BMP2, 4* and *7* in patients with combined pituitary insufficiency has not been performed yet. So, the aim of our study was to investigate whether genetic variants in *BMP2*, *BMP4* and/or *BMP7* are associated with congenital pituitary insufficiency.

Methods
Subjects
In the present study, we included 19 patients (13 males, 6 females) with congenital combined pituitary hormone insufficiency (Table 1). Prior to direct sequencing of *BMP* genes, screening for known mutations in PIT1 and PROP1 has been performed in 19 subjects and did not reveal any aberrant results. Screenings for mutations in further genes are specified in Table 1.

To determine the frequency of newly identified genetic variants in the general population, we included a set of 1046 healthy subjects (Germany) without any history of pituitary disorders [19].

The study was approved by the ethics committee of the University of Leipzig and all subjects provided written informed consent before taking part in the study.

DNA extraction and sequencing
Genomic DNA was extracted from lymphocytes using the Fujifilm (Düsseldorf, Germany) QuickGene DNA whole blood kit according to the manufacturer's protocol. We sequenced all exons, exon-intron boundaries, 5'- and 3'-untranslated regions (UTR) of *BMP2* (Ensembl ENSG00000125845), *BMP4* (Ensembl ENSG00000125378) and *BMP7* (Ensembl ENSG00000101144) in DNA samples from 19 non-related Caucasian subjects. Sequencing was performed using the Big Dye® Terminator (Applied Biosystems, Inc., Foster City, CA) on an automated DNA capillary sequencer (ABI PRISM® 3100 Avant; Applied Biosystems, Inc., Foster City, CA). Sequence information and PCR conditions for all oligonucleotide primers used for variant screening are available in Additional files 1 and 2. Known single nucleotide polymorphisms (SNPs) are designated according to dbSNP (http://www.ncbi.nlm.nih.gov/snp/) reference accession numbers.

Prediction of functional relevance
To predict the potential impact of an identified variant on protein structure and function we used several online tools and databases: SIFT (http://sift.bii.a-star.edu.sg/) [20], PolyPhen (http://genetics.bwh.harvard.edu/pph/) [21], Mutpred (http://mutpred.mutdb.org) [22], FATHMM (http://fathmm.biocompute.org.uk) [23], Mutation Taster (http://www.mutationtaster.org) [24], SNP and Go (http://snps-and-go.biocomp.unibo.it/snps-and-go) [25].

Genotyping of novel variants in control subjects
We genotyped all newly identified variants that predict an amino acid exchange in the cohort of healthy subjects by employing the TaqMan allelic discrimination assay (Applied Biosystems, Inc., Foster City, CA). The genotypes were detected on an ABI PRISM 7500 sequence detector (Applied Biosystems Inc.) according to the manufacturer's protocol. Genotyping success rates for all analyzed SNPs were 99%.

Phylogenetic analysis of the newly identified *BMP4* variant c.899G > C
For the coding region of *BMP4*, the conservation between species was determined by using Phylogenetic Analysis by Maximum Likelihood (PAML) [26]. Specifically, the aim of this analysis was to identify the ratio of non-synonymous to synonymous base substitutions (omega, $\omega=dN/dS$). The coding sequences of 37 *BMP4* orthologues were downloaded from ENSEMBL (http://www.ensembl.org) and the NCBI (http://www.ncbi.nlm.nih.gov) databases.

Results
BMP2
Direct sequencing of *BMP2* revealed 10 that have been previously reported. The non-synonymous SNP rs2273073, found to be heterozygous in one out of 19 analyzed subjects represents a T to G base pair exchange resulting in a serine to alanine amino acid (aa) substitution at protein position 37 (p.Ser37Ala). A second non-synonymous variant (rs235768) also located within the coding region results in an arginine to serine exchange (p.Arg190Ser) and was found with a minor allele frequency (MAF) of 0.34 in our analyzed cohort. Detailed information of all identified SNPs in *BMP2* is presented in Table 2.

BMP4
Sequencing of the *BMP4* gene revealed four SNPs. Three of them have already been described by others (Table 2). The newly identified variant c.899G > C leads to an aa exchange from arginine to proline at position 300 (p.Arg300Pro) within the protein and was found as a heterozygous mutation in one of the 19 analyzed subjects (patient number 5; Table 1). Genotyping of this variant

Table 1 Patient characteristics

Pat	Sex	Genetic screening	Further genetic tests	Lack of GH	Lack of TSH	Lack of LH/FSH	Lack of ACTH	Pituitary gland in MRI-scan	Special aspects	Symptoms leading to diagnosis	Age of diagnosis	Family history
1	m	PIT1, PROP1, HESX1, LHX3	/	+	+	+	+	hypoplastic	/	growth retardation and hypopituitarism	childhood/adolesence	no
2	m	PIT1, PROP1, HESX1, LHX3	SOX2, OTX2	+	+	+	+	hypoplastic	midline defect, right anophthalmia, mental retardation	severe malformations	birth	no
3	f	PIT1, PROP1, HESX1, LHX3	/	+	+	+	+	hypoplastic	brain atrophy	growth retardation	childhood/adolesence	no
4	f	PIT1, PROP1, HESX-1	/	+	+	no	no	hypoplastic	/	growth retardation	childhood/adolesence	no
5	m	PIT1, PROP1, HESX-1, LHX3	LHX4	+	+	+	+	hypoplastic	sclerosed nodules at the hands, short metacarpalia IV, azoospermia,	growth retardation	childhood/adolesence	no
6	m	PIT1, PROP1, HESX1, LHX3	LHX4	+	+	no	+	n.a.	/	unknown	childhood/adolesence	no
7	f	PIT1, PROP1, HESX1, LHX3	/	+	+	no	+	small and ectopic neuropituitary gland	left optic atrophy	growth retardation, postpartal hypoglycaemia	childhood/adolesence	no
8	m	PIT1, PROP1, HESX1, LHX3	GLI2	+	+	no	+	small pituitary and ectopic neuropituitary gland	/	unknown	unknown	no
9	m	PIT1, PROP1, HESX1, LHX3	/	no	+	no	+	ectopic adeno- and neuropituitary gland	/	prolonged jaundice, hypothyroidism	early infancy	no
10	f	PIT1, PROP1, HESX1, LHX3	/	+	+	+	+	hypoplastic	/	hypoglycaemia, hypothyroidism	early infancy	no
11	m	PIT1, PROP1	LHX4, GLI2	+	no	+	+	n.a.	Asperger syndrome	unknown	early infancy	no
12	m	PIT1, PROP1, HESX1, LHX3	/	+	+	+	+	n.a.	/	growth retardation, puberty onset at the age of 18, hypogonadism	childhood/adolesence	yes
13	m	PIT1, PROP1, HESX1, LHX3	/	+	+	no	+	n.a.	/	unknown	unknown	no
14	m	PIT1, PROP1, HESX1, LHX3	/	+	+	+	+	hypoplastic	/	pericardial effusion	adulthood	yes
15	m	PIT1, PROP1, HESX1, LHX3	/	+	+	no	+	normal size, but ectopic neuropituitary gland	/	prolonged jaundice, hypoglycaemia, micropenis, muscular hypotonia, hypothyroidism	early infancy	no
16	f	PIT1, PROP1, HESX1, LHX3	LHX4	+	+	+	+	hypoplastic	/	hypoglycaemia, hyponatraemia, hepatopathy, muscular hypotonia	3rd day of life	n.a.
17	m	PIT1, PROP1, HESX1, LHX3	GLI2, SHH	+	+	+	+	hypoplastic	/	complex facial malformations	childhood/adolesence	no
18	m	PIT1, PROP1, HESX1, LHX3	/	+	+	+	+	small and ectopic neuropituitary gland	arachnodactyly, pulmonalisectasia, cryptorchidism, scoliosis	unknown	childhood/adolesence	no
19	f	PIT1, PROP1, HESX1, LHX3	/	+	+	no	+	hypoplastic	/	growth retardation	childhood/adolesence	no

m = male; f = female; MRI-scan = magnetic resonance imaging; MPHD = screening for PIT1, PROP1, HESX1, LHX3; PIT1 = POU domain, class 1, transcription factor 1; PROP1 = Homeobox protein prophet of Pit-1; HesX-1 = HESX homeobox 1; SOX2 = SRY (sex determining region Y)-box 2; OTX2 = SRY (sex determining region Y)-box 2; LHX4 = LIM/homeobox protein Lhx4; GLI2 = Zinc finger protein GLI2; SHH = Sonic hedgehog homolog; GH = growth hormone; TSH = thyroid stimulating hormone; LH = luteinizing hormone; FSH = follicle stimulating hormone; ACTH = adrenocorticotropic hormone; n.a. = not available.

Table 2 SNPs within *BMP2/4/7* identified by sequencing of 19 subjects with congenital combined pituitary hormone insufficiency

Gene region	Exon/Intron	SNP	MAF according to NCBI	MM/mm in analyzed cohort	aa-exchange	MAF in analyzed cohort
BMP2 (ENST00000378827, NM_001200.2)						
5'-UTR	Exon 1#	rs35123420	C = 0.040	G/C		C = 0.026
	Exon 1	rs141364472	n.a.	G/A		A = 0.026
	Exon 2	rs2273073	G = 0.028	T/G	p.Ser37Ala	G = 0.026
coding	Exon 2	rs1049007	A = 0.250	G/A	synonymous	A = 0.342
region	Exon 3	rs235768	A = 0.240	T/A	p.Arg190Ser	A = 0.342
	Exon 3	rs13037675	T = 0.046	C/T	synonymous	T = 0.026
	Exon 3	rs15705	C = 0.280	A/C		C = 0.368
3'-UTR	Exon 3	rs3178250	C = 0.264	T/C		C = 0.368
	Exon 3	rs235769	A = 0.234	G/A		A = 0.368
	Exon 3	rs170986	A = 0.162	C/A		A = 0.053
BMP4 (ENST00000245451, NM_001202.3)						
5'-UTR	Intron 2	rs2855532	T = 0.427	C/T		T = 0.342
	Intron 2	rs2761880	T = 0.221	C/T		T = 0.053
coding	Exon 4	rs17563	C = 0.373	C/T	p.Val152Ala	T = 0.447
region	**Exon 4**	**c.899G > C**		**G/C**	**p.Arg300Pro**	**C = 0.026**
BMP7 (ENST00000395863, NM_001719.2)						
	Exon 2	rs41274738	T = 0.018	C/T	synonymous	T = 0.026
	Intron 2*	rs192121279	n.a.	G/A	p.Thr105Met	A = 0.026
	Intron 2*	rs6070031	T = 0.281	C/T		T = 0.421
	Intron 2	**c.611 + 3366C > T**		**C/T**		**T = 0.026**
coding	Exon 4	rs61733436	T = 0.005	C/T	synonymous	T = 0.026
region	Intron 4	rs6014948	T = 0.069	C/T		T = 0.053
	Intron 4	rs6070008	T = 0.466	A/T		T = 0.421
	Exon 5	rs61733438	C = 0.005	T/C	p.Asn321Ser	C = 0.026
	Intron 6$	rs2148328	A = 0.466	A/G	p.Ala399Gly	G = 0.474
	Intron 7	rs10375	C = 0.484	C/T		T = 0.447
	Intron 7	rs151255710	n.a.	A/G		G = 0.026
	Intron 7	rs17480735	A = 0.051	G/A		A = 0.105
	Intron 7	rs6025418	G = 0.479	A/G		G = 0.447
3'-UTR	Intron 7	rs6025417	C = 0.478	G/C		C = 0.447
	Intron 7	rs6025416	C = 0.452	T/C		C = 0.447
	Intron 7	rs6014947	T = 0.460	C/T		T = 0.474
	Intron 7	rs6025415	C = 0.478	G/C		C = 0.473
	Intron 7	rs6014946	C = 0.461	A/C		C = 0.473

SNP = single nucleotide polymorphism, BMP = bone morphogenetic protein; MAF = minor allele frequency; MM = major allele, mm = minor allele in analyzed cohort; aa = amino acid; UTR = untranslated region; n.a. = not available; novel identified SNPs are presented in bold; #) only in ENST00000378827 but not in NM_001200 part of exon 1 (5'UTR) ; *) variants are located within an additional exon only present in isoform BMP7 ENST00000433911; $) for transcript variant ENST00000450594 the SNPs is located within the coding region.

in 1046 healthy subjects did not reveal any further heterozygous or homozygous c.899G > C carrier. Additionally, we have found the non-synonymous variant rs17563, resulting in a p.Val152Ala substitution. This SNP was found with a MAF of 0.45 within the cohort.

PAML analyses showed an overall strong conservation of the gene. Positional analyses further indicated that most positions are conserved or strongly conserved. Position number 300 is highly conserved. Regarding each species separately revealed that the human lineage seems to have no synonymous substitutions leading to an infinite omega. The absence of synonymous changes in the data leads to the infinite omega, as there is a positive number divided by zero. A likelihood ratio test (LRT) against the model with the average omega reveals that $P < 0.005$, underlining that we have a strongly conserved gene.

All identified genetic variants in the *BMP4* gene are presented in Table 2.

BMP7

All protein-coding exons that constitute the various transcripts of *BMP7* were sequenced. In total we found 18 genetic variants. One variant (c.611 + 3366C > T) has not been reported so far. The novel intronic SNP at position c.611 + 3366C > T showed a MAF of 0.026. This variation was found in patient number 17 (Table 1). This subject presented a phenotype including a hypoplastic pituitary gland and complex facial malformations. The previously known genetic variant rs61733438 results in the aa exchange p.Asn321Ser and was found in one out of the 19 subjects. Finally, two further previously known SNPs (rs192121279 and rs2148328) resulted in the aa substitutions p.Thr105Met and p.Ala399Gly each in one of the known BMP7 isoforms (ENST00000433911 and ENST00000450594). The results for sequencing of *BMP7* are summarized in Table 2.

Prediction of functional relevance

Potential impacts of all newly identified variants on protein structure and function was investigated by use of several online tools [20-25]. The only variant with consistent evidence for functional consequences was c.899G > C in *BMP4*. Results are summarized in Table 3.

Discussion

The development of the distinct cell lines of the pituitary gland is directed by nuclear mediators of cell type commitment, including the BMP pathway and a number of transcription factors (reviewed in [2]). The role of BMP2, BMP4 and BMP7 as signalling peptides in the programming of pituitary development makes them plausible candidates for pituitary disorders including congenital insufficiency as well as pituitary adenomas. In our study we systematically screened for genetic variation in these genes in a group of patients with CPHD.

Inhibition of *Bmp2/Bmp4* in mice causes loss of the Pit-1 lineage and gonadotropes but not of POMC-expressing cells [8]. In detail, BMP2 is essential for the expression of ventral markers such as the insulin gene enhancer protein ISL-1 and human glycoprotein hormone α-subunit gene and necessary for terminal differentiation of pituitary cell types [8,27]. We could identify two known SNPs, rs2273073 and rs235768, in two

different patients. To predict the potential impact of an identified variant on protein structure and function we used several online tools and databases [20-25]. However, we are aware of limitations of these tools and used comparative considerations and degree of conservation of amino acid residues do not provide functional evidence. The p.Ser37Ala substitution caused by rs2273073 is assumed to be tolerated according to SIFT and PolyPhen whereas it is predicted to be disease associated by Mutation taster and SNP&GO. The carrier of this variant in our study did not present any further phenotype other than CPHD. There is evidence in the literature that variation at rs2273073 affects bone mineral density [28] but we do not possess any clinical data on this phenotype in our study. Additionally, we identified rs235768 predicting the p.Arg190Ser exchange in one subject in our cohort of CPHD patients. An association of p.Arg190Ser substitution with the development of childhood IgA nephropathy has been described [29], the functional relevance cannot be predicted explicit based on SIFT and PolyPhen database search, it described as neutral or tolerated by MutPred and FATHMM but potentially disease associated by SNP&GO. Further functional studies are required to elucidate detailed effects of this variant.

In accordance with previous studies [27] our phylogenetic analyses of the *BMP4* gene revealed a highly conserved sequence of the *BMP4* region which would suggest a potential functional relevance of variation at this locus. We identified a novel variant resulting in a c.899G > C substitution predicting a missense mutation within the protein sequence (p.Arg300Pro). Bioinformatic prediction tools provide substantial evidence to functional consequences and the fact that we have not found a second heterozygous or homozygous c.899G > C carrier in a set of 1046 healthy subjects and the high conservation at this locus furthermore support a potential association with the phenotype. An X-ray of the patient at the age of 17 presents skeletal abnormalities described as vertebral platyspondylia, sclerosis of the metaphyses and a short metacarpalia IV, which would be in line with the diagnosis of spondyloepiphyseal dysplasia tarda. Since *BMP4* is known to increase osteoblast differentiation the affection of the skeletal system would be consistent with a functional relevance of the newly identified c.899G > C substitution. Furthermore, fibrodysplasia ossificans progressiva is characterized by an overexpression of *BMP4* in lymphocytes [30], so detailed functional analyses are required to assess effects on *BMP4* expression and interaction with BMPR1A receptor pathway. A detailed family history or genetic material of the patient's family are unfortunately not available which is a clear limitation of the study. According to the self reported family history all other relatives do not

Table 3 Assessment of potential functional relevance of identified variants

		Sift [20]	PolyPhen [21]	Mutation taster [22]	SNP&GO [23]	FATHMM [24]	MutPred [25]
BMP2							
rs2273073	Ser37Ala	- tolerated	- tolerated	- aas changed - heterozygous in TGP - known disease mutation at this position (HGMD CM034611) - protein features (might be) affected - splice site changes	- aas changed - disease associated variation (probability – 0.527)	- tolerated - score 0.61	- score 0.123 - neutral
rs235768	Arg190Ser	- functional relevance cannot be predicted explicit	- functional relevance cannot be predicted explicit	- aas changed - homozygous in TGP - protein features (might be) affected - splice site changes	- aas changed - disease associated variation (probability – 0.974)	- tolerated - score –0.45	- score 0.293 - neutral
BMP4							
rs17563	Val152Ala	- tolerated	- tolerated	- aas changed - homozygous in TGP - protein features (might be) affected - splice site changes	- aas changed - disease associated variation (probability – 0.755)	- tolerated - score –0.08	- score 0.145 - neutral
c.899G > C	Arg300Pro	- substantial evidence for functional consequences	- substantial evidence for functional consequences	- disease causing - aas changed - protein features (might be) affected - splice site changes	- aas changed - disease associated variation (probability – 0.906)	- tolerated - score –0.78	- score 0.381 - neutral
BMP7							
rs192121279	Thr105Met	- deleterious	- unknown	- not found	n.a.	- No dbSNP mapping(s)	- score 0.466 - neutral
c.611 + 3366C > T	intronic	n.a.	n.a.	n.a.	n.a.	-n.a.	n.a.
rs61733438	Asn321Ser	- tolerated	- tolerated	- disease causing - aas changed - heterozygous in TGP - protein features (might be) affected - splice site changes	- aas changed - disease associated variation (probability – 0.848)	- tolerated - score –0.92	- score 0.278 - neutral
rs2148328	Ala399Gly	- tolerated	- unknown	- aas changed - protein features (might be) affected	- aas changed	- No dbSNP mapping(s)	- score 0.540 - "Actionable Hypotheses"*5

[5]) Loss of relative solvent accessibility (P = 0.0071); Gain of loop (P = 0.0166); Loss of helix (P = 0.0376); Loss of solvent accessibility (P = 0.0442); aas = amino acid sequence, TGP = 1000 Genome Project.

show any affection of the pituitary function. However, it is of note that there is a substantial variability in the clinical presentation of patients with combined pituitary hormone deficiency even if the same gene is affected and even in subjects with identical mutations. Intrafamilial penetrance can range from high to incomplete and it is not possible to draw direct conclusions form the clinical manifestation to the potential genotype. This indicates the remarkable influence of the genetic background, incomplete penetrance, highly variable expressivity, environmental factors and possibly stochastic events. Also co-occuring mutations in interacting genes have to be taken into account.

Additionally to this new variation we found the SNP rs17563 in the coding region of *BMP4*. This variation has been suggested to be involved in the development of otosclerosis [31]. According to the high prevalence in healthy subjects an association with pituitary disorders is rather unlikely.

BMP7, also called Osteogenic Protein 1 has an important function during the embryonic development of the eye, brain and ear [17,18]. In mice, Bmp7 is responsible for the expression of *Pax6* and *Sox2* [32] that are both known to be involved in the development of the pituitary gland [3]. We have identified rs61733438, resulting in p.Asn321Ser substitution. So far, rs61733438 has been described in patients with several eye defects [33]. The male patient identified in our CPHD cohort who is carrier of the heterozygous rs61733438 variant has an ectopic neurohypophysis but no other specific symptoms. Furthermore, there is no family history of CPHD.

Taken together, we identified several genetic variants in *BMP2*, *BMP4* and *BMP7* in a group of patients with CPHD. However, genotyping of further patients and mainly functional analyses are required to clarify the exact role in pituitary insufficiency. Clear limitation of our study is the missing genetic information for family members. These data would significantly support phenotype-genotype associations and would strengthen potential functional relevance of the identified variants. Furthermore, the group of CPHD patients included in our study presents a heterogeneous phenotype and most likely also diverse genetic source. We are also aware that by including only a few genes the data remain inconclusive. However, we believe that even by extending the list of studied genes by further candidates there would be no guarantee that further players will be identified. Thus, a systematic approach including whole genome/exome sequencing strategies would be desirable here.

Conclusions

Our study provides a systematic analysis of *BMP* genes in patients with CPHD. We identified novel variants in *BMP2*, *BMP4* and *BMP7*. Of particular interest is a novel variant in *BMP4* (p.Arg300Pro) found in one patient with skeletal malformation in addition to CPHD. Further functional characterization of the newly identified variant is desirable not only to ultimately pinpoint their biological and clinical consequences but also to better understand the role of bone morphogenetic proteins in the pathophysiology of congenital combined pituitary insufficiency.

Competing interests

The authors declare that they have no competing interests.

Authors' contributions

JB and SM sequenced the genes, analyzed the results, contributed to discussion and drafted the manuscript. JK and RP participated in the design of the study, provided samples and contributed to discussion. KW carried out the evolutionary analyses. DF and MS contributed to the study design and discussion of the results. PK and DS analyzed the results, contributed to discussion and edited the manuscript. AT designed the study, provided samples and contributed to discussion and manuscript writing. All authors read and approved the final manuscript.

Acknowledgements

We thank all those who participated in the studies. We also thank Beate Enigk, Manuela Prellberg and Ines Müller for excellent technical assistance. Peter Kovacs is funded by the Boehringer Ingelheim Foundation. This work was supported by a research grant from Pfizer, Inc.

Author details

[1]Department of Medicine, University of Leipzig, Liebigstrasse 20, Leipzig 04103, Germany. [2]IFB Adiposity Diseases, University of Leipzig, Philipp-Rosenthal-Str. 27, Leipzig 04103, Germany. [3]Hospital for Children & Adolescents, University of Leipzig, Liebigstrasse 22, Leipzig 04103, Germany. [4]Department of Endocrinology, University of Essen, Hufelandstraße 55, Essen 45147, Germany.

References

1. Rizzoti K, Lovell-Badge R: **Early development of the pituitary gland: induction and shaping of Rathke's.** *Rev Endocr Metab Disord* 2005, **6:**161–172.
2. Scully KM, Rosenfeld MG: **Pituitary development: regulatory codes in mammalian organogenesis.** *Science* 2002, **295:**2231–2235.
3. Zhu X, Gleiberman AS, Rosenfeld MG: **Molecular physiology of pituitary development: signaling and transcriptional.** *Physiol Rev* 2007, **87:**933–963.
4. Dattani MT, Robinson IC: **The molecular basis for developmental disorders of the pituitary gland in man.** *Clin Genet* 2000, **57:**337–346.
5. Kelberman D, Dattani MT: **Hypopituitarism oddities: congenital causes.** *Horm Res* 2007, **68**(Suppl 5):138–144.
6. Pfäffle R, Klammt J: **Pituitary transcription factors in the aetiology of combined pituitary hormone.** *Best Pract Res Clin Endocrinol Metab* 2011, **25:**43–60.
7. Ericson J, Norlin S, Jessell TM, Edlund T: **Integrated FGF and BMP signaling controls the progression of progenitor cell.** *Development* 1998, **125:**1005–1015.
8. Treier M, Gleiberman AS, O'Connell SM, Szeto DP, McMahon JA, McMahon AP, Rosenfeld MG: **Multistep signaling requirements for pituitary organogenesis in vivo.** *Genes Dev* 1998, **12:**1691–1704.
9. Zhu X, Lin CR, Prefontaine GG, Tollkuhn J, Rosenfeld MG: **Genetic control of pituitary development and hypopituitarism.** *Curr Opin Genet Dev* 2005, **15:**332–340.
10. Kingsley DM: **The TGF-beta superfamily: new members, new receptors, and new genetic tests of function in different organisms.** *Genes Dev* 1994, **8:**133–146.

Genetic analyses of bone morphogenetic protein 2, 4 and 7 in congenital combined pituitary...

103

11. Hogan BL: **Bone morphogenetic proteins: multifunctional regulators of vertebrate development.** *Genes Dev* 1996, **10:**1580–1594.

12. Massague J, Weis-Garcia F: **Serine/threonine kinase receptors: mediators of transforming growth factor beta.** *Cancer Surv* 1996, **27:**41–64.

13. Chen D, Zhao M, Mundy GR: **Bone morphogenetic proteins.** *Growth Factors* 2004, **22:**233–241.

14. Kishigami S, Mishina Y: **BMP signaling and early embryonic patterning.** *Cytokine Growth Factor Rev* 2005, **16:**265–278.

15. Zhang H, Bradley A: **Mice deficient for BMP2 are nonviable and have defects in amnion/chorion and.** *Development* 1996, **122:**2977–2986.

16. Dunn NR, Winnier GE, Hargett LK, Schrick JJ, Fogo AB, Hogan BL: **Haploinsufficient phenotypes in Bmp4 heterozygous null mice and modification by.** *Dev Biol* 1997, **188:**235–247.

17. Jena N, Martin-Seisdedos C, McCue P, Croce CM: **BMP7 null mutation in mice: developmental defects in skeleton, kidney, and eye.** *Exp Cell Res* 1997, **230:**28–37.

18. Dudley AT, Lyons KM, Robertson EJ: **A requirement for bone morphogenetic protein-7 during development of the.** *Genes Dev* 1995, **9:**2795–2807.

19. Tönjes A, Zeggini E, Kovacs P, Böttcher Y, Schleinitz D, Dietrich K, Morris AP, Enigk B, Rayner NW, Koriath M, Eszlinger M, Kemppinen A, Prokopenko I, Hoffmann K, Teupser D, Thiery J, Krohn K, McCarthy MI, Stumvoll M: **Association of FTO variants with BMI and fat mass in the self-contained.** *Eur J Hum Genet* 2010, **18:**104–110.

20. Ng PC, Henikoff S: **SIFT: Predicting amino acid changes that affect protein function.** *Nucleic Acids Res* 2003, **31:**3812–3814.

21. Adzhubei IA, Schmidt S, Peshkin L, Ramensky VE, Gerasimova A, Bork P, Kondrashov AS, Sunyaev SR: **A method and server for predicting damaging missense mutations.** *Nat Methods* 2010, **7:**248–249.

22. Li B, Krishnan VG, Mort ME, Xin F, Kamati KK, Cooper DN, Mooney SD, Radivojac P: **Automated inference of molecular mechanisms of disease from amino acid substitutions.** *Bioinformatics* 2009, **25:**2744–2750.

23. Shihab HA, Gough J, Cooper DN, Stenson PD, Barker GLA, Edwards KJ, Day INM, Gaunt TR: **Predicting the Functional, Molecular and Phenotypic Consequences of Amino Acid Substitutions using Hidden Markov Models.** *Hum Mutat* 2013, **34:**57–65.

24. Schwarz JM, Rödelsperger C, Schuelke M, Seelow D: **MutationTaster evaluates disease-causing potential of sequence alterations.** *Nat Methods* 2010, **7:**575–576.

25. Calabrese R, Capriotti E, Fariselli P, Martelli PL, Casadio R: **Functional annotations improve the predictive score of human disease-related mutations in proteins.** *Hum Mutat* 2009, **30:**1237–1244.

26. Yang Z: **PAML 4: phylogenetic analysis by maximum likelihood.** *Mol Biol Evol* 2007, **24:**1586–1591.

27. Shore EM, Xu M, Shah PB, Janoff HB, Hahn GV, Deardorff MA, Sovinsky L, Spinner NB, Zasloff MA, Wozney JM, Kaplan FS: **The human bone morphogenetic protein 4 (BMP-4) gene: molecular structure and.** *Calcif Tissue Int* 1998, **63:**221–229.

28. McGuigan F, Larzenius E, Callreus M, Gerdhem P, Luthman H, Akesson K: **Variation in the bone morphogenetic protein-2 gene: effects on fat and lean body.** *Eur J Endocrinol* 2008, **158:**661–668.

29. Suh JS, Hahn WH, Lee JS, Park HJ, Kim MJ, Kang SW, Chung JH, Cho BS: **Coding polymorphisms of bone morphogenetic protein 2 contribute to the.** *Exp Ther Med* 2011, **2:**337–341.

30. Shafritz AB, Shore EM, Gannon FH, Zasloff MA, Taub R, Muenke M, Kaplan FS: **Overexpression of an osteogenic morphogen in fibrodysplasia ossificans.** *N Engl J Med* 1996, **335:**555–561.

31. Schrauwen I, Thys M, Vanderstraeten K, Fransen E, Dieltjens N, Huyghe JR, Ealy M, Claustres M, Cremers CR, Dhooge I, Declau F, Van DHP, Vincent R, Somers T, Offeciers E, Smith RJ, Van CG: **Association of bone morphogenetic proteins with otosclerosis.** *J Bone Miner Res* 2008, **23:**507–516.

32. Wawersik S, Purcell P, Rauchman M, Dudley AT, Robertson EJ, Maas R: **BMP7 acts in murine lens placode development.** *Dev Biol* 1999, **207:**176–188.

33. Wyatt AW, ORJSHRMK: **Bone Morphogenetic protein 7 (BMP7) Mutations are Associated with Variable Ocular, Brain, Ear, Palate, and Skeletal Anomalies.** *Hum Mutat* 2010, **31:**781–787.

15

Optic glioma and precocious puberty in a girl with neurofibromatosis type 1 carrying an R681X mutation of NF1

Mirjana Kocova*, Elena Kochova and Elena Sukarova-Angelovska

Abstract

Background: Neurofibromatosis type 1 (NF1) is a common autosomal dominant genetic disorder with an extremely variable phenotype. In childhood NF1 can be associated with optic glioma and central precocious puberty; the latter is more common when the optic chiasm is affected. The mutational spectrum of the NF1 gene is wide and complex; R681X is a rare severe mutation of the NF1 gene known to cause truncation of neurofibromin, with only ten reported cases in the literature so far.

Case presentation: We describe a girl with NF1 associated with early central precocious puberty appearing at 2.5 years of age and optic glioma affecting the optic chiasm as seen on magnetic resonance imaging (MRI). Genetic analysis confirmed the presence of R681X. Therapy with a gonadotropin-releasing hormone agonist was instituted with good response to therapy. The lesions on MRI were stable and no significant vision impairment was present during the 6 years of follow-up.

Conclusion: Of the ten reported cases of NF1 due to R681X, one has presented with optic glioma and none with precocious puberty. Thus, to our knowledge, this is the first reported case of this mutation presenting with precocious puberty. We believe that this is a contribution to the few reports on the phenotype of this mutation and to the future elucidation of genotype-phenotype correlations of this disease.

Keywords: Neurofibromatosis, NF1, Precocious puberty, Optic glioma, R681X

Background

Neurofibromatosis type 1 (NF1) is one of the most common autosomal dominant genetic disorders, affecting approximately 1 in 3500 individuals worldwide [1]. The primary clinical features are café-au-lait spots which progress throughout life to benign peripheral nerve sheath tumors or neurofibromas and Lisch nodules (iris hamartomas). However, other complications, such as skeletal dysplasias, learning disabilities, mental retardation, seizures, and optic glioma fall within the wide clinical spectrum of the disease. Characteristic of NF1 is extreme clinical variability, even in familial cases [2–4]. The National Institutes of Health (NIH) provide the well known diagnostic criteria; presence of at least two of these criteria is sufficient for the diagnosis [5].

NF1 is caused by defects in the *NF1* tumor suppressor gene located at chromosome 17q11.2 and spanning across approximately 300 kb of genomic DNA. *NF1* is composed of 60 exons with at least 4 alternatively spliced exons which are expressed in a developmental- and tissue-specific pattern [6–9]. The *NF1* gene encodes neurofibromin, a protein containing 2818 amino acids (AA) which harbors a functional GAP (GTPase-activating protein)-related domain (GRD, AA 1205–1536) in its central region. Neurofibromin is ubiquitously expressed and most abundant in the nervous system. The protein is highly conserved among vertebrates and shows 60 % identity with the *Drosophila* homolog [10–12]. The mutational spectrum of the *NF1* gene is complex due to the large number of coding exons

* Correspondence: mirjanakocova@yahoo.com
Department of Endocrinology and Genetics, University Pediatric Clinic, Vodnjanska 17, 1000 Skopje, Macedonia

and the considerable mutational heterogeneity. Most of the mutations occur in eight exons/flanking regions, representing only 16 % of the coding region. Mutations that cause skipping of exon 7, 30, and 29 are very common [13, 14]. Most of the mutations result in truncation and loss of function of neurofibromin. No specific genotype/phenotype correlation has been revealed [15].

The most common NF1-associated tumor is the benign peripheral nerve sheath tumor or neurofibroma. In a small percentage of NF1 patients, plexiform neurofibromas progress to malignant peripheral nerve sheath tumors. While defects in the peripheral nervous system glial cells (Schwann cells) underlie neurofibroma development, NF1 patients are also predisposed to astrocytic brain tumors, spinal tumors, pheochromocytoma, myeloid leukemia and gastrointestinal stromal tumors [1, 16]. Between 15 and 50 % of NF1 patients develop some type of glioma; these are often indolent in nature [17, 18]. Optic nerve gliomas occur in 12–15 % of patients with NF1 usually within the first decade of life [1]. No specific mutation of the NF1 gene has been associated with localization of the glioma at the optic chiasm. Precocious puberty due to optic glioma is not rare in patients with NF1, especially when the optic chiasm is involved [1–4, 19]. In fact, it is among the most common endocrine disorders in these patients and becomes more frequent with long-term follow up [20, 21]. However, very few patients with NF1 associated with optic glioma or precocious puberty have been molecularly characterized.

Here we present a child with NF1 and optic glioma, who presented with precocious puberty at the age of 2.5 years and was found to bear a rare mutation of the NF1 gene, R681X. We have reviewed the available literature and here we summarize the clinical findings in published case reports with this mutation.

Case presentation
Our patient was a Caucasian girl born from a normal, well controlled, uneventful pregnancy, delivered by Caesarean with average anthropometric parameters. No family history of neurofibromatosis was reported. At the age of five months, her parents had noticed café-au-lait spots on the skin that were steadily increasing in size over time. At the age of 2.5 years, breast enlargement was noticed and she was referred for hormonal work-up. Her height and weight were at the 95th percentile according to the charts of Tanner and Whitehouse. Telarche was at stage B2. Numerous café-au-lait spots on the skin were noted, various in size, the largest of which measured 30x40 mm. Axillary freckles were present bilaterally. No Lisch nodules or oculomotor difficulties were detected. Fundoscopy revealed pallor of the optic nerves bilaterally. Blood counts were normal. Peak serum values of LH = 16.4 IU/dl and of FSH = 45.3 IU/dl on the GnRH test confirmed the

diagnosis of precocious puberty of central origin. The growth hormone level after L-dopa stimulation was normal (peak value 12.3 ng/ml) and was completely supressed with the glucose tolerance test (0.6 ng/ml). The IGF-1 value was within the normal range (289 pg/ml), confirming no GH secretion abnormalities. Magnetic resonance imaging (MRI) of the pituitary region showed a normal pituitary gland with significant thickening of both optic nerves and the optic chiasm (optic glioma). The signal was enhanced by Gadolinium (Table 1, Fig. 1). Molecular analysis of the NF1 gene showed presence of the R681X mutation.

Therapy with a GnRH agonist (Triptorelin) at 28-day intervals was instituted and the patient has been receiving this therapy for 6 years thus far. With therapy, growth continued at a normal rate (on the 75th percentile) and the breasts returned to pre-pubertal stage B1. MRI was performed at yearly intervals and did not reveal any enlargement of the optic glioma. The first check-up of the visual field was performed at the age of 6 years and showed minor peripheral loss of vision (Fig. 2).

Although this case initially presented with a complex combination of clinical features, the diagnosis of NF1 was straightforward, due to our significant clinical experience and promptly conducted focused diagnostic procedures, as well as the genetic confirmation of the disease. As such, even though the prognostic characteristics of this particular case are difficult to assess, the long term follow-up of our patient has given some insight into the evolution of the disease.

We searched the Pubmed database using the keywords "neurofibromatosis" "NF1", "mutation", "R681X", and found ten pediatric cases with a reported R618X mutation; all are presented in Table 2. Optic glioma has so far been reported in only one patient with this mutation, however, with no associated precocious puberty [22].

Table 1 Clinical presentation and diagnostic procedures in presented case

Age at diagnosis	2.5 years
Height at diagnosis	+2.5 SDS
Bone age	+1.1 SDS
Puberty	B2, P1
Peak LH value after GnRH stimulation	16.4 IU/dl
GH value after L-Dopa stimulation/glucose tolerance test	12.3 ng/ml / 0.6 ng/ml
IGF-1	289 ng/ml
MRI	Optic glioma spreading to the chiasm
Visual field	Peripheral narrowing of the visual field
Ultrasound of the ovaries	Normal

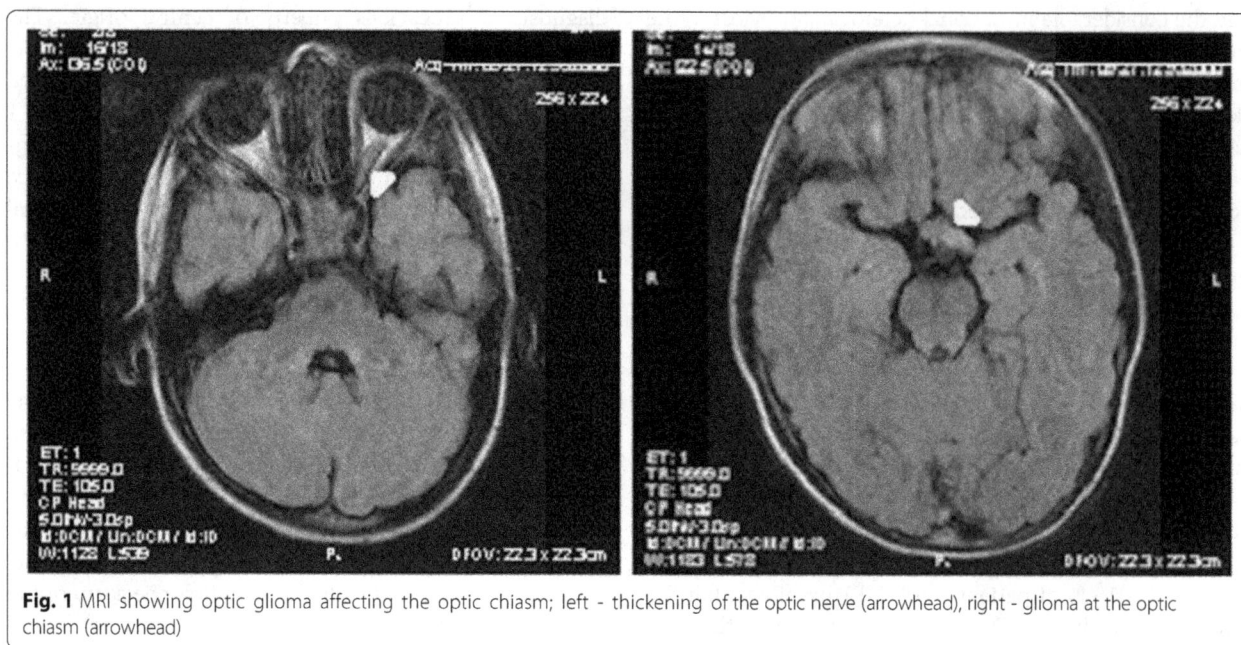

Fig. 1 MRI showing optic glioma affecting the optic chiasm; left - thickening of the optic nerve (arrowhead), right - glioma at the optic chiasm (arrowhead)

NF1 is caused by mutations in the *NF1* gene, one of the largest human genes bearing one of the highest mutation rates in the human genome. Although most of the described mutations are private, several hot spots with a higher mutation rate such as exons 4b, 7, 10b, 13, 15, 20, 29 and 37 have been described. No strict genotype/phenotype correlations have been confirmed in large studies [13–15, 23]. However, some of the signs of NF1, such as plexiform neurofibroma, scoliosis and learning disabilities have been associated with specific mutations [13].

Association of NF1 with optic glioma or precocious puberty is not rare, but has rarely been molecularly characterized [13, 14, 17–19]. Among 20 patients with optic glioma, *NF1* mutations were detected in 12. Most of these mutations were in the first exons of the *NF1* gene and three of them were located in exon 7; all mutations were different and produced truncated proteins [24]. The R681X (2041C > T) mutation is a nonsense mutation in exon 13 producing a truncated protein composed of 680 amino acids. A familial R681X mutation has been found in only two siblings in one family so far [13]. Central nervous system neoplasms can appear in patients with NF1, the most common being a visual pathway glioma involving one or both optic nerves, the chiasm, or other segments of the visual pathway [21, 25, 26]. These tumors can present clinically with unilateral or bilateral proptosis, decreased vision in one or both eyes, optic nerve pallor or restricted extraocular movements. Pure chiasmatic tumors do not cause proptosis; this was also absent in our patient. Tumors of the optic chiasm are usually associated with a variable degree of loss of visual acuity and visual field unilaterally

or bilaterally [27]. However, there is often discrepancy between the tumor size and visual impairment. Many patients will have appropriate vision, but some will be blind [28–30]. In children with so-called asymptomatic optic nerve tumors, careful clinical examination often reveals some degree of optic nerve pallor or restricted ocular movement. Central scotomas, a measurable depression of central vision, occur in approximately 70 % of patients. Peripheral field defects are common, but they are also variable and include quadrantic or hemianopic fields. Bitemporal hemianopic visual field loss occurs in less than one half of patients [29]. Our patient did not have any clinical signs of decreased vision at diagnosis. The ophthalmological examination revealed only a subtle decrease of the peripheral visual field and optic nerve pallor. Long-term follow-up did not show any progression of the optic and chiasmatic glioma, therefore no therapy was indicated. Most of the reported patients in the literature have a similar evolution, i.e. after the age of 6 years no further progression is expected [25, 30].

If the tumor is large enough, hypothalamic dysfunction occurs, and according to some recent data, optic pathway glioma might have stronger causative role for precocious puberty than the presence of NF1 condition [20, 21, 31]. Long-term follow up is necessary since patients with optic glioma and precocious puberty could progress towards gonadotropin deficiency later in life [21].

Reported NF1 patients from the literature carrying the R681X mutation have a variety of clinical presentations (Table 2). The clinical presentation of NF1 associated with optic glioma affecting the optic chiasm together

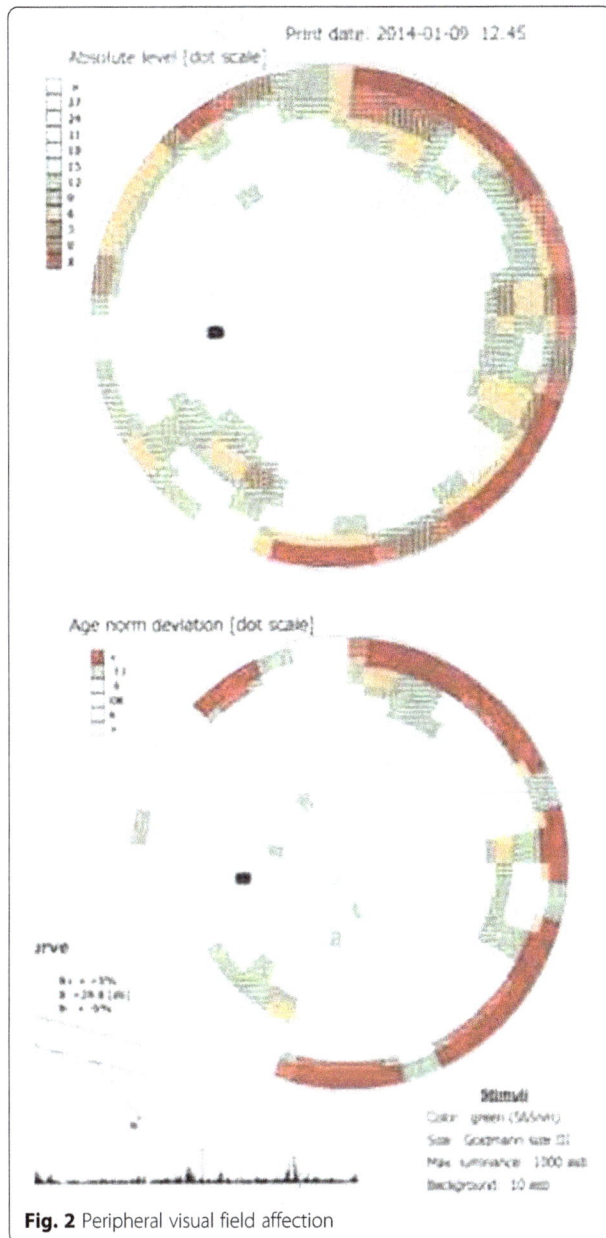

Fig. 2 Peripheral visual field affection

Table 2 Phenotype in published cases with confirmed R681X mutation of *NF1*

N° of patients with R681X/Total N° of study participants	Phenotype	Reference	
		Authors	Journal [Reference N°]
3/189	Learning disability (2 cases)	Ars E et al.	J Med Genet 2003 [13]
1/16	Optic glioma; Stargardt's disease	Gerth C et al.	Graefes Arch Clin Exp Ophtalmol 2002 [22]
4/500	?	Fashold M et al.	Am J Hum Genet 2000 [7]
1/108	?	Origone P et al.	Hum Mut 2002 [14]
1/3	Cutaneous neurofibromas	Maertens O et al.	Hum Genet 2007 [32]
1	Optic glioma + Precocious puberty	Kocova M et al.	BMC Endocr Disord

and other mutations of the *NF1* gene on the resulting phenotypic expression remains to be elucidated.

Consent

All procedures were performed according to the Declaration of Helsinki and approved by the Ethics Committee within the University Pediatric Clinic. Written informed consent was obtained from the patient's parent for publication of this Case report and any accompanying images. A copy of the written consent is available for review by the Editor of this journal.

Abbreviations

AA: Amino acids; GAP: GTP-ase activating protein; GnRH: Gonadotropin-releasing hormone; GRD: GAP-related domain; MRI: Magnetic resonance imaging; NF1: Neurofibromatosis type 1; *NF1*: Neurofibromin-1 gene; NIH: National Institutes of Health.

Competing interests

The authors declare that they have no competing interests.

Authors' contributions

The patient was under the care of MK, who conceived the idea of the report and drafted the manuscript. EK participated in the writing, review of the literature, text editing and finalization of the manuscript. ESA carried out the molecular genetic studies and participated in the review of the literature. All authors read and approved the final manuscript.

with precocious puberty found in our patient is a combination of clinical features that has thus far never been associated with the R681X mutation.

Conclusions

The R681X mutation is a very rare mutation of the *NF1* gene. In the literature we found a total of 10 reported cases of NF1 with this mutation so far, presenting with a heterogeneous phenotype. Optic glioma was reported in only one of these cases. The association of this mutation with precocious puberty present in our patient is the very first to our knowledge. The precise influence of this

References

1. Williams VC, Lucas J, Babcock MA, GButmann DH, Koef B, Maria L. Neurofibromatosis Type 1 Revisited. Pediatrics. 2009;123:124–33.
2. Upadhyaya M. Neurofibromatisis type 1: diagnosis and recent advances. Expert Opin Med Diagn. 2010;4:307–22.

3. Szudek J, Evans DG, Friedman JM. Patterns of associations of clinical features in neurofibromatosis 1 (NF1). Hum Genet. 2003;112:289–97.

4. Szudek J, Joe H, Friedman JM. Analysis of intrafamilial phenotypic variation in neurofibromatosis 1 (NF1). Genet Epidemiol. 2002;23:150–64.

5. Neurofibromatosis. Conference statement. NIH Consensus Development Conference. Arch Neurol. 1988;45:575–8.

6. Marchuk DA, Saulino AM, Tavakkol R, Swaroop M, Wallace MR, Andersen LB, et al. cDNA cloning of the type 1 neurofibromatosis gene: complete sequence of the NF1 gene product. Genomics. 1991;11:931–40.

7. Fahsold R, Hoffmeyer S, Mischung C, Gille C, Ehlers C, Kucukceylan N, et al. Minor Lesion Mutational Spectrum of the Entire NF1 Gene Does Not Explain Its High Mutability but Points to a Functional Domain Upstream of the GAP-Related Domain. Am J Hum Genet. 2000;66:790–818.

8. Viskochil D. Genetics of neurofibromatosis 1 and the NF1 gene. J Child Neurol. 2002;17:562–70.

9. Messiaen LM, Callens T, Mortier G, Beysen D, Vandenbroucke I, Van Roy N, et al. Exhaustive mutation analysis of the NF1 gene allows identification of 95 % of mutations and reveals a high frequency of unusual splicing defects. Hum Mutat. 2000;15:541–55.

10. Xu GF, Lin B, Tanaka K, Dunn D, Wood D, Gesteland R, et al. The catalytic domain of the neurofibromatosis type 1 gene product stimulates ras GTPase and complements ira mutants of S. cerevisiae. Cell. 1990;63:835–41.

11. Bernards A, Snijders AJ, Hannigan GE, Murthy AE, Gusella JF. Mouse neurofibromatosis type 1 cDNA sequence reveals high degree of conservation of both coding and non-coding mRNA segments. Hum Mol Genet. 1993;2:645–50.

12. The I, Hannigan GE, Cowley GS, Reginald S, Zhong Y, Gusella JF, et al. Rescue of a Drosophila NF1 mutant phenotype by protein kinase A. Science. 1997;276:791–4.

13. Ars E, Kruyer H, Morell M, Pros E, Serra E, Ravella A, et al. Recurrent mutations in the NF1 gene are common among neurofibromatosis type 1 patients. J Med Genet. 2003;40:e82.

14. Origone P, De Luca A, Bellini C, Buccino A, Mingarelli R, Costabel S, et al. Ten novel mutations in the human neurofibromatosis type 1 (NF1) gene in Italian patients. Hum Mutat. 2002;20:74–5.

15. Castle B, Baser ME, Huson SM, Cooper DN, Upadhyaya M. Evaluation of genotype-phenotype correlations in neurofibromatosis type 1. J Med Genet. 2003;40:e109.

16. Nishi T, Lee PS, Oka K, Levin VA, Tanase S, Morino Y, et al. Differential expression of two types of the neurofibromatosis type 1 (NF1) gene transcripts related to neuronal differentiation. Oncogene. 1991;6:1555–9.

17. Zoller ME, Rembeck B, Oden A, Samuelsson M, Angervall L. Malignant and benign tumors in patients with neurofibromatosis type 1 in a defined Swedish population. Cancer. 1997;79:2125–31.

18. Muir D, Neubauer D, Lim IT, Yachnis AT, Wallace MR. Tumorigenic properties of neurofibromin-deficient neurofibroma Schwann cells. Am J Pathol. 2001;158:501–13.

19. Habiby R, Silverman B, Listernick R, Charrow J. Precocious puberty in children with neurofibromatosis type 1. J Pediatrics. 1995;126(3):364–7.

20. Viridis R, Street ME, Bandello MA, Tripodi C, Donadio A, Villani AR, et al. Growth and pubertal disorders in neurofibromatosis type 1. J Pediatr Endocrinol Metab. 2003;16 Suppl 2:289–92.

21. Gan HW, Phipps K, Aquilina K, Gaze MN, Hayward R, Spoudeas HA. Neuroendocrine morbidity after pediatric optic gliomas: a longitudinal analysis of 166 children over 30 years. J Clin Endocrinol Metab. 2015;100(10):3787–99.

22. Gerth C, Andrassi-Darida M, Bock M, Preising MN, Weber BH, Lorenz B. Phenotypes of 16 Stargardt macular dystrophy/fundus flavimaculatus patients with known ABCA4 mutations and evaluation of genotype-phenotype correlation. Graefes Arch Clin Exp Ophthalmol. 2002;240:628–38.

23. Ben-Salem S, Al-Shamsi AM, Ali BR, Al-Gazali L. The mutational spectrum of the NF1 gene in neurofibromatosis type I patients from UAE. Childs Nerv Syst. 2014;30:1183–9.

24. Sharif S, Upadhyaya M, Ferner R, Majounie E, Shenton A, Baser M, et al. A molecular analysis of individuals with neurofibromatosis type 1 (NF1) and optic pathway gliomas (OPGs), and an assessment of genotype–phenotype correlations. J Med Genet. 2011;48:256–60.

25. Segal L, Darvish-Zargar M, Dilenge ME, Ortenberg J, Polomeno RC. Optic pathway gliomas in patients with neurofibromatosis type 1: follow-up of 44 patients. J AAPOS. 2010;14:155–8.

26. Rutkowski JL, Wu K, Gutmann DH, Boyer PJ, Legius E. Genetic and cellular defects contributing to benign tumor formation in neurofibromatosis type 1. Hum Mol Genet. 2000;9:1059–66.

27. Avery RA, Ferner RE, Listernick R, Fisher MJ, Gutmann DH, Liu GT. Visual acuity in children with low grade gliomas of the visual pathway: implications for patient care and clinical research. J Neurooncol. 2012;110:1–7.

28. Graff JM, Coombs JM, Pramanik S. Neurofibromatosis Type 1 - Optic Nerve Glioma: 8-year-old white female with acute awareness of complete vision loss., OS. EyeRounds.org. May 15, 2005; Available from: http://www.EyeRounds.org/cases/38-NeurofibromatosisOpticNerveGlioma.htm. Accessed 2014

29. Fisher MJ, Avery RA, Allen JC, Ardern-Holmes SL, Bilaniuk LT, Ferner RF, et al. Functional outcome measures for NF1 associated optic pathway glioma clinical trials. Neurology. 2013;18(21 Suppl1):S15–24.

30. Fisher MJ, Loguidice M, Gutmann DH, Listernick R, Ferner RE, Ullrich NJ, et al. Visual outcomes in children with neurofibromatosis type 1 - associated optic pathway glioma following chemotherapy: a multicenter retrospective analysis. Neuro Oncol. 2012;14:790–7.

31. Virdis R, Sigorini M, Laiolo A, Lorenzetti E, Street ME, Villani AR, et al. Neurofibromatosis type 1 and precocious puberty. J Pediatr Endocrinol Metab. 2000;13:841–4.

32. Maertens O, De Schepper S, Vandesimpele J, Brems H, Heyns I, Janssens S, et al. Molecular dissection of isolated disease features in mosaic neurofibromatosis type 1. Am J Hum Genet. 2007;81:243.

16

Ectopic insulin secreting neuroendocrine tumor of kidney with recurrent hypoglycemia: a diagnostic dilemma

S Ramkumar[1], Atul Dhingra[1], VP Jyotsna[1*], Mohd. Ashraf Ganie[1], Chandan J Das[2], Amlesh Seth[3], Mehar C Sharma[4] and Chandra Sekhar Bal[5]

Abstract

Background: Hypoglycemia secondary to ectopic insulin secretion of non-pancreatic tumors is rare.

Case presentation: We describe a middle aged woman with recurrent hypoglycemia. On evaluation, she was detected to have hyperinsulinemic hypoglycemia and right sided renal mass lesion. 68Ga-Dotanoc and 99mTc-HYNICTOC scans confirmed the intrarenal mass to be of neuroendocrine origin. Right nephrectomy was done and it turned out to be an insulin secreting neuroendocrine tumour. Neuroendocrine nature of this tumour was further confirmed by ultra-structural examination. Her hypoglycemia did not recur after resection of this tumour.

Conclusion: Few cases of ectopic insulin secretion have been reported though some are not proven convincingly. This case addresses all the issues raised in previous case reports and proves by clinical, laboratory, functional imaging and immunohistochemical analysis that ectopic origin of insulin by non-pancreatic tumors does occur. To our knowledge, this is the first reported case of ectopic insulinoma arising from the kidney.

Keywords: Hyperinsulinemic hypoglycemia, Neuroendocrine tumour, Insulinoma, Carcinoid tumor, Renal tumour, 68Ga-Dotanoc scan, 99mTc-HYNICTOC scan

Background

The most common cause of endogenous hypoglycemia is hyperinsulinemia secondary to islet cell tumours of pancreas. Hypoglycemia due to non-pancreatic tumours is infrequently reported. Most of these non-pancreatic tumours secrete factors with insulin like activity. Ectopic insulin secretion has been reported in few cases but not convincingly proved. We report a case of ectopic insulin secretion by neuroendocrine tumour (NET) of kidney. The ectopic origin of the tumour is demonstrated by functional imaging (⁶⁸Ga-Dotanoc and ⁹⁹ᵐTc-HYNICTOC), and by immunohistochemistry for insulin staining. We also extensively reviewed literature for similar cases of ectopic insulin secreting tumours published previously.

Case presentation

This 44-year-old female was admitted for evaluation of recurrent hypoglycemic episodes of 3 years duration. She had complains of forgetfulness, altered behaviour, headache, palpitation, sweating, and giddiness. Most of her symptoms occurred early in the morning and these symptoms improved spontaneously in 15 minutes. She had consulted various physicians including neurologist and psychiatrist and had been diagnosed as pseudoseizure, panic attacks or conversion disorder. One year back, she consulted endocrinologist and was diagnosed to have hypoglycemia and hyperinsulinemia. For suspecting insulinoma, she underwent CT abdomen which showed a right renal mass lesion and possibility of renal cell carcinoma was entertained. She was advised surgery for renal tumour. However, patient did not agree for surgery. There were no complains of hematuria, urinary frequency, urgency, burning micturition, diarrhoea or

---
* Correspondence: vivekapjyotsna@yahoo.com
[1]Department of Endocrinology and Metabolism, All India Institute of Medical Sciences, Ansari Nagar, New Delhi 110029, India
Full list of author information is available at the end of the article

flushing episodes. She was not on antidiabetic treatment and was not hypertensive. For last 2 months, patient was having recurrent hypoglycemic seizures and came to this hospital.

After admission, she had persisted hypoglycemia and required continuous infusion of 10% Dextrose at the rate of 75 – 100 ml/hr in addition to 1-2 hourly feeds. Her hemogram, electrolytes, renal and liver functions were normal. HbA1c was 4.5%. Hormonal assay showed thyroxine (T4) 5.67 (5.1 – 14.1 mcg/dl), TSH 4.42 (0.27 – 4.2 mIU/ml), Insulin like Growth Factor- I(IGF-1) - 165.90 (62 – 205 ng/ml), growth hormone 1.20 ng/ml and cortisol 15.78 mcg/dl. Samples collected during hypoglycemia showed a serum insulin of 134 (2.6 – 24.9 μU/ml) and C-peptide of 13.35 (1.1 – 4.4) ng/ml. During another symptomatic hypoglycemia, she had plasma glucose of 44 mg/dl while her plasma insulin and C-peptide were 49.81 miu/ml and 9.36 ng/ml respectively confirming endogenous hyperinsulinemic hypoglycemia. She underwent high resolution radiological and functional imaging for localisation of insulinoma.

Both multi-phase CT abdomen (Figure 1) and contrast enhanced MRI abdomen demonstrated a mass lesion arising from upper- mid pole of right kidney (Figure 1a, 1b, 1c). No lesion was identified in the pancreas (Figure 1d). Endoscopic ultrasound also did not demonstrate any pancreatic lesion. 68Gallium DOTANOC scan (Figure 2a-c) and 99mTc-HYNICTOC (Figure 2d,e) did not demonstrate any uptake in the pancreas but both demonstrated intense uptake in the mass lesion indicating a NET. She underwent abdominal exploration and right nephrectomy.

Post-operative period was uneventful and she became euglycemic without need for dextrose infusion. Her glucose values were maintained between 120 – 160 mg/dl thus confirming the right sided mass near renal hilum to be the source of ectopic insulin secretion.

Pathologic examination

Gross examination: Grossly the kidney measured 10×7×6 cm and weighed 350 gram. A solid well circumscribed yellowish tumour, measuring 7×6×5 cm, was identified in the upper pole of kidney (Figure 3a). There was no capsule breach or renal sinus infiltration. Rest of the renal parenchyma and pelvicalyceal system were unremarkable. Areas of necrosis or hemorrhage were not identified.

Microscopic Finding: Microscopically, the tumor was composed of solid nests anastomosing cords and trabeculae of low columnar cells separated by a vascular stroma [Figures 3b-d]. The cellular outlines were indistinct with centrally placed oval nuclei, fine chromatin and inconspicuous nucleoli. The cytoplasm was eosinophilic, finely granular and moderate in amount. At places there were intense desmoplasia around the tumor cells (Figure 3e). Mitotic rate was 1 per 10 high power fields (hpf). Areas of tumour necrosis were not identified. Foci of perineural, lymphatic and vascular invasion were not seen. No intra or extra-cellular mucin was identified. Immunohistochemical staining revealed diffuse and intense staining for pancytokeratin, synaptophysin, chromogranin A, neuron specific enolase (NSE) and insulin (Figure 3f, 3g, 3h). MIB I labeling index was 2% (Figure 3i). The lymph nodes dissected from the specimen show metastasis (2/3).

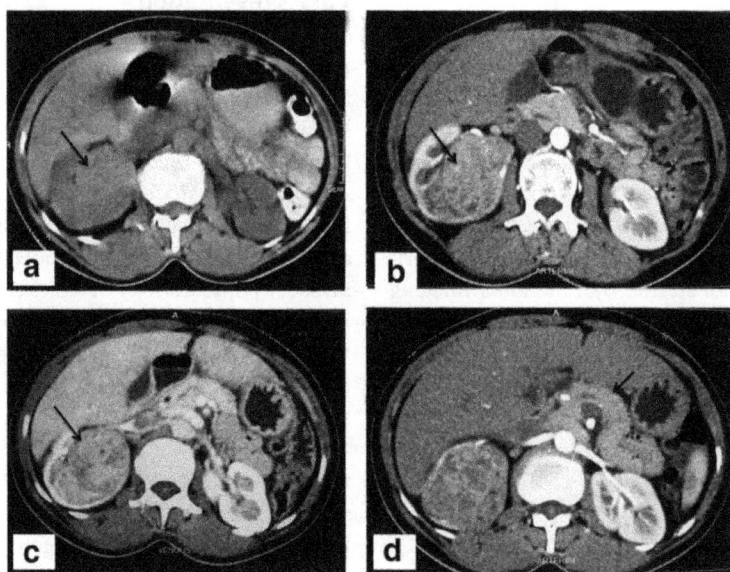

Figure 1 CT scan. Unenhanced CT axial image (**1a**) showing an isodense mass (arrow) to renal parenchyma which show enhancement in arterial phase image (**1b**) but lesser than the renal cortex. The enhancement continued till the venous phase (**1c**). Arterial phase image (**1d**) taken at the level of pancreas (arrow) did not show any arterial enhancing lesion.

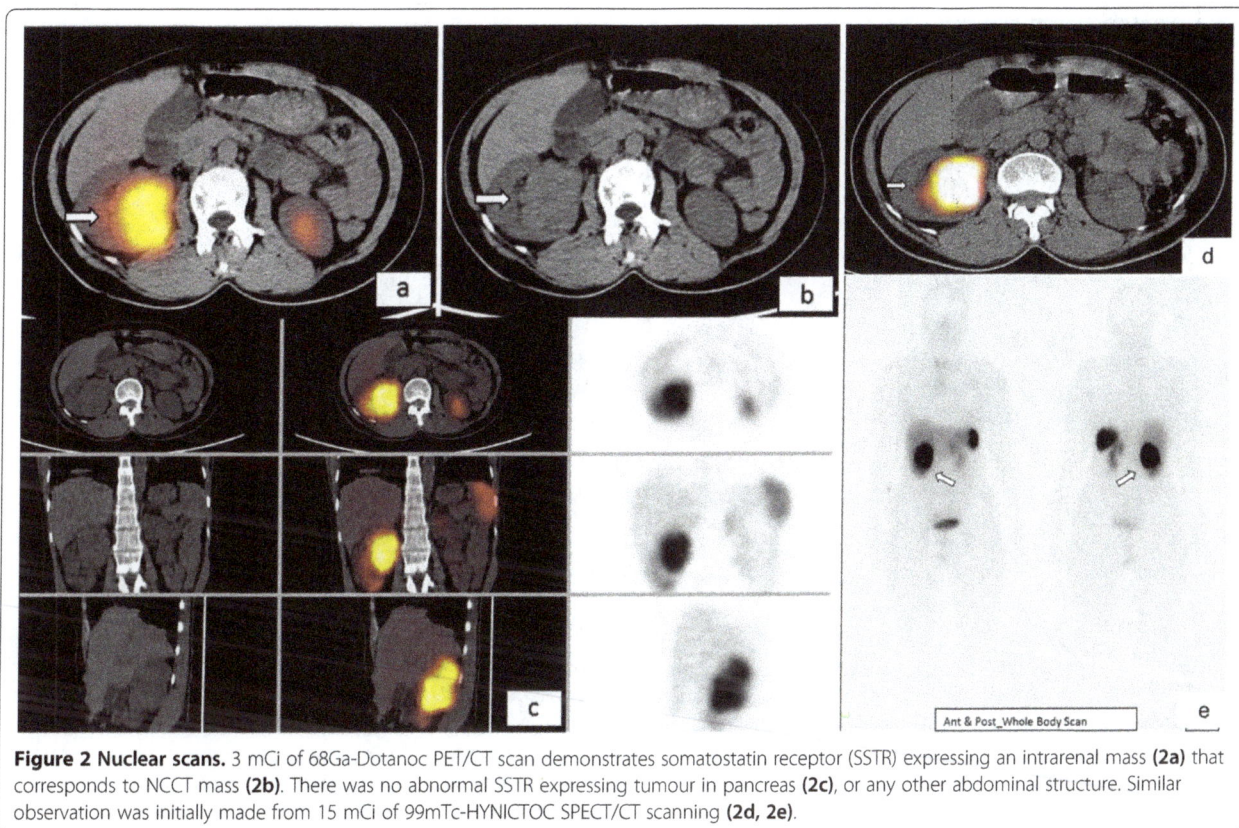

Figure 2 Nuclear scans. 3 mCi of 68Ga-Dotanoc PET/CT scan demonstrates somatostatin receptor (SSTR) expressing an intrarenal mass **(2a)** that corresponds to NCCT mass **(2b)**. There was no abnormal SSTR expressing tumour in pancreas **(2c)**, or any other abdominal structure. Similar observation was initially made from 15 mCi of 99mTc-HYNICTOC SPECT/CT scanning **(2d, 2e)**.

Ultrastructural examination revealed numerous electron dense, membrane bound round to oval shaped granules of variable diameter in the cytoplasm [Figure 3j, 3k]. A narrow peripheral lighter zone was present in some of the granules.

Based on the above features; the diagnosis neuroendocrine tumour grade G1; pathological stage IV was entertained. Serum chromogranin A measured in the samples collected before surgery and stored in -40 degree was 2126.1 (N < 90.1 ng/ml).

Follow up

No metastasis was detected. Our patient got discharged in stable condition on 10th post-operative day. The patient is asymptomatic, euglycemic and disease free at last follow-up at 3 months.

Discussion

Islet cell tumours of pancreas produce insulin which cause hypoglycemia. Hypoglycemia due to non-pancreatic tumours is infrequently reported and poorly understood. Various mechanisms were proposed [1] are: (a) insulin or insulin-like activity produced by the tumour, (b) decreased gluconeogenesis, (c) disruption of glucagon metabolism, and (d) increased utilization of glucose by the tumour. The non-suppressible Insulin like Activity (NSILA) has been purposed to be secondary to Insulin like Growth Factor-2. The non-islet cell tumours which

commonly cause hypoglycaemia are of mesenchymal, epithelial or hematopoietic cell lines. Fibrosarcomas, mesotheliomas, leiomyosarcomas, and hemangiopericytomas are the most frequent types of tumours which cause hypoglycemia. Hepatoma, gastric, pancreatic, exocrine gland and lung carcinomas are epithelial cancers with frequent hypoglycemic potential. Mesenchymal and epithelial tumors, which generally present as large masses, are located in the mediastinum or the abdomen. These tumours are known to cause hypoglycemia via secretion of IGF-2 that leads to stimulation of insulin receptors [2]. In a series of 78 cases of non-islet-cell tumour, hypoglycemia (NICTH) due to IGF-2 production, hepatocellular carcinoma and gastric carcinoma were the common causes [3].

Ectopic insulin secreting tumours are rare, comprising only 1% to 2% of all insulinomas [4] and are commonly located in the peripancreatic or periduodenal region where most heterotopic pancreatic tissue is located. Ectopic insulin producing tumours located away from pancreatic beds are infrequently reported in literature. Only few cases were described in literature due to hyperinsulinemic hypoglycemia and non-pancreatic tumour and these tumors are described in Table 1.

The patient under discussion had presented with right renal mass lesion and hyperinsulinemic hypoglycemia. We initially considered the possibility of incidentally

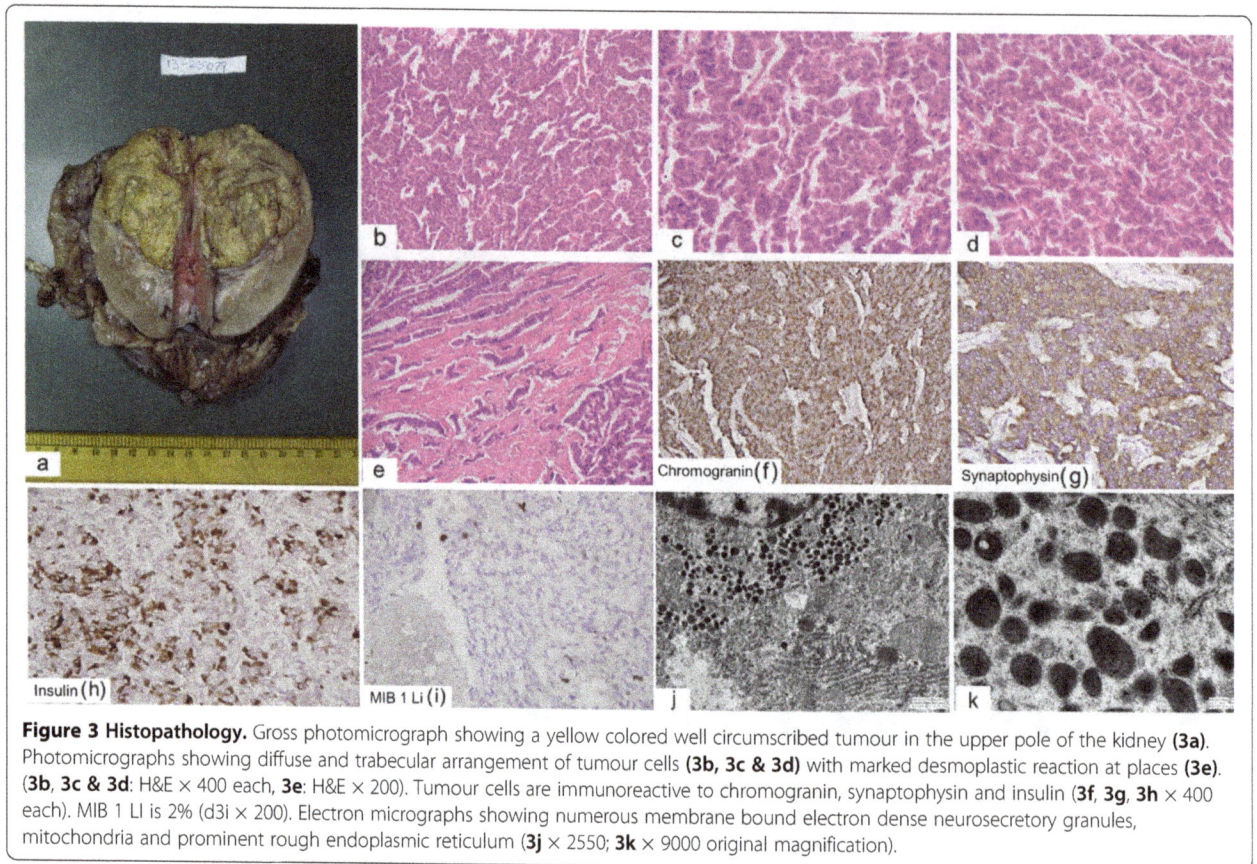

Figure 3 Histopathology. Gross photomicrograph showing a yellow colored well circumscribed tumour in the upper pole of the kidney **(3a)**. Photomicrographs showing diffuse and trabecular arrangement of tumour cells **(3b, 3c & 3d)** with marked desmoplastic reaction at places **(3e)**. **(3b, 3c & 3d**: H&E × 400 each, **3e**: H&E × 200). Tumour cells are immunoreactive to chromogranin, synaptophysin and insulin **(3f, 3g, 3h** × 400 each). MIB 1 LI is 2% (d3i × 200). Electron micrographs showing numerous membrane bound electron dense neurosecretory granules, mitochondria and prominent rough endoplasmic reticulum **(3j** × 2550; **3k** × 9000 original magnification).

detected right renal cell carcinoma in patient with insulinoma. In our Institute, we have both PET and SPECT imaging agents for octreoscan available for the localisation of insulinoma. Somatostain receptor scintigraphy (SRS) is an established functional imaging method for patients with NETs. The sensitivity of SRS for insulinoma is 50 – 60% [12]. We did both ^{68}Ga-Dotanoc and ^{99m}Tc-HYNICTOC scans for the localisation of insulinoma which unexpectedly revealed increased uptake in the right renal mass lesion itself confirming it to be a NET. To the best of our knowledge, this is the first case of ectopic insulin secretion confirmed *in vivo* by ^{68}Ga-Dotanoc and ^{99m}Tc-HYNICTOC scan. Further, the neuroendocrine and insulin secreting nature of the tumour was confirmed *ex vivo* by histopathological examination, immunohistochemistry and ultra-structural examination. Paraganglioma and pheochromoctyoma were also reported to cause hyperinsulinemic hypoglycemia and also show tracer uptake by SRS and are immunoreactive for chromogranin A and syanptophysin. Though the mass lesion was arising from upper pole of right kidney, it was intra-renal and hisopathological examination was suggestive of NET.

NETs are neoplasms that arise from cells of dispersed neuroendocrine system. Although there are many kinds of NETs but they are treated as a group of tumours as these neoplasms share common features such as histology,

immunoreactivity for neuroendocrine markers (chromogranin A, synaptophysin, neuron specific enolase), presence of neurosecretory granules, and secretion of biogenic amines and polypeptide hormones. Neuroendocrine tumours arising from pancreas are classified by the hormone most commonly secreted. Neuroendocrine tumours arising from the intestine, respiratory system and rest of the body were known as carcinoids but under the recent nomenclature they are all know as neuroendocrine neoplasm (NEN) of tumour. Primary carcinoid tumours of kidney are extremely rare and around 90 cases has been reported in literature [13]. None of the reported cases including two cases were reported from our institute previously [14, 15] were insulin secreting.

The cell of origin of renal carcinoid is unclear as neuroendocrine cells are not normally found in adult renal parenchyma. Carcinoid tumours of kidney are usually asymptomatic. In symptomatic cases, these tumours present with abdominal pain or abdominal mass with hematuria or fever. Evidence of carcinoid syndrome with serotonin-related flushing, generalized edema and diarrhoea, and occasional elevation of urine 5-hydroxyindoleaceticacid are uncommon and are seen in less than 10% of cases [14]. Our patient did not have these symptoms prior to presentation, although she had flushing, edema and blanching of the skin intraoperatively. Rarely, these tumours may present with neuroendocrine syndromes like cushing syndrome, vipoma, or glucagonoma [16]. Our case presented as insulinoma. Macroscopically, renal carcinoid tumours are usually solitary and unilateral. They are well circumscribed with a lobulated and bulging appearance. The cut surface the tumour is yellow-tan, or red brown as also observed in the case under discussion. Renal carcinoids exhibit histological features that are typical of carcinoids at other sites. Primary carcinoid tumors as well as metastasis possess high affinity receptors for somatostatin in 87% of cases [17]. Localization of gastrointestinal tract carcinoid tumours and pancreatic endocrine tumors has been achieved by the use of radiolabeled octreotide, a synthetic and slowly degraded somatostatin analogue that has a high affinity for somatostatin receptors. Use of indium-111 pentetreotide scanning in the diagnosis of carcinoid tumors had been reported [18]. In the present case, functional imaging with ^{68}Ga-Dotanoc and ^{99m}Tc-HYNICTOC was done for the localisation of insulinoma. Both showed uptake in the right renal mass lesion and no uptake in pancreas (Figure 2a-e). All available modalities for diagnosis of carcinoid tumors were employed namely Electron microscopy, immunohistochemistry, both PET and SPECT octreotide scan along with conventional radiographic imaging techniques were used in preoperative diagnosis this tumour.

Prognosis of NET depends upon the grade and stage of the tumour. Although the grade of the tumour was low, however stage was high as there was metastasis in the regional lymph nodes. There was no recurrence of hypoglycaemia on till this time of reporting, however, long-term close follow up is needed for the malignant behaviour.

Conclusions

Ectopic insulin secreting extra-pancreatic tumours are rare. Confirmation of the source of hyperinsulinemia is often difficult. To our knowledge, this is the first case of extra-pancreatic insulin secreting neuroendocrine tumour fully characterised by biochemical, radiological & functional imaging, histopathology and immunohistochemistry. Our patient had successful post-operative outcome and maintained euglycaemia after three months of follow-up.

Consent

Written informed consent was obtained from the patient for publication of this Case report and any accompanying images. A copy of the written consent is available for review by the Editor of this journal.

Table 1 Insulin secreting extra-pancreatic tumors reported in literature

Case		Evidence of hyperinsulinemia[a] in tumour	Resolution of hypoglycemia after resection of tumour	Evidence of neuro-endocrine origin	Mechanism of hypoglycemia -proposed
1	Ovarian carcinoid [5]	Insulin staining (5%), EM – beta cell granules, absence of pancreatic tumor at autopsy	Not demonstrated	HPE	Direct tumoral secretion of insulin
2	Carcinoma cervix [6]	Insulin staining, absence of pancreatic tumor at autopsy	Not demonstrated	HPE	Liver metastasis[b], Direct tumoral secretion of insulin
3	Bronchial carcinoid [7]	Insulin staining	Not demonstrated	HPE	Liver metastasis[c], Direct tumoral secretion of insulin
4	Paraganglioma [8]	None	Yes	HPE	No conclusive evidence of direct tumoral secretion of insulin
5	Paraganglioma [9]	Insulin staining (3%)	Yes	HPE	Direct tumoral secretion of insulin
6	Pheochromocytoma [10]	Insulin stain negative, absence of pancreatic tumor at autopsy	Not demonstrated	HPE	Beta adrenoceptor mediated release of insulin from pancreas
7	Neuroendocrine tumor of liver [11]	Insulin staining, absence of any extrahepatic tumor at autopsy, Selective arterial calcium stimulation	Not demonstrated	HPE	Direct tumoral secretion of insulin[d]
8	Neuroendocrine tumour kidney (carcinoid) (present case)	Insulin staining, EM – beta cell granules,	Yes	HPE, 68Gallium DOTANOC, HYNICTOC imaging	Direct tumoral secretion of insulin

[a]Includes evidences other than biochemical documentation of hyperinsulinemia in critical samples(collected at the time of hypoglycemia).
[b]Liver functions are reportedly normal in this patient.
[c]70% of the liver was replaced by tumor at autopsy in this patient.
[d]This patient developed hypoglycemia after left hepatectomy.
HPE – Histo-pathological examination, EM – Electron Microscopy.

Abbreviations
SRS: Somatostain receptor scintigraphy; NEN: Neuroendocrine neoplasm;
NICTH: Non-islet-cell tumour hypoglycemia; NET: Neuroendocrine tumor.

Competing interests
The authors declare that they have no competing interests.

Authors' contributions
1) RS, JVP, DA, GMA have managed the case clinically with the help of DCJ
(radiology), BCS (Nuclear Medicine), SMC (pathology) and SA (Uro-Surgery)
for diagnosis and management. DCJ has done and reported the CT scans,
BCS has done and reported the Nuclear scans (68Ga-Dotanoc PET/CT and
99mTc-HYNICTOC SPECT/CT scans), SMC has done the ultrastructural examination
and immunostaining while SA has performed the definitive surgery which was
curative in this case. 2) RS And DA have been involved in drafting the manuscript
and JVP in revising it critically for important intellectual content. 3) All authors have
given final approval of the version to be published.

Author details
[1]Department of Endocrinology and Metabolism, All India Institute of Medical
Sciences, Ansari Nagar, New Delhi 110029, India. [2]Departments of Radiology,
All India Institute of Medical Sciences, New Delhi, India. [3]Departments of
Urology, All India Institute of Medical Sciences, New Delhi, India.
[4]Departments of Pathology, All India Institute of Medical Sciences, New
Delhi, India. [5]Departments of Nuclear Medicine, All India Institute of Medical
Sciences, New Delhi, India.

References
1. Immerman SC, Sener SF, Khandekar JD: **Causes and evaluation of tumor-induced hypoglycemia.** *Arch Surg* 1982, **117**:905–908.
2. Daughaday WH, Trivedi B: **Measurement of derivatives of proinsulin-like growth factor-II in serum by a radioimmunoassay directed against the E-domain in normal subjects and patients with nonislet cell tumor hypoglycemia.** *J Clin Endocrinol Metab* 1992, **75**:110–115.
3. Fakuda I, Hizuka N, Ishikawa Y, Yasumoto K, Murakami Y, Sata A, Morita J, Kurimoto M, Okubo Y, Takano K: **Clinical features of insulin-like growth factor-II producing non-islet-cell tumor hypoglycemia.** *Growth Horm IGF Res* 2006, **16**:211–216.
4. Filipi CJ, Higgins GA: **Diagnosis and management of insulinoma.** *Am J Surg* 1973, **125**:231–239.
5. Morgello S, Schwartz E, Horwith M, King ME, Gorden P, Alonso DR: **Ectopic insulin production by a primary ovarian carcinoid.** *Cancer* 1988, **61**:800–805.
6. Seckl MJ, Mulholland PJ, Bishop AE, Teale JD, Hales CN, Glaser M, Watkins S, Seckl JR: **Hypoglycemia due to an insulin-secreting small-cell carcinoma of the cervix.** *N Engl J Med* 1999, **341**:733–736.
7. Shames JM, Dhurandhar NR, Blackard WG: **Insulin-secreting bronchial carcinoid tumor with widespread metastases.** *Am J Med* 1968, **44**:632–637.
8. Fujino K, Yamamoto S, Matsumoto M, Su-nada M, Ota T: **Paraganglioma associated with hypoglycemia.** *Intern Med* 1992, **31**:1239–1241.
9. Uysal M, Temiz S, Gul N, Yarman S, Tanakol R, Kapran Y: **Hypoglycemia due to ectopic release of insulin from a Paraganglioma.** *Horm Res* 2007, **67**:292–295.
10. Frankton S, Baithun S, Husain E, Davis K, Grossman AB: **Pheochromocytoma crisis presenting with profound hypoglycemia and subsequent hypertension.** *Hormones* 2009, **8**:65–70.
11. McCaffrey JA, Reuter VV, Herr HW, Macapinlac HA, Russo P, Motzer RJ: **Carcinoid tumor of the kidney the use of somatostatin receptor scintigraphy in diagnosis and management.** *Urol Oncol* 2005, **5**:108–111.
12. Sundin A, Garske U, Orlefors H: **Nuclear imaging of neuroendocrine tumours.** *Best Pract Res Clin Endocrinol Metab* 2007, **21**(1):69–85.
13. Armah HB, Parwani AV: **Primary carcinoid tumor arising within mature teratoma of the kidney. Report of a rare entity and review of the literature.** *Diagn Pathol* 2007, **2**:15.
14. Jain D, Sharma MC, Singh K, Gupta NP: **Primary carcinoid tumor of the kidney: case report and brief review of the literature.** *Indian J Pathol Microbiol* 2010, **53**(4):772.
15. Singh PP, Malhotra AS, Kashyap V: **Carcinoid tumor of the kidney: an unusual renal tumor.** *Indian J Urol* 2009, **25**:537–538.
16. Korkmaz T, Seber S, Yavuzer D, Gumus M, Turhal NS: **Primary renal carcinoid: treatment and prognosis.** *Crit Rev Oncol Hematol* 2013, **87**:256–264.
17. Reubi JC, Kvols LK, Waser B, Nagorney DM, Heitz PU, Charboneau JW, Reading CC, Moertel C: **Detection of somatostatin receptors in surgical and percutaneous needle biopsy samples of carcinoids and islet cell tumors.** *Cancer Res* 1990, **50**:5969–5973.
18. McCaffrey JA, Reuter VV, Herr HW, Macapinlac HA, Russo P, Motzer RJ: **Carcinoid tumor of the kidney the use of somatostatin receptor scintigraphy in diagnosis and management.** *Urol Oncol* 2005, **5**:108–111.

17

How should we interrogate the hypothalamic-pituitary-adrenal axis in patients with suspected hypopituitarism?

Aoife Garrahy[1] and Amar Agha[1,2*]

Abstract

Hypopituitarism is deficiency of one or more pituitary hormones, of which adrenocorticotrophic hormone (ACTH) deficiency is the most serious and potentially life-threatening. It may occur in isolation or, more commonly as part of more widespread pituitary failure. Diagnosis requires demonstration of subnormal cortisol rise in response to stimulation with hypoglycemia, glucagon, ACTH(1-24) or in the setting of acute illness. The choice of diagnostic test should be individualised for the patient and clinical scenario. A random cortisol and ACTH level may be adequate in making a diagnosis in an acutely ill patient with a suspected adrenal crisis e.g. pituitary apoplexy. Often however, dynamic assessment of cortisol reserve is needed. The cortisol response is both stimulus and assay-dependent and normative values should be derived locally. Results must be interpreted within clinical context and with understanding of potential pitfalls of the test used.

Background

Hypopituitarism is a clinical syndrome of deficiencies in one or more pituitary hormones of which adrenocorticotrophic hormone (ACTH) deficiency resulting in adrenal failure is the most serious and potentially life-threatening feature. ACTH deficiency can present as a part of generalized pituitary failure (multiple pituitary hormone deficiency, MPHD) or less commonly as an isolated entity. In the most severe cases, it can manifest acutely and dramatically as a life-threatening adrenal crisis with vascular collapse especially during an intercurrent illness while in other cases, the features are more subtle and the onset is gradual. It may also be diagnosed during assessment of pituitary axes as part of routine practice in those with pituitary tumours or following pituitary surgery or radiation therapy in otherwise well patients with little or no symptoms.

Physiology

ACTH is a 39 amino acid peptide produced in the anterior pituitary by proteolytic cleavage of the much larger precursor polypeptide proopiomelanocortin (POMC).

POMC gene expression, processing to ACTH and ACTH secretion are stimulated by corticotropin releasing factor (CRF) which is secreted in the hypothalamus [1]. These processes are under negative feedback by glucocorticoids. ACTH secretion can be suppressed by exogenous glucocorticoids via this negative feedback mechanism and this represents the most common cause of ACTH deficiency.

ACTH acts on the G protein coupled melanocortin 2 receptor in the zona fasiculata of the adrenal cortex to stimulate the synthesis of cortisol. In addition to this rapid effect, ACTH induces steroidogenic gene transcription and causes adrenal hypertrophy leading to an increase in the long-term capacity of the adrenal gland to generate cortisol [2]. This results in the adrenal hypertrophy seen in chronic ACTH excess. In contrast, in chronic ACTH deficiency adrenal atrophy can occur. Cortisol circulates in the blood bound to cortisol binding globulin (CBG) and free cortisol binds to the glucocorticoid receptor in target tissues to regulate gene transcription as well as exerting rapid, non-genomic effects [1, 3].

ACTH also stimulates the production of adrenal androgens, primarily dehydroepiandrosterone (DHEA), from the zona reticularis. These represent the main source of circulating androgen in females. Mineralocorticoid production is spared in central hypoadrenalism as

* Correspondence: amaragha@beaumont.ie
[1]Division of Endocrinology, Beaumont Hospital, Dublin, Ireland
[2]RCSI Medical School, Dublin, Ireland

mineralocorticoid secretion is primarily mediated by the renin-angiotensin system [4].

Clinical context

ACTH deficiency can be congenital or acquired due to structural or functional diseases of the pituitary or hypothalamus. It can occur in isolation or as part of more widespread pituitary failure. The most common cause of ACTH deficiency is ACTH suppression and subsequent adrenal atrophy due to chronic glucocorticoid use. Other causes are outlined in Table 1.

Interrogation of the hypothalamic pituitary axis may be required acutely or in a more routine setting. The

Table 1 Causes of central hypoadrenalism

Congenital	Acquired
Genetic	Tumor
Isolated ACTH deficiency	Non-functioning pituitary adenoma
POMC mutation/cleavage defect	Functional pituitary adenoma
Mutations in POMC transcription factors (TBX19)	Craniopharyngioma
	Pituitary metastases
Associated with other pituitary deficiencies	Germinoma
PROP1, LHX3, LHX4, HESX1, OTX2 mutations	Other tumours including astrocytoma, meningioma.
Midline Defects	Iatrogenic
Septo-optic dysplasia (without HESX1 mutation)	Exogenous glucocorticoids
	Pituitary surgery
	Cranial irradiation
	Post-treatment for hypercortisolism
	Opiates
	Infiltrative
	Neurosarcoidosis
	Histiocytosis X
	Haemochromatosis
	Inflammatory/Infective
	Hypophysitis (lymphocytic, granulomatous)
	Post-basal meningitis, abscesses, encephalitis.
	Traumatic/vascular
	Traumatic brain injury
	Subarachnoid haemorrhage
	Sheehan's syndrome
	Miscellaneous
	Idiopathic
	Pituitary apoplexy
	Empty sella syndrome
	Rathkes cleft cyst

clinical scenario can mandate which test is performed. For example a random cortisol and ACTH level may be adequate in making a diagnosis in an acutely ill patient with a suspected adrenal crisis e.g. pituitary apoplexy. In other situations a low morning cortisol level in an at risk patient may also be sufficient in diagnosing ACTH/cortisol deficiency. Often however, dynamic assessment of cortisol reserves is needed (see below).

In hypopituitarism, there is generally a specific sequential failure of pituitary hormones with GH being the most common pituitary hormone affected followed by gonadotrophins and culminating in loss of ACTH and thyroid stimulating hormone (TSH) [5]. ACTH however can be the first or only pituitary hormone affected in certain situations such as lymphocytic hypophysitis [6] or suppression of the hypothalamic-pituitary-adrenal (HPA) axis by exogenous glucocorticoids.

Detection and treatment of central hypoadrenalism is important as it has been shown to be associated with increased morbidity and mortality [7, 8].

Testing for central hypoadrenalism

Interrogation of the HPA axis is performed as part of a formal screening process for hypopituitarism in patients with organic hypothalamic-pituitary disease such as those with sellar/parasellar tumours, post pituitary surgery or apoplexy, history of cranial irradiation or traumatic brain injury. In other situations the assessment may be triggered by suggestive symptoms such as fatigue, unexplained weight loss, spontaneous hypoglycaemia or hyponatraemia.

Timing of assessment
ACTH suppression from exogenous steroids

ACTH suppression and subsequent cortisol deficiency can result from chronic glucocorticoid use, can be unpredictable regardless of dose and duration of glucocorticoid and recovery can take weeks to years [4, 9]. Patients on long-term glucocorticoids for inflammatory conditions are frequently referred to specialist endocrine services for assessment of possible ACTH suppression. As prednisone can cross-react with the cortisol assay we suggest waiting until the patient is tapered to a dose of 5 mg at which point they are switched to an equivalent dose hydrocortisone 10 mg twice daily and a dynamic test can be carried out with the dose held the afternoon before and morning of the test.

Pituitary surgery/apoplexy

All patients with sellar/parasellar tumours should be subjected to an assessment of HPA axis function, with perhaps the exception of those with pituitary microadenomas who are at a very low risk of ACTH deficiency. Patients should undergo post-operative interrogation of the HPA axis regardless of whether they had pre-operative

ACTH deficiency as there is potential for these patients to gain functional recovery providing that viable normal pituitary tissue remains in situ [10].

ACTH deficiency is the most common deficit observed in pituitary apoplexy occurring in 50–80 % of cases [11]. Due to its high frequency and potentially life-threatening effects, empiric parenteral corticosteroid is administered, when possible preceeded by blood drawing for serum cortisol levels. Pituitary function can recover following surgical decompression [12, 13]. Therefore post-operative re-assessment of the HPA axis is required.

A 08.00 h plasma cortisol can be measured on day 1–3 post-operatively in patients not treated with glucocorticoids and day 3–5 in patients covered with glucocorticoids once the dose is tapered down to physiological replacement [14] with the second dose of hydrocortisone given early in the afternoon (if hydrocortisone is used) and the morning dose of hydrocortisone not given until after the sample is drawn. However, there are conflicting opinions regarding what constitutes a safe level of 08.00 h plasma cortisol [15–17]. Patients with a 08.00 h unstressed cortisol of >400 nmol/L have an extremely low risk of ACTH deficiency and no further dynamic testing of the HPA axis is required [18, 19]. Conversely, patients with a post-operative 08.00 h cortisol of <100 nmol/L are invariably ACTH deficient and glucocorticoid replacement should be commenced. Patients with a 08.00 h cortisol between these values require definitive testing [17].

The alternative, and our preferred, approach is to routinely perform a dynamic test of HPA axis function 6–8 weeks post-operatively. This has the advantage of facilitating early discharge of patients post-operatively on empiric glucocorticoid replacement rather than waiting for day 3–5 cortisol values and may better identify those patients with later recovery of cortisol secretion.

Traumatic brain injury

Hypopituitarism is a common occurrence among survivors of severe or moderate traumatic brain injury (TBI) with an estimated prevalence of 11–35 % among adult long term survivors [20]. Acute post TBI central hypoadrenalism is potentially life-threatening [21] and has shown to be associated with increased mortality [7]. In the acute post-traumatic phase morning cortisol measurements should be carried out on those with moderate (GCS 9-12) or severe TBI (GCS ≤ 8) or those with clinical features suggestive of ACTH deficiency ie. hypotension, hypoglycaemia or hyponatraemia. Patients should also be tested in the post-acute phase between 3–6 months after the event as early abnormalities can recover while new deficiencies may become apparent later [22].

Post cranial radiation

Hypopituitarism is a recognised consequence of cranial radiation both for pituitary and non-pituitary brain tumours. Its onset is dose and time dependent. The HPA axis seems to be the most radio-resistant site in patients who have undergone irradiation for non-pituitary disorders. Clinically apparent ACTH deficiency is uncommon (3 %) in patients receiving a total radiation dose of less than 50Gy to the hypothalamic-pituitary (HP) axis. The incidence dramatically increases in those receiving more intensive radiotherapy [23, 24] and is highest in those receiving pituitary radiotherapy for pituitary tumors [25]. It is our practice to routinely screen patients from 1 year post cranial radiation and annually thereafter unless a diagnosis of ACTH deficiency is made.

Choice of test

The choice of the most appropriate test for the assessment of alterations in the HPA axis remains an area of considerable debate. The "ideal test" is one which is convenient, non-expensive, without side-effects while having a high degree of reproducibility and diagnostic sensitivity and specificity. Morning cortisol may be useful if it is clearly low or clearly healthy. In the appropriate clinical context, an early morning cortisol less than 100 nmol/L suggests a requirement for glucocorticoid replacement, while a level greater than 390–400 nmol/L strongly suggests an intact HPA axis [26, 27]. Most patients however require a dynamic assessment of the HPA axis (see Table 2).

Insulin tolerance test

The insulin tolerance test (ITT) is regarded by many endocrinologists as the gold standard for interrogation of the hypothalamic pituitary axis. Hypoglycemic stress is a major stimulant of the HPA axis. In a seminal study in 1969, Plumpton and Besser showed that a normal cortisol response to ITT predicts an appropriate cortisol response during major surgery in both healthy and corticosteroid-treated patients [28]. Therefore normal response to ITT is highly reassuring (Fig. 1).

The ITT is performed under supervision by intravenous injection of 0.15 units/kg (0.1 units/kg if high suspicion of hypocortisolism, 0.2units/kg in insulin resistant states such as diabetes mellitus or acromegaly) soluble insulin with measurement of plasma cortisol at 0, 30, 45, 60, 90 and 120 min. Adequate hypoglycemia (blood glucose <2.2 mmol/L) with symptoms must be achieved to validate the test. The test has the advantage of also robustly assessing growth hormone (GH) production [29].

Contraindications to the ITT include history of seizures (particularly relevant in assessment of patients post TBI, subarachnoid haemorrhage (SAH) or with structural brain abnormalities who may have increased risk of

Table 2 Evaluating the utility of the insulin stress test (ITT), glucagon stimulation test (GST) and the short synacthen (corticotropin) test (SST)

Test	Strengths	Drawbacks
Insulin tolerance test	1. Very high sensitivity 2. Assessment of ACTH and GH axes	1. Requires experience and medical supervision 2. Labour intensive and time consuming 3. Contraindicated in ischemic heart disease and seizure disorders 4. Hypoglycaemia not always achieved 5. Unpleasant for patients
Glucagon stimulation test	1. Assessment of ACTH and GH axes 2. Can be used in cases where ITT is contra-indicated	1. Nausea in up to 30 % cases 2. False positive (fail) rate 8 % 3. Time consuming
Short synacthen (corticotropin) test	1. Simple and well tolerated 2. Can be used in cases where ITT is contraindicated 3. Reliably excludes clinically significant ACTH deficiency	1. Does not assess GH axis 2. Unreliable if recent pituitary insult e.g. surgery, apoplexy 3. Theoretical concerns of false negative (pass) rate (when compared with ITT)

seizures) and ischaemic heart disease (baseline ECG is required before performing test).

Some advocate against using the ITT in patients with a baseline cortisol of <100 nmol/L. However, Finucane et al showed the ITT to be safe in these patients and also an important diagnostic tool as 4 of 14 patients who had morning serum cortisol concentrations <100 nmol/L passed the ITT and remained well during long-term follow-up without glucocorticoid replacement [26]. Some centres recommend against the use of ITT in patients over age of 65 years due to safety concerns but in the previous paper none of the 9 % of patients who were over the age of 65 years had any adverse reactions to the test and we therefore do not use age as a contraindication to ITT in otherwise healthy individuals as long as the other exclusion criteria are taken into account.

Glucagon stimulation test
The glucagon stimulation test (GST) can be used to assess both the HPA and GH axes if the ITT is contraindicated, for example in those with heart disease. However the test is not usually used for the sole assessment of the HPA axis if GH assessment is not needed. Because of the false positive results, confirmatory tests (see below) are needed if the result is abnormal. 1 mg of glucagon (1.5 mg in those over 100 kgs) is given intramuscularly and samples taken for glucose, cortisol and GH at 0, 90, 120, 150 and 180 min. While the test is generally safe, up to 30 % of patients report nausea and occasional vomiting [30, 31]. Glucagon induced cortisol release has been shown to be ACTH dependent [32] but the precise mechanism of this physiological effect is not well-defined.

Short Synacthen (SST, corticotrophin)Test
Originally introduced to assess cortisol reserve in suspected primary adrenal failure (Addison's disease), this test has also gained favour among many endocrinologists for the indirect assessment of the HPA axis [33–37] in cases of suspected secondary hypoadrenalism. Its diagnostic value relies on the assumption that chronic ACTH deficiency results in adrenal atrophy and therefore diminished response to exogenous acute ACTH stimulation [38]. The SST should not be used to assess for central hypoadrenalism therefore for at least 4–6 weeks post pituitary insult (e.g. surgery or apoplexy).

The high dose SST (HDSST) test involves the intravenous or intramuscular administration of 250 mcg of Synacthen (cosyntropin, ACTH (1-24)) a truncated ACTH peptide that has full biological activity but longer half-life than native ACTH (1-39). Baseline morning serum cortisol and ACTH (if central aetiology of the suspected hypoadrenalism is not clear) are taken and then cortisol measurement repeated 30 min after ACTH is administered. Another variant of the test is the administration of low dose (1 mcg) ACTH instead aiming for better sensitivity but comparing the performances of the two doses showed them to be equivalent [39]. Furthermore 1 mcg ACTH preparations are not available hence most centres use the high dose test.

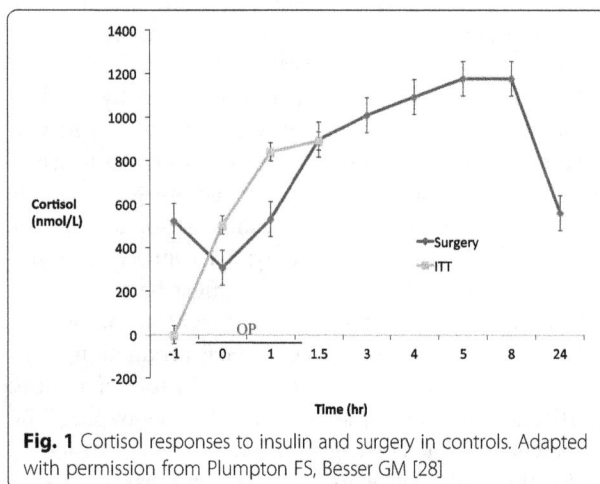

Fig. 1 Cortisol responses to insulin and surgery in controls. Adapted with permission from Plumpton FS, Besser GM [28]

CRF test

The CRF test has been proposed for the diagnosis of central adrenal insufficiency and for the distinction between secondary and tertiary adrenal insufficiency. CRF (100mcg) is injected intravenously and ACTH and cortisol measured every 15 min for 90 min. Patients with secondary adrenal failure have low ACTH levels that fail to respond to CRF while patients with tertiary (hypothalamic) failure show a prolonged and exaggerated rise in ACTH levels following CRF. The CRF test is not widely used to assess the HPA axis due to its unacceptably low sensitivity [40].

Overnight metyrapone test

The overnight metyrapone test assesses the negative feedback rather than stress related cortisol responses by utilizing the capacity of metyrapone to inhibit 11β-hydroxylase, the enzyme responsible for the conversion of 11-deoxycortisol to cortisol, thereby stimulating ACTH production and consequently increasing 11-deoxycortisol levels. While some studies have reported the metyrapone test to be reliable [41], other authors raised concerns about its sensitivity and specificity when using the traditional post-metyrapone 11-deoxycortisol level >200 nmol/L to define normality [42]. The diagnostic accuracy of the metyrapone test can be improved by integrating cortisol and ACTH levels with 11-deoxycortisol measurements [42]. Nevertheless, the assay for 11-deoxycortisol is a manual assay and is not available in most laboratories which limits the use of this test particularly as first line in the assessment of the HPA axis.

Clinical and analytical considerations and caveats

As mentioned above, the SST should be avoided in the acute phase after a pituitary insult. The 30 min cortisol response to synacthen is the one which correlates with the peak cortisol response to hypoglycaemia [39]. The increment response to either the ITT or SST is less important than the absolute post-stimulation response which should be used to define normality.

Defining a normal cortisol response to hypoglycemia is a matter of contention. The study by Plumpton and Besser used a fluorimetric (Mattingly) method to measure serum cortisol and suggested a cut-off value of 580 nmol/L (20 ug/dl) for a normal response [28]. However, it is recognised that the fluorometric method reported a cortisol concentration that is 20 % higher than more modern immunoassays. More recent studies using contemporary cortisol assays redefined the normal cutoff for cortisol response to the ITT to closer to 500 nmol/L [43, 44] with one recent study suggesting a peak cortisol level of 414 nmol (14.8 ug/dl) to ITT to be the minimum acceptable cut-off value for healthy individuals [45]. In our institution we use a cut-off value of 500 nmol/L (18 ug/L) to define a normal response to ITT.

Normative cut-off values for peak cortisol in the GST are not easy to define but values between 450–500 nmol/l are appropriate. The GST is associated with an 8 % false positive (false fail) rate [31] especially when the baseline cortisol > 400 nmol/l.

Over the years, some endocrinologists have raised concerns that the SST may not be sensitive enough to diagnose central hypoadrenalism leading to missed diagnoses. This was based on studies comparing the cortisol response to hypoglycaemia with synacthen and finding that some patients who "failed" the ITT passed the SST. Unfortunately these studies have many limitations including failure to define normative cut-offs for ITT and or the SST locally in some studies (see below), issues regarding poor reproducibility with the ITT and use of the 60 min rather the 30 min response for the SST. In addition, it is well known that the ITT errs on the side of caution and probably overdiagnoses adrenal insufficiency as some patients do not show a normal cortisol response to hypoglycaemia but show a healthy response to major surgery [28].

However, studies looking at the outcome in patients who pass the SST and therefore were not given glucocorticoid replacement are reassuring. In a study of 148 hypothalamic-pituitary patients who passed the SST and were not treated with hydrocortisone, only 2 patients subsequently developed adrenal insufficiency, one with suspected evolving hypopituitarism and one who had a borderline response [36]. These results confirmed those of another similar study [37]. Therefore, when time-related clinical outcome is taken as the "gold standard" the SST rarely misses clinically significant adrenal insufficiency provided sufficient time has lapsed between the pituitary insult and testing [44].

For the SST, the cut-off for normality has been shown to be assay dependent, and therefore should be determined in each unit based on responses in healthy controls [46]. In our institution, we use 500 nmol/l as cutoff for normal cortisol response, with peak levels of 500–550 nmol/L interpreted to be safe for the purpose of withholding routine glucocorticoid therapy but these patients are prescribed stress dose glucocorticoids in times of intercurrent illness [36].

Dynamic tests assess ACTH/cortisol reserves rather than the adequacy of cortisol production from day-to-day under normal physiological conditions. Hence patients with partial or borderline responses may not need day-to-day glucocorticoid replacement as they have been shown to have normal cortisol production under unstressed physiological conditions [47]. As a precaution they should receive sick days glucocorticoid therapy [36].

Borderline results are often difficult to interpret. The ITT and the SST are not mutually exclusive and in some cases both tests can be used to rule in or rule out adrenal insufficiency when one test alone is borderline or when the test result does not support the clinical context. For example a patient with a pituitary tumour or after pituitary surgery with healthy morning cortisol level but a sub-optimal cortisol response to hypoglycaemia and otherwise normal anterior pituitary function is unlikely to have adrenal insufficiency and therefore a SST can be useful to verify or vice versa.

Analytical issues are also important when interpreting the result of a dynamic test. Reproducibility of the ITT has been shown to be 79 % compared with 88 and 83 % for the GST and the low dose ACTH stimulation test respectively [48]. Mean coefficient of variation of cortisol response to ITT is between 7–10 % and repeat cortisol values may differ by over 100 nmol/L [49–51]. No test correctly identifies all cases and borderline results should be interpreted in the clinical context. Failing to diagnose ACTH deficiency can have potentially life threatening consequences leading to adrenal crisis but over-zealous diagnosis can lead to unnecessary or over-treatment which has negative consequences for bone and metabolic health [52, 53].

Normative values should be derived locally as the cortisol response is both stimulus and assay-dependent. In one study by Clark et al, the 5th percentile 30 min cortisol response to the SST ranged from 510 to 626 nmol/L depending on which of four different assays was used [46]. In a study of 129 patients comparing ITT, GST and low dose synacthen testing Simsek et al would have to treat 75, 65 and 40 % of the patients with glucocorticoids if they used the same cut-off of 500 mmol/L to diagnose central hypoadrenalism using these tests [48]. Furthermore, in clinical practice, laboratories measure total rather than the biologically active free cortisol. In situations where significant alterations in binding proteins exist, total cortisol measurement can be grossly misleading leading to misdiagnosis. For example septic patients have low levels of CBG and albumin hence their total cortisol measurement is much lower relative to their free cortisol measured by equilibrium dialysis [54] while patients taken estrogen will have an elevation in their total cortisol relative to free cortisol due to increased levels of binding proteins [55].

Conclusion

The choice of test used to interrogate the HPA axis should be individualised for each patient and the results interpreted within clinical context and with understanding of potential pitfalls of the test used. An alternative test should be performed if the result is borderline and clinical suspicion is high. Clinical vigilance is required and patients should be made aware of the symptoms and signs of adrenal insufficiency so that assessment can be repeated if necessary. The results should be interpreted rationally and those with apparent borderline normal/abnormal results or values suggestive of partial ACTH deficiency could be treated with short courses of stress dose of glucocorticoids during incurrent illness only.

Abbreviations

ACTH, adrenocorticotropic hormone; CBG, cortisol binding globulin; CRF, corticotropin releasing factor; DHEA, dehydroepandrosterone; ECG, electrocardiogram; GH, growth hormone; GST, glucagon stimulation test; HDSST, high dose short synacthen test; HP, hypothalamic pituitary; HPA, hypothalamic pituitary adrenal; ITT, insulin tolerance test; MPHD, multiple pituitary hormone deficiencies; POMC, proopiomelanocortin; SAH, subarachnoid haemorrhage; SST, short synacthen test; TBI, traumatic brain injury; TSH, thyroid stimulating hormone

Acknowledgements

None.

Funding

Not applicable.

Authors' contributions

AG performed a literature review of the topic, prepared the manuscript and approved the final manuscript. AA provided a critical review of the the the manuscript and approved the final manuscript.

Competing interests

The authors declare that they have no competing interests.

References

1. Raffin-Sanson ML, de Keyzer Y, Bertagna X. Proopiomelanocortin, a polypeptide precursor with multiple functions: from physiology to pathological conditions. Eur J Endocrinol. 2003;149(2):79–90.
2. Lehoux JG, Fleury A, Ducharme L. The acute and chronic effects of adrenocorticotropin on the levels of messenger ribonucleic acid and protein of steroidogenic enzymes in rat adrenal in vivo. Endocrinology. 1998;139(9):3913–22.
3. Grossman AB. Clinical Review#: The diagnosis and management of central hypoadrenalism. J Clin Endocrinol Metab. 2010;95(11):4855–63.
4. Dinsen S, Baslund B, Klose M, Rasmussen AK, Friis-Hansen L, Hilsted L, et al. Why glucocorticoid withdrawal may sometimes be as dangerous as the treatment itself. Eur J Intern Med. 2013;24(8):714–20.
5. Molitch ME. Nonfunctioning pituitary tumors and pituitary incidentalomas. Endocrinol Metab Clin N Am. 2008;37(1):151–71. xi.
6. Caturegli P, Newschaffer C, Olivi A, Pomper MG, Burger PC, Rose NR. Autoimmune hypophysitis. Endocr Rev. 2005;26(5):599–614.
7. Hannon MJ, Crowley RK, Behan LA, O'Sullivan EP, O'Brien MM, Sherlock M, et al. Acute glucocorticoid deficiency and diabetes insipidus are common after acute traumatic brain injury and predict mortality. J Clin Endocrinol Metab. 2013;98(8):3229–37.
8. Sherlock M, Reulen RC, Alonso AA, Ayuk J, Clayton RN, Sheppard MC, et al. ACTH deficiency, higher doses of hydrocortisone replacement, and

radiotherapy are independent predictors of mortality in patients with acromegaly. J Clin Endocrinol Metab. 2009;94(11):4216–23.

9. Livanou T, Ferriman D, James VH. Recovery of hypothalamo-pituitary-adrenal function after corticosteroid therapy. Lancet (London, England). 1967;2(7521):856–9.

10. Arafah BM, Kailani SH, Nekl KE, Gold RS, Selman WR. Immediate recovery of pituitary function after transsphenoidal resection of pituitary macroadenomas. J Clin Endocrinol Metab. 1994;79(2):348–54.

11. Briet C, Salenave S, Bonneville JF, Laws ER, Chanson P. Pituitary Apoplexy. Endocr Rev. 2015;36(6):622–45.

12. Arafah BM, Harrington JF, Madhoun ZT, Selman WR. Improvement of pituitary function after surgical decompression for pituitary tumor apoplexy. J Clin Endocrinol Metab. 1990;71(2):323–8.

13. Bujawansa S, Thondam SK, Steele C, Cuthbertson DJ, Gilkes CE, Noonan C, et al. Presentation, management and outcomes in acute pituitary apoplexy: a large single-centre experience from the United Kingdom. Clin Endocrinol. 2014;80(3):419–24.

14. Inder WJ, Hunt PJ. Glucocorticoid replacement in pituitary surgery: guidelines for perioperative assessment and management. J Clin Endocrinol Metab. 2002; 87(6):2745–50.

15. Hout WM, Arafah BM, Salazar R, Selman W. Evaluation of the hypothalamic-pituitary-adrenal axis immediately after pituitary adenomectomy: is perioperative steroid therapy necessary? J Clin Endocrinol Metab. 1988;66(6):1208–12.

16. Auchus RJ, Shewbridge RK, Shepherd MD. Which patients benefit from provocative adrenal testing after transsphenoidal pituitary surgery? Clin Endocrinol. 1997;46(1):21–7.

17. Courtney CH, McAllister AS, McCance DR, Bell PM, Hadden DR, Leslie H, et al. Comparison of one week 0900 h serum cortisol, low and standard dose synacthen tests with a 4 to 6 week insulin hypoglycaemia test after pituitary surgery in assessing HPA axis. Clin Endocrinol. 2000;53(4):431–6.

18. Jayasena CN, Gadhvi KA, Gohel B, Martin NM, Mendoza N, Meeran K, et al. Day 5 morning serum cortisol predicts hypothalamic-pituitary-adrenal function after transsphenoidal surgery for pituitary tumors. Clin Chem. 2009;55(5):972–7.

19. Klose M, Lange M, Kosteljanetz M, Poulsgaard L, Feldt-Rasmussen U. Adrenocortical insufficiency after pituitary surgery: an audit of the reliability of the conventional short synacthen test. Clin Endocrinol. 2005;63(5):499–505.

20. Schneider HJ, Kreitschmann-Andermahr I, Ghigo E, Stalla GK, Agha A. Hypothalamopituitary dysfunction following traumatic brain injury and aneurysmal subarachnoid hemorrhage: a systematic review. JAMA. 2007; 298(12):1429–38.

21. Agha A, Sherlock M, Thompson CJ. Post-traumatic hyponatraemia due to acute hypopituitarism. QJM. 2005;98(6):463–4.

22. Agha A, Phillips J, O'Kelly P, Tormey W, Thompson CJ. The natural history of post-traumatic hypopituitarism: implications for assessment and treatment. Am J Med. 2005;118(12):1416.

23. Agha A, Sherlock M, Brennan S, O'Connor SA, O'Sullivan E, Rogers B, et al. Hypothalamic-pituitary dysfunction after irradiation of nonpituitary brain tumors in adults. J Clin Endocrinol Metab. 2005;90(12):6355–60.

24. Constine LS, Woolf PD, Cann D, Mick G, McCormick K, Raubertas RF, et al. Hypothalamic-pituitary dysfunction after radiation for brain tumors. N Engl J Med. 1993;328(2):87–94.

25. Rush S, Cooper PR. Symptom resolution, tumor control, and side effects following postoperative radiotherapy for pituitary macroadenomas. Int J Radiat Oncol Biol Phys. 1997;37(5):1031–4.

26. Finucane FM, Liew A, Thornton E, Rogers B, Tormey W, Agha A. Clinical insights into the safety and utility of the insulin tolerance test (ITT) in the assessment of the hypothalamo-pituitary-adrenal axis. Clin Endocrinol. 2008;69(4):603–7.

27. Hagg E, Asplund K, Lithner F. Value of basal plasma cortisol assays in the assessment of pituitary-adrenal insufficiency. Clin Endocrinol. 1987;26(2): 221–6.

28. Plumpton FS, Besser GM. The adrenocortical response to surgery and insulin-induced hypoglycaemia in corticosteroid-treated and normal subjects. Br J Surg. 1969;56(3):216–9.

29. Biller BM, Samuels MH, Zagar A, Cook DM, Arafah BM, Bonert V, et al. Sensitivity and specificity of six tests for the diagnosis of adult GH deficiency. J Clin Endocrinol Metab. 2002;87(5):2067–79.

30. Agha A, Rogers B, Sherlock M, O'Kelly P, Tormey W, Phillips J, et al. Anterior pituitary dysfunction in survivors of traumatic brain injury. J Clin Endocrinol Metab. 2004;89(10):4929–36.

31. Rao RH, Spathis GS. Intramuscular glucagon as a provocative stimulus for the assessment of pituitary function: growth hormone and cortisol responses. Metab Clin Exp. 1987;36(7):658–63.

32. Littley MD, Gibson S, White A, Shalet SM. Comparison of the ACTH and cortisol responses to provocative testing with glucagon and insulin hypoglycaemia in normal subjects. Clin Endocrinol. 1989;31(5):527–33.

33. Stewart PM, Corrie J, Seckl JR, Edwards CR, Padfield PL. A rational approach for assessing the hypothalamo-pituitary-adrenal axis. Lancet (London, England). 1988;1(8596):1208–10.

34. Crowley RK, Argese N, Tomlinson JW, Stewart PM. Central hypoadrenalism. J Clin Endocrinol Metab. 2014;99(11):4027–36.

35. Kazlauskaite R, Evans AT, Villabona CV, Abdu TA, Ambrosi B, Atkinson AB, et al. Corticotropin tests for hypothalamic-pituitary- adrenal insufficiency: a metaanalysis. J Clin Endocrinol Metab. 2008;93(11):4245–53.

36. Agha A, Tomlinson JW, Clark PM, Holder G, Stewart PM. The long-term predictive accuracy of the short synacthen (corticotropin) stimulation test for assessment of the hypothalamic-pituitary-adrenal axis. J Clin Endocrinol Metab. 2006;91(1):43–7.

37. Gleeson HK, Walker BR, Seckl JR, Padfield PL. Ten years on: Safety of short synacthen tests in assessing adrenocorticotropin deficiency in clinical practice. J Clin Endocrinol Metab. 2003;88(5):2106–11.

38. Lindholm J, Kehlet H. Re-evaluation of the clinical value of the 30 min ACTH test in assessing the hypothalamic-pituitary-adrenocortical function. Clin Endocrinol. 1987;26(1):53–9.

39. Dorin RI, Qualls CR, Crapo LM. Diagnosis of adrenal insufficiency. Ann Intern Med. 2003;139(3):194–204.

40. Schmidt IL, Lahner H, Mann K, Petersenn S. Diagnosis of adrenal insufficiency: Evaluation of the corticotropin-releasing hormone test and Basal serum cortisol in comparison to the insulin tolerance test in patients with hypothalamic-pituitary-adrenal disease. J Clin Endocrinol Metab. 2003;88(9):4193–8.

41. Fiad TM, Kirby JM, Cunningham SK, McKenna TJ. The overnight single-dose metyrapone test is a simple and reliable index of the hypothalamic-pituitary-adrenal axis. Clin Endocrinol. 1994;40(5):603–9.

42. Berneis K, Staub JJ, Gessler A, Meier C, Girard J, Muller B. Combined stimulation of adrenocorticotropin and compound-S by single dose metyrapone test as an outpatient procedure to assess hypothalamic-pituitary-adrenal function. J Clin Endocrinol Metab. 2002;87(12):5470–5.

43. Gonzalbez J, Villabona C, Ramon J, Navarro MA, Gimenez O, Ricart W, et al. Establishment of reference values for standard dose short synacthen test (250 microgram), low dose short synacthen test (1 microgram) and insulin tolerance test for assessment of the hypothalamo-pituitary-adrenal axis in normal subjects. Clin Endocrinol. 2000;53(2):199–204.

44. Hurel SJ, Thompson CJ, Watson MJ, Harris MM, Baylis PH, Kendall-Taylor P. The short Synacthen and insulin stress tests in the assessment of the hypothalamic-pituitary-adrenal axis. Clin Endocrinol. 1996;44(2):141–6.

45. Cho HY, Kim JH, Kim SW, Shin CS, Park KS, Kim SW, et al. Different cut-off values of the insulin tolerance test, the high-dose short Synacthen test (250 mug) and the low-dose short Synacthen test (1 mug) in assessing central adrenal insufficiency. Clin Endocrinol. 2014;81(1):77–84.

46. Clark PM, Neylon I, Raggatt PR, Sheppard MC, Stewart PM. Defining the normal cortisol response to the short Synacthen test: implications for the investigation of hypothalamic-pituitary disorders. Clin Endocrinol. 1998; 49(3):287–92.

47. Paisley AN, Rowles SV, Brandon D, Trainer PJ. A subnormal peak cortisol response to stimulation testing does not predict a subnormal cortisol production rate. J Clin Endocrinol Metab. 2009;94(5):1757–60.

48. Simsek Y, Karaca Z, Tanriverdi F, Unluhizarci K, Selcuklu A, Kelestimur F. A comparison of low-dose ACTH, glucagon stimulation and insulin tolerance test in patients with pituitary disorders. Clin Endocrinol. 2015;82(1):45–52.

49. Nye EJ, Grice JE, Hockings GI, Strakosch CR, Crosbie GV, Walters MM, et al. The insulin hypoglycemia test: hypoglycemic criteria and reproducibility. J Neuroendocrinol. 2001;13(6):524–30.

50. Pfeifer M, Kanc K, Verhovec R, Kocijancic A. Reproducibility of the insulin tolerance test (ITT) for assessment of growth hormone and cortisol secretion in normal and hypopituitary adult men. Clin Endocrinol. 2001;54(1):17–22.

51. Vestergaard P, Hoeck HC, Jakobsen PE, Laurberg P. Reproducibility of growth hormone and cortisol responses to the insulin tolerance test and the short ACTH test in normal adults. Horm Metab Res. 1997;29(3): 106–10.

52. Suliman AM, Freaney R, Smith TP, McBrinn Y, Murray B, McKenna TJ. The impact of different glucocorticoid replacement schedules on bone

turnover and insulin sensitivity in patients with adrenal insufficiency. Clin Endocrinol. 2003;59(3):380–7.

53. Sherlock M, Behan LA, Hannon MJ, Alonso AA, Thompson CJ, Murray RD, et al. The modulation of corticosteroid metabolism by hydrocortisone therapy in patients with hypopituitarism increases tissue glucocorticoid exposure. Eur J Endocrinol. 2015;173(5):583–93.

54. Hamrahian AH, Oseni TS, Arafah BM. Measurements of serum free cortisol in critically ill patients. N Engl J Med. 2004;350(16):1629–38.

55. Brien TG. Human corticosteroid binding globulin. Clin Endocrinol. 1981; 14(2):193–212.

18

A modified M-stage classification based on the metastatic patterns of pancreatic neuroendocrine neoplasms

Xianbin Zhang[1,2*†] (iD), Jiaxin Song[3†], Peng Liu[1], Mohammad Abdul Mazid[1], Lili Lu[3], Yuru Shang[1], Yushan Wei[4], Peng Gong[5] and Li Ma[3,6*]

Abstract

Background: The present study aims to improve the M-stage classification of pancreatic neuroendocrine neoplasms (pNENs).

Methods: Two thousand six hundred sixty six pNENs were extracted from the Surveillance, Epidemiology, and End Results database to explore the metastatic patterns of pNENs. Metastatic patterns were categorized as single, two, or multiple (three or more) distant organ metastasis. The mean overall survival and hazard rate of different metastatic patterns were calculated by Kaplan-Meier and Cox proportional hazards models, respectively. The discriminatory capability of the modified M-stage classification was evaluated by Harrell's concordance index.

Results: The overall survival time significantly decreased with an increasing number of metastatic organs. In addition, pNENs with only liver metastasis had better prognosis when compared to other metastatic patterns. Thus, we modified the M-stage classification (mM-stage) as follows: mM_0-stage, tumor without metastasis; mM_1-stage, tumor only metastasized to liver; mM_2-stage, tumor metastasized to other single distant organ (lung, bone, or brain) or two distant organs; mM_3-stage, tumor metastasized to three or more distant organs. Harrell's concordance index showed that the modified M-stage classification had superior discriminatory capability than both the American Joint Committee on Cancer (AJCC) and the European Neuroendocrine Tumor Society (ENETS) M-stage classifications.

Conclusions: The modified M-stage classification is superior to both AJCC and ENETS M-stage classifications in the prognosis of pNENs. In the future, individualized treatment and follow-up programs should be explored for patients with distinct metastatic patterns.

Keywords: Metastasis, Survival, Prognosis, Pancreas, Cancer

Background

Pancreatic neuroendocrine neoplasms (pNENs) are relatively rare tumors. However, a recent population study showed that the incidence of pNENs increased more than 4-fold from 1973 to 2012 [1]. Moreover, pNENs are considered the most serious neuroendocrine neoplasms (NENs), due to the patients have a shorter median overall survival times (3.6 years) when compared to those with tumors located in lung (5.5 years), rectum (24.6 years), and appendix (more than 30.0 years) [1].

Cancer staging classification systems are used to codify the extent of cancer. They allow clinicians to quantify prognosis and plan treatment for individual patients. Two widely used tumor staging classification systems, which are proposed by the American Joint Committee on Cancer (AJCC) and the European Neuroendocrine Tumor Society (ENETS), describe M_0-stage as having no distant metastasis and M_1-stage as having at least one

* Correspondence: zhangxianbin@hotmail.com; mali_lele@sina.com
†Xianbin Zhang and Jiaxin Song contributed equally to this work.
[1]The First Affiliated Hospital of Dalian Medical University, Zhongshan 222, Dalian 116011, China
[3]Department of Epidemiology, Dalian Medical University, Lvshun West 9, Dalian 116044, China
Full list of author information is available at the end of the article

distant metastasis [2, 3]. However, several studies demonstrated that pNENs with liver metastasis have better prognosis than other metastatic patterns [4–6].

Therefore, we utilized the Surveillance, Epidemiology, and End Result (SEER) database to explore the prognosis of different metastatic patterns of pNENs and propose a modified M-stage classification. This modified M-stage classification proves to be superior to both AJCC and ENETS M-stage classifications in prognosis.

Methods
Study cohort
As published previously [3], we utilized the topography codes (C25.0 to C25.9) and histology codes (8150, 8151, 8152, 8153, 8154, 8155, 8156, 8157, 8240, 8241, 8242, 8243, 8244, 8245, 8246, and 8249) of the International Classification of Diseases for Oncology (third edition) to identify pNENs.

Outcomes and variables
The primary outcome was overall survival. Demographic data included age, sex, and race; tumor characteristics included tumor size, primary site, differentiation, 7th AJCC T-stage, and N-stage; treatment information included surgery and radiotherapy. Single organ metastasis was defined as the tumor spreading from pancreas to another single distant organ [7]. Similarly, two organ metastases were defined as the tumor spreading from pancreas to two distant organs. Tumors spreading from pancreas to three or more distant organs were defined as multiple metastases.

Inclusion and exclusion criteria
Patients microscopically diagnosed as pNENs were included in the present study. We excluded cases with

unclear or incomplete information about metastasis. In addition, we also excluded cases without information about survival time.

Statistical analyses
To compare the constituent ratio of variables among patients, we broke the continuous variables (age, tumor size) into binary variables. Survival time was plotted using the Kaplan-Meier estimator and Cox proportional hazards model. The results were presented as mean and hazard ratio, respectively, each with a 95% confidence interval (CI). Harrell's concordance index was used to evaluate the discriminatory capability of the modified M stage classification. An index value of greater than 0.70 suggests the classification has an acceptable discriminatory capability [8]. Differences with $P \leq 0.05$ divided by the number of meaningful comparisons, Bonferroni correction, were considered to be significant. Differences with $P \leq 0.1$ divided by the number of meaningful comparisons, were considered to indicate a tendency. All statistical analyses were performed using SPSS 19.0 (IBM, New York, USA) or R (version 3.5.0).

Results
Patient characteristics
In total, 2666 patients (mean age 60.9 years ±13.6 years; 55.7% male, 78.8% white) were included in the present study (Fig. 1). Many patients (55.4%) underwent surgery, and some (4.7%) were treated with radiation. The constituent ratios of tumor size, location, differentiation, T-stage, and N-stage were significantly ($P < 0.05$) different between patients with and without metastasis (Table 1).

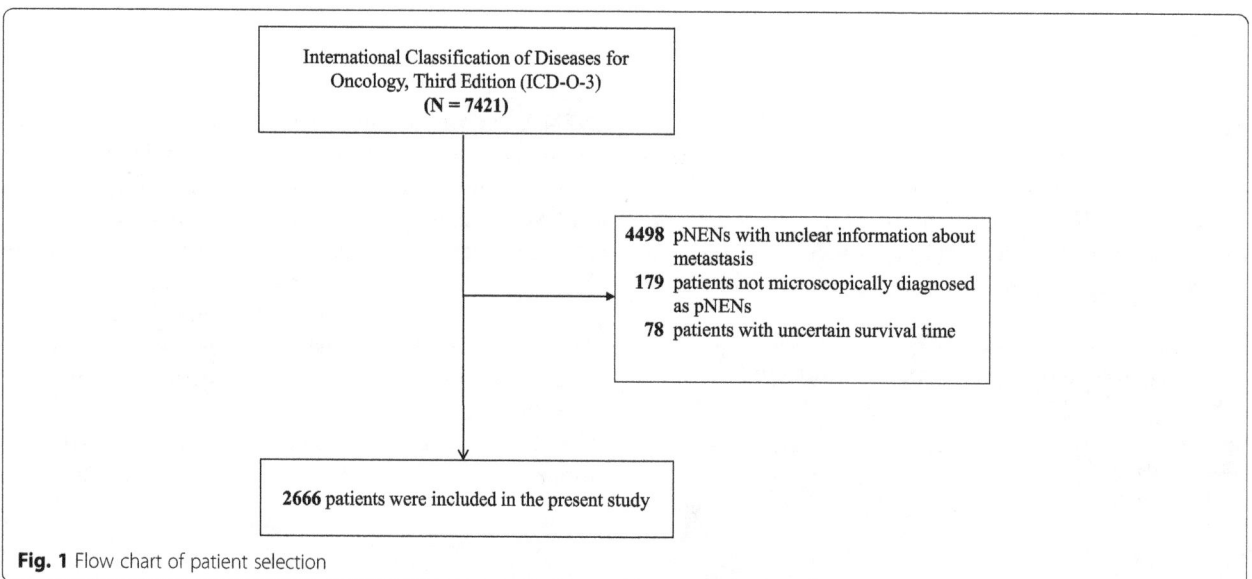

Fig. 1 Flow chart of patient selection

Table 1 Clinicopathological Characters

	Without Metastasis N = 1679	Metastasis N = 987	P
Age (years)			0.221[b]
≤ 60	793 (47.2%)	442 (44.8%)	
> 60	886 (52.8%)	545 (55.2%)	
Sex			0.338[a]
Male	924 (55.0%)	562 (56.9%)	
Female	755 (45.0%)	425 (43.1%)	
Race			0.011[a]
White	1314 (78.3%)	787 (79.7%)	
Black	191 (11.4%)	130 (13.2%)	
Other	174 (10.3%)	70 (7.1%)	
Size (cm)			< 0.001[b]
≤ 2	670 (39.9%)	68 (6.9%)	
> 2	934 (55.6%)	699 (70.8%)	
Unclear	75 (4.5%)	220 (22.3%)	
Primary Site			< 0.001[b]
Head	502 (29.9%)	258 (26.2%)	
Body	295 (17.6%)	106 (10.7%)	
Tail	542 (32.3%)	314 (31.8%)	
Other	340 (20.2%)	309 (31.3%)	
Differentiation			< 0.001[b]
Well	1043 (62.1%)	189 (19.1%)	
Moderately	221 (13.2%)	86 (8.7%)	
Poorly	64 (3.8%)	95 (9.6%)	
Undifferentiated	17 (1.0%)	28 (2.8%)	
Unclear	334 (19.9%)	589 (59.7%)	
T-sage			< 0.001[b]
T_1	602 (35.9%)	37 (3.7%)	
T_2	538 (32.0%)	276 (28.0%)	
T_3	389 (23.2%)	271 (27.5%)	
T_4	67 (4.0%)	102 (10.3%)	
Tx	83 (4.9%)	301 (30.5%)	
N-stage			< 0.001[b]
N_0	1247 (74.3%)	463 (46.9%)	
N_1	401 (23.9%)	338 (34.3%)	
Nx	31 (1.8%)	186 (18.8%)	
Surgery			< 0.001[b]
Yes	1313 (78.2%)	164 (16.6%)	
No	339 (20.2%)	813 (82.4%)	
Unclear	27 (1.6%)	10 (1.0%)	
Radiation			< 0.001[b]
Yes	52 (3.1%)	74 (7.5%)	
No	1609 (95.8%)	905 (91.7%)	
Unclear	18 (1.1%)	8 (0.8%)	

[a]Chi-square test; [b]Kruskal-Wallis test

Metastatic patterns and survival

At the time of diagnosis, 1679 (62.98%) patients showed no metastasis. As shown in Fig. 2a, single organ metastases comprised 850 (31.88%) patients, including 817 liver (30.64%), 22 lung (0.83%), nine bone (0.34%), and two brain (0.07%) cases. One hundred and twelve patients (4.20%) showed two-organ metastases, including 52 liver plus bone (1.95%), 53 liver plus lung (1.99%), four bone plus lung (0.15%), two liver plus brain (0.08%), and one bone plus brain (0.04%) cases. Twenty-five patients (0.94%) presented multiple organ metastases, including 19 cases of liver plus lung plus bone (0.71%), three cases of liver plus lung plus brain (0.11%), and three cases of liver plus lung plus brain plus bone (0.11%).

To assess survival time of different metastatic patterns, we compared the survival time of patients without metastasis to those with single distant organ metastasis, two-organ metastases, and multiple organ metastases. As the number of metastatic organs increased, survival time was significantly ($P < 0.001$) reduced (Fig. 2b). In addition, patients with only liver metastasis had a longer survival time than did other single-organ metastases (Fig. 2c), whereas patients with bone, lung or two-organ metastasis had similar mean survival time (bone, 18.32 months ± 5.27 months; lung, 17.77 months ± 3.54 months, two organs metastases, 15.79 months ± 1.70 months).

Modified M-stage classification and discriminatory capability

Thus, based on the observed metastatic patterns and survival times, we modified the M-stage classification (mM-stage) as shown in Table 2. Tumor without metastasis was defined as mM_0-stage. Tumor spread from pancreas only to liver was defined as mM_1-stage. Tumor spreading from pancreas to other single distant organ or to two distant organs was defined as mM_2-stage. Tumor spreading to three or more distant organs was defined as mM_3-stage.

To evaluate survival time among mM-stage classifications, survival curves were plotted using the Kaplan-Meier estimator and then compared with the log-rank test. We observed that all survival curves were well separated (Fig. 2d). Patients with advanced mM stages (mM_1, mM_2, mM_3) had significantly ($P < 0.001$) shorter survival times than patients with mM_0-stage (Fig. 2e). Moreover, the modified M-stage classification was an independent prognostic factor for pNENs, after adjusting for other clinical and pathological characteristics (Table 3).

To explore discriminatory capability of the modified M-stage classification, Harrell's concordance index was calculated. The mM-stage classification had a better discriminatory capability (Harrell's concordance index, 0.712; 95% CI, 0.692–0.732) than AJCC M-stage and

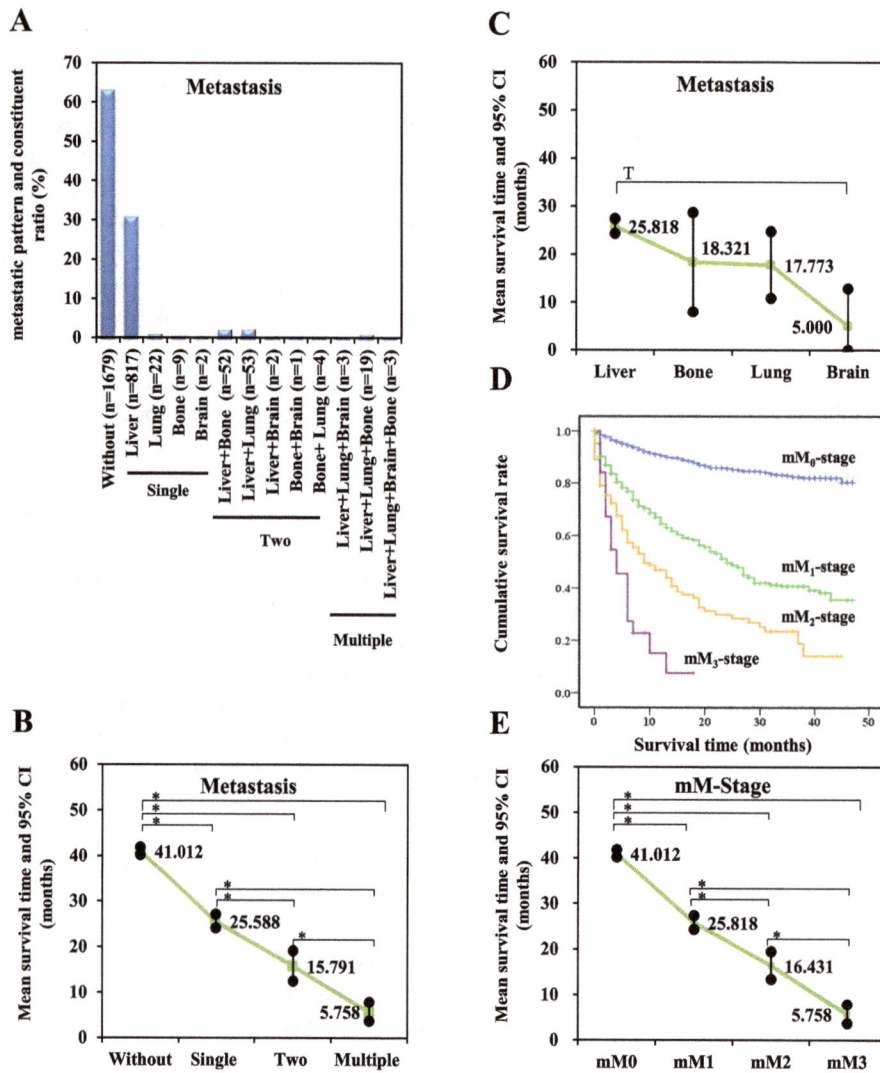

Fig. 2 a Metastatic patterns of pNENs. **b** Survival time of patients different metastatic patterns. **c** Survival time of patients with single distant organ metastasis. **d** Kaplan-Meier curve of overall survival of patients with modified M-stage classification. **e** Survival time of patients with modified M-stage classification. * Significant difference: $P < 0.008$; ^{T} Tendentious difference: $P < 0.017$

ENETS M-stage (Harrell's concordance index, 0.697; 95% CI, 0.678–0.717).

Discussion

In agreement with previous studies [9–11], the present study also demonstrated that nearly one quarter of patients (37.02%, 987/2666) presenting metastasis at the time of pNEN diagnosis. In addition, liver metastasis was the majority metastatic pattern, followed by lung, bone and brain metastasis. The hematogenous mode of metastasis might contribute to the metastatic pattern, which we have observed in the present study. Usually, carcinoma cells seed in the liver via the portal venous system. Then, these cells would spread to lung via the inferior vena cava and pulmonary arteries. Finally, the carcinoma cells from lung metastases would seed in other organs via arterial blood [12].

Table 2 Definition of M-stage classifications

AJCC and ENTES M-stage classifications	Modified M-stage classifications
M_0-stage, no distant metastasis	mM_0-stage, no distant metastasis
M_1-stage, distant metastasis	mM_1-stage, only liver metastasis
	mM_2-stage, other single distant organ or two organs metastases
	mM_3-stage, three or more organs metastases

AJCC American Joint Committee on Cancer; *ENETS* European Neuroendocrine Tumor Society

Table 3 Independent Prognostic Factors

	Univariate		Multivariate	
	HR and 95% CI	*P*-value	HR and 95% CI	*P*-value
Age (years)				
≤ 60	Reference		Reference	
> 60	1.875 (1.595–2.204)	< 0.001	1.744 (1.479–2.055)	< 0.001
Sex				
Male	Reference		Reference	
Female	0.808 (0.691–0.945)	0.008	0.850 (0.726–0.996)	0.044
Race				
White	Reference		Reference	
Black	1.345 (1.082–1.670)	0.007	1.247 (0.998–1.558)	0.052
Other	0.715 (0.527–0.970)	0.031	0.767 (0.565–1.043)	0.090
Size (cm)				
≤ 2	Reference		Reference	
> 2	2.889 (2.241–3.724)	< 0.001	1.322 (1.009–1.731)	0.043
Unclear	6.799(5.110–9.047)	< 0.001	1.547(1.129–2.119)	0.007
Primary Site			a	
Head	Reference			
Body	0.684(0.530–0.884)	0.004		
Tail	0.682(0.556–0.836)	< 0.001		
Other	1.128(0.929–1.368)	0.223		
Differentiation				
Well	Reference		Reference	
Moderately	1.557 (1.095–2.215)	0.014	1.049 (0.735–1.498)	0.791
Poorly	7.414 (5.608–9.803)	< 0.001	3.349 (2.498–4.489)	< 0.001
Undifferentiated	9.494 (6.113–14.743)	< 0.001	3.166 (2.000–5.011)	< 0.001
Unclear	5.136 (4.179–6.311)	< 0.001	1.626 (1.290–2.048)	< 0.001
T-stage			a	
T_1	Reference			
T_2	3.434(2.474–4.766)	< 0.001		
T_3	3.353(2.399–4.688)	< 0.001		
T_4	7.082(4.867–10.306)	< 0.001		
Tx	9.288(6.696–12.882)	< 0.001		
N-stage				
N_0	Reference		Reference	
N_1	1.679 (1.415–1.993)	< 0.001	1.304 (1.092–1.557)	0.003
Nx	3.732 (3.019–4.613)	< 0.001	1.452 (1.152–1.829)	0.002
Surgery				
Yes	Reference		Reference	
No	8.556 (6.941–10.548)	< 0.001	3.901 (3.013–5.050)	< 0.001
Unclear	1.991 (0.812–4.883)	0.133	1.487 (0.601–3.680)	0.391
Radiation			a	
Yes	Reference			
No	1.984(1.511–2.603)	< 0.001		
Unclear	0.939(0.420–2.098)	0.878		

Table 3 Independent Prognostic Factors *(Continued)*

	Univariate		Multivariate	
	HR and 95% CI	*P*-value	HR and 95% CI	*P*-value
mM-stage				
mM$_0$-stage	Reference		Reference	
mM$_1$-stage	4.520 (3.789–5.393)	< 0.001	1.643 (1.339–2.016)	< 0.001
mM$_2$-stage	8.199(6.380–10.537)	< 0.001	2.249(1.704–2.968)	< 0.001
mM$_3$-stage	16.356 (10.266–26.059)	< 0.001	5.034 (3.110–8.150)	< 0.001

[a]variables excluded by multivariate forward stepwise cox regression

The present study found that with an increasing number of metastatic organs, there was a significant decrease in survival time. In addition, pNENs with liver metastasis had longer overall survival than other single-organ metastatic patterns. However, AJCC and ENETS classify both pNENs with liver metastasis and pNENs with the other metastasitic patterns as M$_1$-stage. Our modified M-stage classification distinguishes that tumor spreading from pancreas only to liver should be separated from the other metastatic patterns, and that it is necessary to design individualized treatment and follow-up programs for patients with lung, bone, or brain metastasis.

Usually, pancreatic resection is not performed when the pancreatic malignant tumor has spread to other organs [13]. However, considering the indolent behavior of pNENs and the high frequency of liver metastasis, several clinicians suggested surgical management could give rise to benefit to pNENs with liver metastasis [4, 14]. Birnbaum et al. pancreatic resection could slow down tumor growth and reduce hormone production [14], possibly resulting in considerable benefit for patients with liver metastasis [4].

Consistent with previous studies, the tumor size, primary site, differentiation, AJCC T-stage and AJCC N-stage were identified as predictors of distant organ metastasis (Additional file 1: Table S1). Unfortunately, SEER database did not record Ki-67 status and graded the primary tumor only on the basis of morphological description (ICD-O-3) in the pathology report. Thus, we failed to evaluate the predictive role of Ki-67 status and WHO 2010 grading classification (NET G1, NET G2, NET G3 and NEC) in distant organ metastasis.

It seems the primary tumor site is a particularly useful predictor because it is available before any operation occurs. Hao et al. reported that compared to tumors located in the head and neck of the pancreas, tumors in the body and tail showed a decreased risk of liver metastasis in pancreatic adenocarcinoma [15]. In contrast, the present study showed that pNENs located in the pancreatic tail are actually 1.728 times more likely (*P* < 0.001) to develop metastasis, as compared to tumors located in the pancreatic head. This may be due to the fact that patients with pNENs, especially non-functioning pNENs,

in the tail of the pancreas are less likely to experience obstructive signs and hormonal symptoms until tumors spread to the peritoneum, spleen, and distant organs [16, 17]. Thus, at the time of diagnosis, distant organ metastases exist in most of these patients.

Some limitations of the present study should be noted. First, the SEER database only provides information on pNEN metastasis to liver, lung, bone, and brain. The frequency of pNEN metastasis might be underestimated. Second, Hlatky et al. noted that multiple metastatic lesions may be related to a short survival time [18]. However, the SEER database did not collect data on the number of metastatic lesions in each distant organ.

Conclusions

In conclusion, this is the first population-based study to investigate the metastatic patterns and predictors in advanced pNENs. We found significant differences in survival time across different metastatic patterns. Thus, the modified M-stage classification show a better discriminatory capability than the AJCC and ENETS M-stage classifications. In the future, clinicians should determine individualized treatment and follow-up programs for pNENs with different metastatic patterns.

Abbreviations

AJCC: American Joint Committee on Cancer; ENETS: European Neuroendocrine Tumor Society; OS: Overall survival; pNENs: Pancreatic neuroendocrine neoplasms; SD: Standard deviation; SEER: Surveillance, Epidemiology, and End Result

Acknowledgments

We thank the Surveillance, Epidemiology, and End Results (SEER) program providing the original data. We also thank Prof. Wenli Zhang and Prof. Houli Zhang gave us critical comments during the revision of the manuscript.

Funding

This work was supported by the National Natural Science Foundation of China [grant number 81473504, 81200989]; China Scholarship Council [grant number 201608080195]. The funders had no any role in the manuscript.

Authors' contributions

XZ identified the pNENs from SEER database, designed the study and wrote the manuscript; XZ, JS, MM, PL, LL, YS analyzed and interpreted the data; YW is responsible for the statistical analyses; PG and LM contributed to conception, design and funding. All authors have been involved in revising and proofreading of the manuscript. All authors listed have approved the manuscript.

Competing interests

The authors declare that they have no competing interests.

Author details

[1]The First Affiliated Hospital of Dalian Medical University, Zhongshan 222, Dalian 116011, China. [2]Institute for Experimental Surgery, Rostock University Medical Center, Schillingallee 69a, 18057 Rostock, Germany. [3]Department of Epidemiology, Dalian Medical University, Lvshun West 9, Dalian 116044, China. [4]Department of Evidence-based Medicine and Statistics, the First Affiliated Hospital of Dalian Medical University, Zhongshan 222, Dalian 116011, China. [5]Department of General Surgery, the Shenzhen University General Hospital and Shenzhen University School of Medicine, Xueyuan 1098, Shenzhen 518055, China. [6]Department of Epidemiology, Dalian Medical University, Zhongshan Road 222, Dalian 116011, China.

References

1. Dasari A, Shen C, Halperin D, et al. Trends in the incidence, prevalence, and survival outcomes in patients with neuroendocrine tumors in the United States. JAMA Oncol. 2017;3:1335–42.
2. Panzuto F, Boninsegna L, Fazio N, et al. Metastatic and locally advanced pancreatic endocrine carcinomas: analysis of factors associated with disease progression. J Clin Oncol. 2011;29:2372–7.
3. Zhang X, Lu L, Shang Y, et al. The number of positive lymph node is a better predictor of survival than the lymph node metastasis status for pancreatic neuroendocrine neoplasms: a retrospective cohort study. Int J Surg. 2017;48:142–8.
4. Jin K, Xu J, Chen J, et al. Surgical management for non-functional pancreatic neuroendocrine neoplasms with synchronous liver metastasis: a consensus from the Chinese study Group for Neuroendocrine Tumors (CSNET). Int J Oncol. 2016;49:1991–2000.
5. Garcia-Carbonero R, Rinke A, Valle JW, et al. ENETS consensus guidelines for the standards of care in neuroendocrine neoplasms. Systemic therapy 2: chemotherapy. Neuroendocrinology. 2017;105:281–94.
6. Chamberlain RS, Canes D, Brown KT, et al. Hepatic neuroendocrine metastases: does intervention alter outcomes? Am Coll Surg. 2000;190:432–45.
7. Vatandoust S, Price TJ, Karapetis CS. Colorectal cancer: metastases to a single organ. World J Gastroenterol. 2015;21:11767–76.
8. Bando E, Makuuchi R, Tokunaga M, et al. Impact of clinical tumor–node–metastasis staging on survival in gastric carcinoma patients receiving surgery. Gastric Cancer. 2017;20:448–56.
9. Niederle MB, Hackl M, Kaserer K, et al. Gastroenteropancreatic neuroendocrine tumours: the current incidence and staging based on the WHO and European neuroendocrine tumour society classification: an analysis based on prospectively collected parameters. Endocr Relat Cancer. 2010;17:909–18.
10. Lawrence B, Gustafsson BI, Chan A, et al. The epidemiology of gastroenteropancreatic neuroendocrine tumors. Endocrinol Metab Clin N Am. 2011;40:1–18.
11. Pavel M, Costa F, Capdevila J, et al. ENETS consensus guidelines update for the management of distant metastatic disease of intestinal, pancreatic, bronchial neuroendocrine neoplasms (NEN) and NEN of unknown primary site. Neuroendocrinology. 2016;103:172–85.
12. Weiss L, Grundmann E, Torhorst J, et al. Haematogenous metastatic patterns in colonic carcinoma: an analysis of 1541 necropsies. J Pathol. 1986;150:195–203.
13. Partelli S, Bartsch DK, Capdevila J, et al. ENETS consensus guidelines for standard of care in neuroendocrine tumours: surgery for small intestinal and pancreatic neuroendocrine tumours. Neuroendocrinology. 2017;105:255–65.
14. Birnbaum DJ, Turrini O, Vigano L, et al. Surgical management of advanced pancreatic neuroendocrine tumors: short-term and long-term results from an international multi-institutional study. Ann Surg Onco. 2015;22:1000–7.
15. S D LW, GY B, et al. Risk factors of liver metastasis from advanced pancreatic adenocarcinoma: a large multicenter cohort study. World J Surg Oncol. 2017;15:120.
16. Freelove R, Walling AD. Pancreatic cancer: diagnosis and management. Am Fam Physician. 2006;73:485–92.
17. Zhang X, Ma L, Bao H, et al. Clinical, pathological and prognostic characteristics of gastroenteropancreatic neuroendocrine neoplasms in China: a retrospective study. BMC Endocr Disord. 2014;14:54.
18. Hlatky R, Suki D, Sawaya R. Carcinoid metastasis to the brain. Cancer. 2004; 101:2605–13.

Clinicopathological features and prognosis of gastroenteropancreatic neuroendocrine neoplasms in a Chinese population

Meng Zhang[1], Ping Zhao[1], Xiaodan Shi[1], Ahong Zhao[2], Lianfeng Zhang[1] and Lin Zhou[1]*

Abstract

Background: Gastroenteropancreatic neuroendocrine neoplasms (GEP-NENs) are the most common type of neuroendocrine tumors, accounting for more than half of neuroendocrine neoplasms (NENs). We performed a retrospective study in our center to investigate the clinicopathological features, risk factors of metastasis, and prognosis of GEP-NENs in a Chinese population.

Methods: Four hundred forty patients with GEP-NENs treated at the First Affiliated Hospital of Zhengzhou University between January 2011 and March 2016 were analyzed retrospectively. Multivariate logistic regression was performed to identify independent risk factors for metastasis of the tumors. The Kaplan-Meier method was used for survival analysis, and log-rank tests for comparisons among groups.

Results: Primary sites were the stomach (24.3%), rectum (24.1%), pancreas (20.5%), esophagus (12.3%), unknown primary origin (UPO-NEN) (8.0%), duodenum (6.1%). Three hundred eighty-nine of the 440 GEP-NENs cases (88.4%) were non-functional tumors, and patients had non-specific symptoms, which could have led to delay in diagnosis and treatment. Neuroendocrine tumor, neuroendocrine carcinoma, and mixed adenoendocrine carcinoma were 56. 8%, 33.2% and 3.2%, respectively, of the cases. One hundred thirty (29.5%) of the tumors were G1, 120 (27.3%) G2, and 190 (43.2%) G3. The immunohistochemical positive rate of synaptophysin was 97.7% and of chromogranin 48. 7%. Logistic regression analysis revealed that the diameter and pathological classification of tumors were the most important predictors for metastasis. The median survival time was 34 months for patients with well-differentiated neuroendocrine tumors grade G3 and 11 months for poorly differentiated neuroendocrine carcinoma. The median survival time of patients with localized disease, regional disease, and distant disease was 36 months, 15 month, and 6 months, respectively.

Conclusions: This study constitutes a comprehensive analysis of the clinicopathological features of GEP-NENs in a Chinese population. GEP-NENs may occur at any part of the digestive system. The diameter and pathological classification of tumor are the most important predictors for metastasis. The prognosis is poor for patients with poorly differentiated neuroendocrine cancers and distant metastases.

Keywords: Neuroendocrine neoplasms, Neuroendocrine tumors, Gastro enteropancreatic neuroendocrine tumors, Neuroendocrine cancers, Carcinoid tumor, Gastrinoma, Islet cell tumor

* Correspondence: ZL372@126.com
[1]Department of Gastroenterology, the First Affiliated Hospital of Zhengzhou University, No.1, East Jianshe Road, Zhengzhou 450052, China
Full list of author information is available at the end of the article

Background

Neuroendocrine neoplasms (NENs), which originate from neuroendocrine cells, comprise a heterogeneous family with a broad spectrum of clinical behavior [1]. The neoplasms occur in diverse sites throughout the body, and more than half are gastroenteropancreatic NENs (GEP-NENs) [2]. According to the Surveillance, Epidemiology, End Results database (SEER), which has the largest epidemiologic series, the incidence of NENs has risen substantially over the past 30 years [2]. Although the prevalence of GEP-NENs seems to be increasing in China, there is no accurate database of the characteristics of GEP- NENs in Chinese patients.

In 2010, the World Health Organization [3] proposed a new classification of NENs, with comparisons of clinical, pathological, therapeutic, and prognostic factors. In western countries, the epidemiology, treatment, and survival rates of NENs have been well-studied [1, 2], but comparable information in Asian populations is limited [4, 5]. In order to investigate the clinical pathological characteristics, risk factors of metastasis, and prognosis of NENs in a Chinese population, we performed a comprehensive retrospective review of the recent 5-year experience with this disease in our center.

Methods

Patients

The study was conducted on 440 patients from the First Affiliated Hospital of Zhengzhou University between January 2011 and March 2016. The study was approved by the hospital's Ethics Committee, and informed consent was obtained from all patients. All patients had received a pathological diagnosis of GEP-NENs according to the World Health Organization classification [3] and the China Consensus Guideline [6]. Collected information consisted of clinical characteristics (gender, age, location of tumors, and symptoms); diagnostic procedures (endoscopic and radiographic); tumor characteristics (size, grading, histopathology of primary tumor, metastases); treatments; and follow-up.

The pathological diagnosis of the NENs depended on typical morphological findings and immunohistochemical staining of chromogranin (CgA) and/or synaptophysin (Syn) [7]. Grading was based on morphological criteria and tumor proliferative activity. According to the Ki-67 index, the grading was G1, G2 and G3 $\leq$ 2%, 3 $\sim$ 20%, >20%, respectively. Similarly, tumors with mitotic rates of less than two in 10 high-power fields (HPF) were classified as G1, 2 $\sim$ 20/HPF as G2, and >20/HPF as G3. If the grading of the Ki-67 index differed from that of the mitotic rate, the higher of the two was given priority. Therefore, GEP-NENs were classified as neuroendocrine tumor (NET) (G1 and G2), neuroendocrine carcinoma (NEC) (G3), and mixed adenoendocrine carcinoma (MANEC) (G3) [3, 4]. The well-differentiated G3 NENs (Ki-67 positive index >20%; generally less than 60%) were classified as well-differentiated NET (NET G3) [8, 9].

Statistical analysis

All statistical analyses were performed using SPSS 17.0 for Windows (IBM Corporation. Armonk, NY, USA). Normally distributed continuous variables were expressed as mean and standard deviation, and statistical differences between groups were assessed with the independent samples t-tests. Differences in categorical variables were compared with chi-square test or Fisher 's exact test. Multivariate logistic regression was performed to identify independent risk factors for tumor metastasis. Overall survival was defined as the time from diagnosis to death or, in living patients, the time to last follow-up. Survival curves were drawn according to the Kaplan-Meier method, and differences between subgroups were assessed with the log-rank test. P-values<0.05 were considered statistically significant.

Results

Clinical features

Among the 440 patients with GEP-NENs, 259 (58.9%) were men and 181 (41.1%) were women; the male to female ratio was 1.43. Ages ranged from 9 to 86 years, and the mean age was (54.3 $\pm$ 13.5) years. The mean age of men was (55.5 $\pm$ 13.5), women was (52.7 $\pm$ 13.3). The most common tumor site was the stomach (24.3%, 107/440), followed by the rectum (24.1%, 106/440), pancreas (20.5%, 90/440), esophagus (12.3%, 54/440), unknown primary origin (UPO-NEN) (8.0%, 35/440), duodenum (6.1%, 27/440), and other sites: appendix, jejunum/ileum, and colon (4.7%, 21/440).

Non-functional tumors comprised the majority of GEP-NENs (389/440, 88.4%); the other 51 (11.6%) were functional. The most frequent initial presentation was abdominal pain (101/440, 23%), which was not specific for the diagnosis of tumor, followed by dysphagia (45/440, 10.2%), bleeding (38/440, 8.6%), diarrhea (19/440, 4.3%), jaundice (16/440, 3.6%), and abdominal distention. Forty-one (9.3%) cases were found during routine physical examination. Insulinoma comprised 90.2% (46/51) of functional tumors, all of which were located in the pancreas, and typical symptoms were those of hypoglycemia and epileptic seizure. Seven patients with insulinoma were treated as epilepsy before the diagnosis of NENs, and 2 cases were initially treated as psychiatric disorders. The other functional tumors were gastrinoma (3/51, 5.9%) and glucagonoma (2/51, 3.9%), expressed as multiple refractory peptic ulcer, diarrhea, secondary diabetes mellitus and cutaneous erythema. There was no patient presented with carcinoid syndrome in our study.

Imaging studies

The results of imaging examinations are summarized in Table 1. All imaging examinations can be found in any grade of tumors. Endoscopy, endoscopic ultrasound (EUS) and positron emission computed tomography imaging (PET-CT, using with 18F-FDG) were positive in >90% of cases. Magnetic resonance imaging was the least often positive (79.5%). But MRI and PET-CT, was performed in only about 10% of patients, respectively. MRI is mainly used for the detection of pancreatic and liver tumors and PET-CT for tumors in any part of the digestive system. EUS was performed on 41 patients, of which a lesion was found in 38 patients. At endoscopy, which is used for the detection of gastrointestinal tract tumors, the GEP-NENs usually appeared as ulcers or polypoid prominences. Ultrasound and endoscopic ultrasound (EUS) usually revealed the GEP-NENs as hypoechoic and well-vascularized masses. By computed tomography (CT) and magnatic resonance imaging (MRI), the tumors appeared as local space-occupying lesions, with heterogeneous enhancement on contrast-enhanced CT. PET-CT usually revealed high glucose metabolism in GEP-NENs, especially in poorly differentiated NENs. Seven tumors, initially identified in the liver, were found located in the pancreas by EUS-guided fine-needle biopsy.

Histopathologic characteristics

The histopathologic characteristics (size, World Health Organization 2010 classification, and metastases) of the 440 GEP-NENs are given in Table 2. The most common tumor type was NET (250, 56.8%), followed by NEC (146, 33.2%) and MANEC (14, 3.2%); the other 30 cases of G3 were classified as NET G3. Local infiltration and lymphatic metastasis occurred in 63% (277/440) and 12.3% (54/440) of patients, respectively. Distant metastases were found in 90 (20.5%) patients at initial diagnosis; during follow-up, the number increased to 109 (24.8%). Distant metastases were present at initial diagnosis in 38.4% (73/190) of patients with G3 tumors. The most

frequent site of distant metastasis was liver (67/109, 61.5%), followed by peritoneum (18.3%, 20/109), lung (10.1%, 11/109) and bone (6.4%, 7/109). Among the 67 patients with liver metastases, 55 presented with synchronous lesions and 12 with metachronous lesions during follow-up. The positive rates of immunohistochemistry of Syn and CgA were 97.7% (416/426) and 48.7% (135/277, respectively.

The clinicopathologic characteristics related to metastasis were listed in Table 3. The risk factors of GEP-NENs metastases were then analyzed by the logistic regression method. Multivariate logistic regression analysis revealed that the diameter and pathological classification of tumors were the most important predictors for metastasis (Table 4).

Therapeutic interventions

About two-thirds of the patients (62.5%; 275/440) underwent an operation with curative intent or palliation; 50 patients were treated with endoscopic radical surgery, mainly for rectal lesions. Seventy-three patients received chemotherapy, 34 of whom received postoperative adjuvant chemotherapy. The combination of cisplatin and etoposide was the most widely used chemotherapeutic agents. Six patients received octreotide, a somatostatin analogue, as a biological therapy combined with surgery or chemotherapy. Local-regional therapies, such as transcatheter hepatic arterial chemoembolization, radiofrequency, or other ablative techniques were used in eight patients.

Survival and prognostic factors

Four hundred fourteen of the 440 patients were followed for periods of 3–60 months. Due to the short follow-up time and a low number of deaths in NET (G1 and G2) patients, median survival time was not obtained for them during the observation period. The 1-, 3- and 5- year survival rates of all patients were 78.7%, 60.8% and 54.5, respectively. The 1-, 3- and 5- year survival rates of patients with G3 lesions were 54.3%, 19.4% and 7.8%, respectively. The major causes of death were tumor-related complications (82.7%), treatment-related adverse events (13.4%), and other diseases (3.9%). For patients with G3 NENs, age, gender, primary tumor site, differentiation, and characterization of metastasis were analyzed in order to identify prognostic factors for survival (Table 5). Univariate analysis confirmed that patients with NET G3 and patients without regional or distant metastasis survived longer than did other patients with NENs G3, but age, gender, and primary tumor site had no discernable impact on overall survival. Median overall survival among all the patients with G3 NENs was 13.0 months, and survival was significantly longer for these patients (median 34 months) than for those with NEC (median 11 months). Median overall survival of patients with

Table 1 Characteristics of imaging studies

Imaging study	Site	Cases tested (n)	Positive tests	
			n	%
Endoscopy	gastrointestinal	226	224	99.1%
EUS	pancreas, duodenum, stomach	41	38	92.7%
Ultrasound	pancreas, liver, biliary tree	165	143	86.7%
CT scan	all of above	321	274	85.4%
MRI	pancreas, liver	39	31	79.5%
FDG PET-CT	all of above	29	27	93.1%

EUS endoscopic ultrasonography, *CT* computed tomography, *MRI* magnetic resonance imaging, *FDG PET-CT* fluorodeoxyglucose positron emission computed tomography imaging

Table 2 Histopathological characteristics of the GEP-NENs ($n = 440$)

	Stomach $n = 107$	Esophagus $n = 54$	Duodenum $n = 27$	Jejunum/ileum $n = 8$	Colon $n = 5$	Appendix $n = 8$	Rectum $n = 106$	UPO-NEN $n = 35$	Pancreas $n = 90$	Total $n = 440(\%)$
Size										
<2 cm	24	5	15	1	0	3	67	4	37	156(35.5)
2 ~ 4 cm	12	10	3	2	0	0	2	6	16	51(11.6)
>4 cm	31	12	3	3	2	1	1	8	11	72(16.4)
Unclear	40	27	6	2	3	4	36	17	26	161(36.6)
WHO2010										
G1	17	0	6	1	1	5	70	3	27	130(29.5)
G2	21	1	11	2	0	2	26	7	50	120(27.3)
G3	69	53	10	5	4	1	10	25	13	190(43.2)
Metastases										
Local	43	16	18	4	2	8	94	19	73	277(63)
Loco-regional	28	14	1	2	1	0	3	4	1	54(12.3)
Distant	36	24	8	2	2	0	9	12	16	109(24.8)

Table 3 Clinicopathological characteristics related to metastasis

Pathologic characteristics	Total	Metastasis	Non-metastasis	χ^2	P
Sex					
Male	259	112(43.2%)	147(56.8%)	10.370	<0.01
Female	181	51(28.2%)	130(71.8%)		
Age					
≤ 50	158	33 (20.9%)	125 (79.1%)	27.602	<0.01
>50	282	130 (46.1%)	152 (53.9%)		
Site					
Stomach	107	64(59.8%)	43(40.2%)	67.249	<0.01
Rectum	106	12(11.3%)	94(88.7%)		
Pancreas	90	17(18.9%)	73(81.1%)		
Functional status					
Functional	51	2 (3.9%)	49 (96.1%)	25.556	<0.01
Nonfunctional	389	161 (41.4%)	228 (58.6%)		
Tumor diameter					
≤ 2 cm	156	14(9.0%)	142(91.0%)	80.879	<0.01
2-4 cm	51	23(45.1%)	28(54.9%)		
≥ 4 cm	72	47(65.3%)	25(34.7%)		
Tumor grading					
G1	130	4(3.1%)	126(96.9%)	182.475	<0.01
G2	120	22(18.3%)	98(81.7%)		
G3	190	137(72.1%)	53(27.9%)		
Tumor type					
NET	250	26(10.4%)	224(89.6%)	182.746	<0.01
NEC	146	113(77.4%)	33(22.6%)		
MANEC	14	8 (57.1%)	6 (42.9%)		

Table 4 The logistic regression for the relationship between the clinicopathological characteristics and metastasis

Variable	Coefficient	Standard Error	Wald χ^2	P	Odds ratio	95%CI	
Tumor diameter	0.790	0.239	10.909	0.001	2.203	1.379	3.521
Grading	1.998	0.326	37.510	<0.01	7.373	3.890	13.974
Constant	−6.887	0.811	72.106	<0.01	0.001	–	–

localized G3 NENs was 36 months, 15 months for patients with regional disease, and 6 months for patients with distant disease. Survival curves are displayed in Fig. 1, a-f.

Discussion

This retrospective study explored the clinicopathological characteristics, risk factors of metastasis, treatment, and prognosis of GEP-NENs in a relatively large population of Chinese patients. Tumors located at any possible site within the digestive system were analyzed. In addition, the NENs G3 were classified as NET G3 (well-differentiated NET with a G3 grading) or NEC, and the prognoses of these were compared. The study will contribute to establishing a database of the epidemiology, clinical pathological features, treatment, and prognosis of GEP-NENs in Chinese or Asian patients. It also will permit comparisons between GEP-NENS in these populations and those in western nations.

As others have reported [2], we found that most NENs are present in the gastrointestinal tract. The distribution of GEP-NENs in our population (stomach > rectum > pancreas > duodenum) was similar to that found in Korean [10], Japanese [11], and other Chinese populations [4, 12, 13]. A large-scale analysis of GEP-NENs in the SEER database from the United States in North America found that the rectum and jejunum/ileum were the most common sites for NENs [2]. Ethnic, regional and sample-size differences may lead to differences in the reported distribution of the primary sites of GEP-NENs.

NENs can be classified as functional and non-functional tumors according to the presence or absence of symptoms associated with hormone overproduction [14]. In this study, the majority of tumors were non-functional, which may have led to misdiagnosis or delay in making the diagnosis and treating the patients promptly. The study found also that insulinoma comprised the largest number of functional NENs and accounted for about one-half of all NENs. None of the patients presented with carcinoid syndrome due to overproduction of 5-hydroxytryptamine, a finding similar to a low reported frequency of these tumors in Asian

Table 5 Overall survivals of G3-NENs

Factors	Overall survival				
	Number	Mean(months)	95%CI	χ^2	P
All patients	180	13	10.9-15.1		
Sex				2.386	0.122
Male	123	14	11.7-16.3		
Female	57	11	6.4-15.6		
Age				0.466	0.495
≤ 50	32	16	11.2-20.8		
>50	148	13	11.0-15.0		
Site				0.520	0.771
Gastrointestinal tract	143	13.5	11.8-15.2		
Pancreas	13	8	5.0-11.0		
Others	24	12	2.9-21.1		
Differentiation				9.186	0.002
NEC	137	11	8.5-13.5		
NET G3	30	34	10.7-57.3		
Metastasis				85.305	0.000
Local	48	36	25.9-46.1		
Loco-reginal	45	15	13.9-16.2		
Distant	71	6	4.7-7.3		

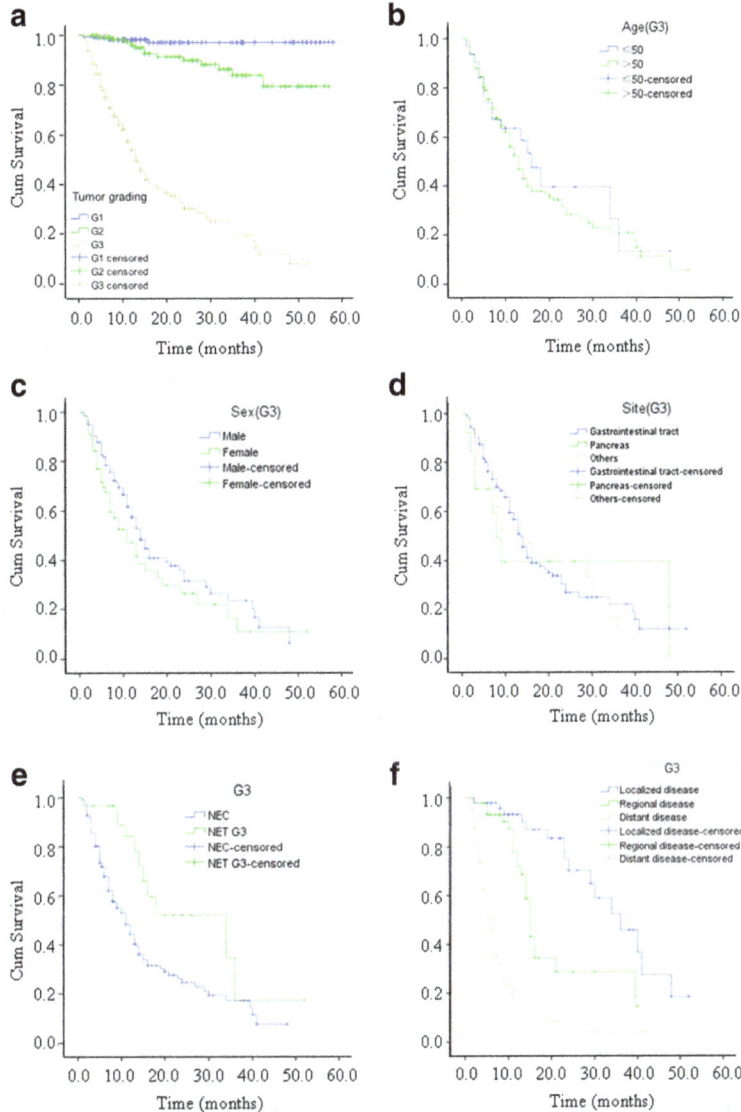

Fig. 1 Kaplan-Meier analysis of overall survival. **a** Overall survival by histological grading. **b** Overall survival by age of of patients with G3 tumors. **c** Overall survival by sex of patient with G3 tumors. **d** Overall survival by site of G3 tumors. **e** Overall survival by differentiation of G3 tumors. **f** Overall survival by characteristics of metastasis of G3 tumors

populations [4, 12, 13]. However, the incidence of carcinoid syndrome (11.5% to 31.1%) in the Western population is relatively high [15–17]. Carcinoid syndrome occurs mainly in the neuroendocrine neoplasms of jejunum/ileum. In the western population, the proportion of neuroendocrine neoplasms of jejunum/ileum is high, which is only 1.8% in our study. These data also indicated that functional NENs were mainly located in the pancreas, and the gastrointestinal neuroendocrine neoplasms were mainly non-functional. Several studies have used serum CgA as a circulating biomarker of GEP-NENs, with sensitivity and specificity rates in the range of 60% to 100% [18]. Serum CgA was mot measured in our series, but we favor measuring it since it is a simple

screening test and can shorten the time needed to make the diagnosis of a NEN.

Since non-functional GEP-NENs in the early stage often have no specific symptoms, imaging examinations are especially important in locating the tumors and assessing their extent. CT scan was the most frequently used imaging modality, whereas endoscopy had the highest yield of tumor detection (99.1%). Because of its convenience and non-invasive nature, ultrasound was chosen as the first screening method for solid organs, where the detection rate was 87%. EUS provides unique advantages in evaluating the upper gastrointestinal tract and pancreas, especially for tumors less than 1.0 cm in diameter and micrometastases [19]. The 92.3% detection rate of GEP-NENs in our series is within the range (91.9% to 97.4%) reported by others [4, 13]. The most common primary site of metastatic liver NENs is the pancreas, so EUS-guided fine-needle biopsy of the pancreas in patients with metastatic liver NENs is helpful for early detection of the primary lesion. Somatostatin receptor scintigraphy is considered a comprehensive imaging modality for many neuroendocrine tumors [20, 21], but, unfortunately, this method is not available in our institution.

The definitive diagnosis of GEP-NENs depends on the pathological analysis of biopsy, including cell morphology and immunohistochemical staining. The World Health Organization revised its nomenclature and classification of GEP-NENs in 2010 [3], and China reported its own classification system soon thereafter [6]. Rates of positive immunohistochemical staining for Syn (97.7%) and CgA (48.7%) in our series indicate that Syn has high sensitivity, and CgA has high specificity [22].

In our series, the rate of distant metastases (20.5% initially and 24.8% during follow-up) was modestly lower than the rate reported from Spain (44%) [23] but in the range reported from the United States (21%) [2] and in other Chinese series (10.4% to 23.0%) [4, 12, 13]. The liver was the most frequent site of metastatic tumors. The rate of distant metastases at diagnosis was high, which indicates that GEP-NENs, especially the nonfunctional tumors, were occult, a characteristic that could have led to delayed diagnosis and increased risk of metastasis. The rate of transfer factors of GEP-NENs was related to location of the primary tumors, with the metastasis rate of gastric NENs significantly higher than that of pancreatic or rectal tumors. The reported rate of metastasis of pancreatic NENs (69.2%) in a Western population [24] was higher than in our series (18.9%); the possible reasons for this difference could be differences in the ratio of non-functional to functional pancreatic NENS, with differences in time duration between onset of symptoms and diagnosis, or sample size. Also, we admit that the rate of missed diagnosis of pancreatic NENs in China may be high.

Surgical treatment is the first choice for GEP-NENs, even if there are nodal or distant metastases. When possible, the primary tumor should be removed, lymph nodes dissected, and distant metastases excised [25]. In this study, 275 patients underwent surgical treatment, including radical surgery and palliative surgery, with 50 patients treated by endoscopy. Early diagnosis is crucial in order that resection can be performed before local invasion or distant disease occurs.

Chemotherapy is the first treatment option for poorly differentiated or rapidly progressive, advanced GEP-NENs. In our series, as in other reports [26], the combination of cisplatin and etoposide was the most widely used chemotherapy regimen. Radiofrequency ablation, transcatheter hepatic arterial chemoembolization, or other ablative treatments, which can be used to treat liver lesions, were used in only 8 patients in our series, and only 6 patients were treated with biological therapy. Limited financial resources in our area may have contributed to the infrequent use of newer or experimental therapies for GEP-NENs such as peptide receptor radionuclide therapy and targeted agents.

The prognosis of GEP-NENs is more favorable than that of adenocarcinomas of the digestive system. In our series, the overall 5-year survival rate was 54.5%, which is similar to that quoted the SEER registry and in Chinese data [2, 4], but lower than the rate in some Europe countries [23]. These differences may be due to the ethnic, regional, or simple-size differences. Due to the short follow-up time and a low number of deaths in NET (G1 and G2) patients, we did not determine median survival times during the observation period, and limited our survival estimates to patients with NENs G3; their 5-year survival rate was 7.8%, which is similar to rates of 6%–11% in European series [27]. Very few data comparing NET G3 and NEC are available [8, 9]. In our series, there was a significant difference in the survival time between the G3 NET and NEC (34 months vs 11 months), which are similar results to those of other series [9, 28, 29]. While most NENs G3 are poorly differentiated, a subgroup of well-differentiated NET with G3 grading is not reflected in the latest Word Health Organization classification. It has been suggested that these two high-grade cancers differ in prognosis, somatostatin receptor scintigraphy uptake and response to chemotherapy regimens [29, 30] and therefore should be classified separately. The small size of our series of NET G3 tumors precluded doing a multivariate analysis to estimate their independent prognostic factors; evaluation in a larger population of such tumors is needed. Unsurprisingly, we found that distant metastasis of GEP-NENs was associated with a poor outcome; thus, early diagnosis of the tumors is very important in improving patients' prognosis.

Conclusions

The results of this study provide a comprehensive analysis of the clinicopathological features of GEP-NENs in a Chinese population. It was found that GEP-NENs may originate from any part of the digestive system, and the majority are non-functional tumors, whose early symptoms are occult, thus often resulting in delay in the diagnosis being made. Tumor diameter and classification are important factors in predicting metastasis. The prognosis of GEP-NENs is more favorable than that of gastrointestinal carcinomas, but the prognosis is poor for patients with high-grade poorly differentiated NEC and distant metastases. It is our hope that this extensive analysis of GEP-NENs will improve physicians' knowledge of the tumors and result in earlier recognition and treatment for Chinese patients. And limited financial resources in our area may lead to the infrequent use of newer or experimental therapies for GEP-NENs. Perhaps this could be a probable explanation on poorer prognosis compared to Western data.

Abbreviations
CgA: Chromogranin; CT: Computed tomography; EUS: endoscopic ultrasound; GEP-NENs: Gastroenteropancreatic neuroendocrine neoplasms; HPF: High-power fields; MANEC: Mixed adenoendocrine carcinoma; MRI: Magnatic resonance imaging; NEC: Neuroendocrine carcinoma; NENs: Neuroendocrine neoplasms; NET G3: Well-differentiated NET with a G3 grading; NET: Neuroendocrine tumor; PET-CT: positron emission computed tomography imaging; SEER: Surveillance, Epidemiology, End Results database; Syn: Synaptophysin; WHO: World Health Organization

Acknowledgements
Not applicable.

Funding
This work was support by National Nature Science Foundation of China (81,472,325; 81,001,103), and Health, Science and Technology Chuang-Xin Talent Program of Henan Province, and Youth Innovation Fund of the First Affiliated Hospital of Zhengzhou University.

Authors' contributions
LZ conceived and designed the study. MZ, AHZ and LFZ collected pathological data and analyzed the data. MZ, PZ and XDS collected clinical data. MZ wrote the original draft of the manuscript. All co-authors revised and approved the current manuscript.

Competing interests
The authors declare that they have no competing interests.

Author details
[1]Department of Gastroenterology, the First Affiliated Hospital of Zhengzhou University, No.1, East Jianshe Road, Zhengzhou 450052, China. [2]Department of Pathology, the First Affiliated Hospital of Zhengzhou University, No.1, East Jianshe Road, Zhengzhou 450052, China.

References
1. Modlin IM, Lye KD, Kidd M. A 5-decade analysis of 13,715 carcinoid tumors. Cancer. 2003;97(4):934–59.
2. Yao JC, Hassan M, Phan A, Dagohoy C, Leary C, Mares JE, Abdalla EK, Fleming JB, Vauthey JN, Rashid A. One hundred years after "carcinoid": epidemiology of and prognostic factors for neuroendocrine tumors in 35,825 cases in the United States. J Clin Oncol. 2008;26(18):3063–72.
3. Bosman FT, Carneiro F, Hruban RH, Theise ND. WHO classification of tumours of the digestive system; 2010. p. 1089.
4. Wang Y-h, Lin Y, Xue L, Wang J-h, Chen M-h, Chen J. Relationship between clinical characteristics and survival of gastroenteropancreatic neuroendocrine neoplasms: A single-institution analysis (1995-2012) in South China. BMC Endocr Disord. 2012;12(1):1–9.
5. Lim T, Lee J, Kim JJ, Lee JK, Lee KT, Kim YH, Kim KW, Kim S, Sohn TS, Dong WC. Gastroenteropancreatic neuroendocrine tumors: Incidence and treatment outcome in a single institution in Korea. Asia Pac J Clin Oncol. 2011;7(7):293–9.
6. Chinese Pathologic Consensus Group for Gastrointestinal and Pancreatic Neuroendocrine N. Chinese pathologic consensus for standard diagnosis of gastrointestinal and pancreatic neuroendocrine neoplasm. Chinese Journal of Pathology. 2011;40(4):257–62.
7. Erickson LA, Lloyd RV. Practical markers used in the diagnosis of endocrine tumors. Adv Anat Pathol. 2004;11(4):175–89.
8. Coriat R, Walter T, Terris B, Couvelard A, Ruszniewski P. Gastroenteropancreatic Well-Differentiated Grade 3 Neuroendocrine Tumors: Review and Position Statement. Oncologist. 2016;21(10):1191–9.
9. Heetfeld M, Chougnet CN, Olsen IH, Rinke A, Borbath I, Crespo G, Barriuso J, Pavel M, O'Toole D, Walter T. Characteristics and treatment of patients with G3 gastroenteropancreatic neuroendocrine neoplasms. Endocr Relat Cancer. 2015;22(4):657–64.
10. Cho MY, Kim JM, Jin HS, Kim MJ, Kim KM, Kim WH, Kim H, Kook MC, Park DY, Lee JH. Current Trends of the Incidence and Pathological Diagnosis of Gastroenteropancreatic Neuroendocrine Tumors (GEP-NETs) in Korea 2000-2009: Multicenter Study. Chin J Cancer Res. 2012;44(3):157–65.
11. Ito T, Sasano H, Tanaka M, Osamura RY, Sasaki I, Kimura W, Takano K, Obara T, Ishibashi M, Nakao K. Epidemiological study of gastroenteropancreatic neuroendocrine tumors in Japan. J Gastroenterol. 2010;45(2):234–43.
12. Jiao X, Li Y, Wang H, Liu S, Zhang D, Zhou Y. Clinicopathological features and survival analysis of gastroenteropancreatic neuroendocrine neoplasms: a retrospective study in a single center of China. Chin J Cancer Res. 2015; 27(3):258–66.
13. Zeng YJ, Liu L, Wu H, Lai W, Cao JZ, Xu HY, Wang J, Chu ZH. Clinicopathological features and prognosis of gastroenteropancreatic neuroendocrine tumors: analysis from a single-institution. Asian Pac J Cancer Prev. 2013;14(10):5775–81.
14. Klimstra DS, Modlin IR, Adsay NV, Chetty R, Deshpande V, Gonen M, Jensen RT, Kidd M, Kulke MH, Lloyd RV. Pathology reporting of neuroendocrine tumors: application of the Delphic consensus process to the development of a minimum pathology data set. Am J Surg Pathol. 2010;34(3):300–13.
15. Pape UF, Böhmig M, Berndt U, Tiling N, Wiedenmann B, Plöckinger U. Survival and Clinical Outcome of Patients with Neuroendocrine Tumors of the Gastroenteropancreatic Tract in a German Referral Center. Ann N Y Acad Sci. 2004;1014(1):222–33.
16. Pape UF, Berndt U, Müllernordhorn J, Böhmig M, Roll S, Koch M, Willich SN, Wiedenmann B. Prognostic factors of long-term outcome in gastroenteropancreatic neuroendocrine tumours. Endocr Relat Cancer. 2008; 15(4):1083–97.
17. Ploeckinger U, Kloeppel G, Wiedenmann B, Lohmann R. The German NET-registry: an audit on the diagnosis and therapy of neuroendocrine tumors. Neuroendocrinology. 2009;90(4):349–63.
18. Diaz Perez JA, Curras Freixes M. Chromogranin A and neuroendocrine tumors. Endocrinologia y nutricion: organo de la Sociedad Espanola de Endocrinologia y Nutricion. 2013;60(7):386–95.
19. Iug S, Solodinina EN, Egorov AV, Shishkin KV, Novozhilova AV, Kurushkina NA. Endoscopic ultrasonography in the diagnosis of neuroendocrine tumors of the pancreas. Eksp Klin Gastroenterol. 2009;10:37–45.
20. Hofman MS, Lau WF, Hicks RJ. Somatostatin receptor imaging with 68Ga DOTATATE PET/CT: clinical utility, normal patterns, pearls, and pitfalls in interpretation. Radiographics. 2015;35(2):500–16.
21. Geijer H, Breimer LH. Somatostatin receptor PET/CT in neuroendocrine tumours: update on systematic review and meta-analysis. Eur J Nucl Med Mol Imaging. 2013;40(11):1770–80.
22. O'Toole D, Grossman A, Gross D, Delle FG, Barkmanova J, O'Connor J, Pape UF, Plöckinger U. ENETS Consensus Guidelines for the Standards of Care in Neuroendocrine Tumors: biochemical markers. Neuroendocrinology. 2009; 90(2):194–202.
23. Garcia-Carbonero R, Capdevila J, Crespo-Herrero G, Diaz-Perez JA, Martinez Del Prado MP, Alonso Orduna V, Sevilla-Garcia I, Villabona-Artero C, Beguiristain-Gomez A, Llanos-Munoz M. Incidence, patterns of care and prognostic factors for outcome of gastroenteropancreatic neuroendocrine tumors (GEP-NETs): results from the National Cancer Registry of Spain (RGETNE). Ann Oncol. 2010;21:1794–803.
24. Panzuto F, Nasoni SM, Corleto VD, Capurso G, Cassetta S, Di FM, Tornatore V, Milione M, Angeletti S, Cattaruzza MS. Prognostic factors and survival in endocrine tumor patients: comparison between gastrointestinal and pancreatic localization. Endocr Relat Cancer. 2005;12(4):1083–92.

25. Falconi M, Bettini R, Scarpa A, Capelli P, Pederzoli P: Surgical strategy in the treatment of gastrointestinal neuroendocrine tumours. Ann Oncol 2001, 12 **suppl 2**(12 Suppl 2):S101-S103.

26. Garciacarbonero R, Jimenezfonseca P, Teulé A, Barriuso J, Sevilla I. SEOM clinical guidelines for the diagnosis and treatment of gastroenteropancreatic neuroendocrine neoplasms (GEP-NENs) 2014. Clin Transl Oncol. 2014;16(12):1025-34.

27. Lepage C, Ciccolallo LAR, Bouvier AM, Faivre J, Gatta G. European disparities in malignant digestive endocrine tumours survival. Int J Cancer. 2010; 126(12):2928-34.

28. Basturk O, Yang Z, Tang LH, Hruban RH, Adsay V, Mccall CM, Krasinskas AM, Jang KT, Frankel WL, Balci S. The high-grade (WHO G3) pancreatic neuroendocrine tumor category is morphologically and biologically heterogenous and includes both well differentiated and poorly differentiated neoplasms. Am J Surg Pathol. 2015;39(5):683-90.

29. Vélayoudom-Céphise FL, Duvillard P, Foucan L, Hadoux J, Chougnet CN, Leboulleux S, Malka D, Guigay J, Goere D, Debaere T. Are G3 ENETS neuroendocrine neoplasms heterogeneous? Endocr Relat Cancer. 2013; 20(5):649-57.

30. Vilar E, Salazar R, Pérez-García J, Cortes J, Oberg K, Tabernero J. Chemotherapy and role of the proliferation marker Ki-67 in digestive neuroendocrine tumors. Endocr Relat Cancer. 2007;14(2):221-32.

20

Prolonged preoperative treatment of acromegaly with Somatostatin analogs may improve surgical outcome in patients with invasive pituitary macroadenoma (Knosp grades 1–3): a retrospective cohort study conducted at a single center

Lian Duan[1], Huijuan Zhu[1], Bing Xing[2] and Feng Gu[1*]

Abstract

Background: This study aimed to investigate preoperative somatostatin analogs (SSAs) treatment on the surgical outcome in patients with acromegaly.

Methods: An analysis of 358 patients with acromegaly was conducted. The preoperative medical therapy group (81 patients) received SSA treatment for at least 3 months prior to surgery, while the primary surgery group (277 patients) underwent transsphenoidal surgery directly. Follow-up duration was ≥3 months. Tumor invasion was evaluated by magnetic resonance imaging (MRI) and classified according to the Knosp grading system.

Results: Most patients were diagnosed with macroadenoma. Among all patients (Knosp grades 0–4), preoperative SSA therapy did not significantly improve the curative effect of surgery, according to the levels of growth hormone (GH) and/or insulin-like growth factor 1 (IGF-1) markers. In patients with macroadenoma (Knosp grades 1–3), the remission rates were significantly higher in the SSA group compared to the surgery group when considering GH (56.4% vs. 37.3%, $P = 0.048$) and IGF-1 (43.2% vs. 17.6%, $P = 0.004$). In the preoperative medical therapy group, long-term use of SSAs (>6 months) led to higher remission rates (GH, 72.2% vs. 51.0%; and IGF-1, 61.1% vs. 29.8%; $P = 0.12$ and 0.02, respectively].

Conclusions: The long-term preoperative SSAs treatment may improve the surgical curative rate in acromegalic patients with invasive macroadenomas (Knosp grades 1–3).

Keywords: Acromegaly, Preoperative treatment, Somatostatin analogs, Invasive macroadenoma, Remission rate

Background

Acromegaly is a chronic disease that is caused, in the great majority of cases, by growth hormone (GH)-producing pituitary tumors. Hypersecretion of GH leads to excessive production of insulin-like growth factor 1 (IGF-1), leading to a multisystem disease characterized by somatic overgrowth, multiple comorbidities, premature mortality, and physical disfigurement. The main complications of untreated acromegaly are cardiovascular disease and malignancy, leading to high mortality [1, 2]. A multidisciplinary approach is critical for the management of this disorder and may decrease the incidence of these complications [1–3].

Transsphenoidal surgery (TSS) is the accepted first-line treatment for acromegaly in most patients. Surgical results are dependent on the preoperative serum GH and IGF-1 levels, extent of tumor invasion, and the skill

* Correspondence: gufeng@gusmedsci.cn
[1]Key Laboratory of Endocrinology, Ministry of Health; Department of Endocrinology, Peking Union Medical College Hospital, Peking Union Medical College and Chinese Academy of Medical Sciences, Beijing 100730, China
Full list of author information is available at the end of the article

of the neurosurgeon. Overall surgical remission rates are estimated to 75–90% for microadenomas and 40–60% for non-invasive macroadenomas, but this rate falls to 10–20% for invasive macroadenomas [4].

Consequently, additional therapy is required in order to reduce the symptoms associated with macroadenomas and to control the GH and IGF-1 levels following initial TSS. Medical therapeutic interventions such as the use of dopamine agonists and somatostatin analogs (SSAs) as adjuvant therapy are associated with favorable outcomes [5, 6]. SSAs are commonly used to control symptoms and hormonal hypersecretion in patients after unsuccessful primary surgery. SSA treatment can be extended for a long-term period and in combination with radiotherapy.

Primary SSAs therapy is used in patients with low probability of surgical remission and when TSS is not feasible. Primary SSAs therapy causes a decline in the hormone levels in most patients, but the individual patient response variation is high. About two thirds of SSA-naïve patients experience significant tumor shrinkage during SSA treatment [5–8]. Preoperative SSA treatment has been shown to result in improved symptomatic and metabolic control (particularly glucose tolerance and blood pressure), reduced soft tissue swelling, reduced tumor size/grade and, occasionally, altered and/or improved tumor consistency [9].

The guidelines from the European Society of Endocrinology and the American Association of Clinical Endocrinologists in 2014 recommended that preoperative SSA treatment should not be used routinely to improve the postoperative biochemical remission rate of acromegaly [10, 11]. Although preoperative SSA treatment alleviates the symptoms and reduces the risk of complications during surgery, this approach remains controversial [12]. To date, four prospective cohort studies suggest that preoperative SSA treatment may increase the recovery rate following surgery for macroadenoma [13–16]. Nevertheless, the postoperative remission rates of the patients with macroadenoma following direct surgery (without SSA treatment) ranged between 10% and 20% in these four studies [13–16].

These studies [13–16] suggested that preoperative SSA treatment could be used to increase the surgical recovery rate of patients with macroadenoma, including those with invasive disease. In addition, the duration of SSA treatment in the literature ranges from 3 to 6 months, while the efficacy of prolonged preoperative SSA treatment (>6 months) on surgical recovery remains unclear. Therefore, the aim of the present retrospective study was to investigate whether the course and preoperative administration of SSAs improve the outcome of surgery for acromegaly.

Methods

Study design

The present study was a retrospective cohort analysis of patients who underwent the resection of GH-secreting pituitary tumors at the Peking Union Medical College Hospital between 2009 and 2014. This study was approved by the Ethics Committee of the Chinese Academy of Medical Sciences and Peking Union Medical College Hospital. The need for individual consent was waived by the committee due to the retrospective nature of the study.

Patients

The inclusion criteria were: 1) 18–80 years of age; 2) confirmed diagnosis of acromegaly based on biochemical tests (fasting GH >2.5 μg/L, lowest GH >1 μg/L in glucose GH inhibition tests, and IGF-1 levels higher than the normal range for age- and sex-matched healthy subjects); 3) confirmed pituitary tumor in the sellar area as determined by magnetic resonance imaging (MRI) or CT scan; and 4) initial diagnosis of acromegaly and pituitary tumor resection at our hospital.

The exclusion criteria were: 1) prior surgical treatment or radiotherapy for a pituitary tumor; 2) the duration of preoperative SSA treatment was <3 months; 3) the interval between the preoperative SSA treatment and surgery was >3 months; 4) treatment with dopamine receptor agonists before surgery; 5) postoperative follow-up <3 months; 6) secondary surgery or radiotherapy within 3 months following the operation; and 7) treatment with SSAs or dopamine receptor agonists within 3 months following the operation.

The selection of the treatment approach was decided by the physicians and the patients, based on the Chinese diagnostic and treatment guidelines for acromegaly [17, 18] and on the patients' capacity to pay for SSAs (medical insurance or not). The patients were divided into two groups: 1) the preoperative medical therapy group (received preoperative SSAs treatment); and 2) the primary surgery group (underwent direct surgical treatment, without SSA therapy before surgery).

Intervention

All the operations were conducted by the surgeons from the Neurosurgery Department of the Peking Union Medical College Hospital. The patients in the preoperative medical therapy group underwent preoperative SSA treatment using octreotide long-acting repeatable (LAR) (20 mg, every 28 days; the dosage was increased to 40 mg, every 28 days when GH and IGF-1 were not adequately controlled) or somatuline (40 mg, every 14 days; dose interval was reduced to 10 days when the biochemical target index could not be achieved). The dose was adapted according to the clinical symptoms of the remission rates in patients with macroadenoma according to preoperative SSA therapy duration

	SSAs ≤6 months (n = 49)	SSAs >6 months (n = 18)	P
diagnosis (µg/L)	46.11 ± 16.40	35.96 ± 14.69	0.383
nosis (µg/L)	874.9 ± 309.7	789.3 ± 257.1	0.702
duration (month)	3.6 ± 0.98	18.1 ± 11.0	<0.001
GH	25/49 (51.0)	13/18 (72.2)	0.121
%)	10/15 (66.7)	5/6 (83.3)	0.623
(%)	15/28 (53.6)	7/11 (63.6)	0.725
%)	0/6 (0)	1/1 (100)	0.143
IGF-1	14/47 (29.8)	11/18 (61.1)	0.020
%)	4/15 (26.7)	4/6 (66.7)	0.146
(%)	10/26 (38.5)	6/11 (54.5)	0.018
%)	0/6 (0)	1/1 (100)	0.143

erapy in pituitary tumors has traditionally o the adjuvant setting, first-line treatment n be used in selected patients, including rasive tumors, those at risk of complica- d with anesthesia, those with severe com- cromegaly, those who refuse surgery, and sire to retain intact pituitary function. It sted that tumor removal during surgery is SA pretreatment [27, 28]. Previous studies operative SSAs and subsequent surgical conflicting [32–37]. In the present study, e SSA treatment increased the postopera- vs. 62.1%) and IGF-1 (60% vs. 35.7%) re- n patients with microadenoma, although re significantly different for the GH and GF-1 levels. In addition, the preoperative nent did not increase the overall surgical s in patients with macroadenoma.

rates of TSS decline substantially in pa- g large and invasive tumors and alterna- c modalities are required when TSS fails e study, male sex and parasellar extension invasion) were the most powerful predic- ent disease [30, 31]. Knosp grade (0–2) (<45 ng/mL) have been shown to correl- y remission in patients with GH-secreting red with preoperative demographics and eristics (which did not exhibit an associ- The present study showed that the post- and IGF-1 remission rates in patients with macroadenoma who underwent surgery 5.5% and 60.4%, respectively, but that the GH and IGF-1 remission rates decreased increasing CS invasion. No cases of bio- ssion were noted among the patients with tumors.

treatment with SSAs reduced the GH and fectively and decreased the tumor size to some extent. Based on these observations, the involvement of the preoperative SSAs treatment in the increase of the surgical recovery rate in patients with invasive macroadenoma was investigated. The subgroup analysis indicated that in the Knosp grade 0 subgroup, the preoperative SSA treatment did not increase the surgical efficacy. In contrast to this finding, the postoperative GH and IGF-1 remission rates in the patients who received preoperative SSAs treatment and exhibited invasive macroadenoma (Knosp grade ≥ 1) were significantly greater compared with those in the patients who underwent surgery directly. The overall postoperative remission rate among the patients with Knosp grade 4 macroadenoma was very low, possibly due to the limited number of cases included in the present study. As a consequence, this group was not included in the analysis. In the subsequent analysis, the preoperative SSAs treatment significantly increased the surgical curative rates in the remaining patients with invasive macroadenoma (Knosp grades 1–3). The aforementioned findings indicate that the preoperative SSAs treatment provides beneficial effects in invasive macroadenoma patients with tumors that do not progress with complete CS invasion.

A review of published studies evaluating SSAs as first-line therapy has reported that octreotide LAR therapy for a period of 6–24 months conferred significant (20–30%) tumor volume reduction in 73–85% of patients, with an overall mean reduction in tumor volume of 35–68% [40]. In a prospective, multicenter study of 98 patients treated with octreotide LAR at a dose of 10–30 mg every 4 weeks, a reduction in tumor volume exceeding 20% tumor was reported in 63% and 75% of patients following 24 and 48 weeks of treatment, respectively. Furthermore, it has been shown that tumor shrinkage increases with time, with the largest decreases in tumor volume generally occurring in the first year of treatment [41]. To date, the studies that have addressed the effects of preoperative SSA treatment on the surgical outcomes have adopted a

patients and the remission rates [19, 20]. Surgery was conducted via the endonasal transsphenoidal approach for the treatment of pituitary tumors [4, 10, 11].

Indicators and measurements

The patients were followed-up for at least 3 months following surgery. Postoperative remission was determined according to the Chinese biochemical remission criteria for acromegaly (2013) [17, 18]: random serum GH <2.5 µg/L, glucose GH inhibition test that exhibited GH levels lower than 1 µg/L, and/or IGF-1 levels that were decreased to normal levels according to the age and the sex of the patients. An oral glucose tolerance test (OGTT) has been proposed as an alternative method to assess remission in acromegaly [21, 22], but several studies have supported the use of GH and IGF-1 biomarkers in assessing remission in acromegaly [23–26]. The disease was evaluated at diagnosis, at 3 months following surgery, and at the last visit (≥3 months following surgery).

GH and IGF-1 levels were measured from fasting venous blood samples using a chemiluminescence method (IMMULITE2000 Growth Hormone (hGH) and IMMULITE2000 IGF-I, Siemens Healthcare Diagnostics, USA). For the glucose GH inhibition test, the patients were asked to ingest 75 g glucose in the morning without food, and the venous blood was obtained prior to and at 30, 60, 90, and 120 min following glucose ingestion.

Tumor invasiveness classification by MRI

A total of 202 patients with macroadenoma (67 in the preoperative medical therapy group and 135 in the primary surgery group) underwent sellar MRI scans at the Peking Union Medical College Hospital during at diagnosis. None of the patients had received any treatment (including drug therapy or surgery). Tumor invasion was evaluated by the doctors in the Radiology Department according to the Knosp criteria. The patients with invasive macroadenoma were grouped as the Knosp 1–3 and Knosp 4 subgroups. This selection was carried out because of the limited number of Knosp 4 patients, while both Knosp 1 and 2 tumors demonstrate considerably low percentage of invasion [27, 28].

The Knosp grading system comprises five categories [19, 20]: (0) no invasion with all of the lesion medial to the cavernous carotid artery (CCA); (1) invasion extending to, but not beyond, the medial aspect of the CCA; (2) invasion extending to, but not beyond, the lateral aspect of the CCA; (3) invasion past the lateral aspect of the CCA, but not completely filling the cavernous sinus (CS); and (4) completely filling the CS both medial and lateral to the CCA. Invasive macroadenoma was defined as macroadenoma with CS extension (Knosp ≥1).

Statistical analysis

Statistical analysis was carried out using the SPSS 16.0 software package (IBM, Armonk, NY, USA). Continuous data were expressed as mean ± standard deviation (SD). The chi-square test and Fisher's exact test were used to compare remission rates. Two-sided P-values <0.05 were considered statistically significant.

Results

Characteristics of the patients

A total of 520 patients were screened and 358 patients were eligible and met the study criteria (Fig. 1). Among these patients, the male (n = 166) to female (n = 192) ratio was 1:1.16, the mean age at disease onset was 34.7 years (range, 15–70 years), and the mean age at disease diagnosis was 40.3 years (range, 18–71 years). The Knosp grade system was used as an alternative stratification method.

The preoperative medical therapy group included 81 patients, 10 of which were diagnosed with microadenoma (adenoma diameter ≤ 1 cm), while 71 were diagnosed with macroadenoma (adenoma diameter > 1 cm). The preoperative drug treatment lasted 3–36 months, and the median treatment duration was 4 months. Only one patient had taken drug therapy for 36 months prior to surgery, with octreotide LAR 20 mg.

A total of 29 out of 277 patients who underwent initial surgery were diagnosed with microadenoma while the remaining 248 were diagnosed with macroadenoma. The patient characteristics at baseline are shown in Table 1.

Age at disease onset, disease duration, baseline biochemical parameters, and percentage of patients with macroadenoma were not significantly different between the two groups.

Among the patients with macroadenoma, 67 were in the preoperative medical therapy group, among which 21, 6, 19, 14, and 7 exhibited Knosp disease of grade 0, 1, 2, 3, and 4, respectively. This corresponded to an estimated percentage of 31.3%, 9.0%, 28.4%, 20.9%, and 10.4%, respectively. A total of 135 of the patients with macroadenoma were included in the primary surgery group. Among those patients 49, 12, 42, 29, and 3 corresponding to 36.3%, 8.9%, 31.1%, 21.5%, and 2.2%, respectively, exhibited disease Knosp grade 0, 1, 2, 3, and 4, respectively (Table 1).

A total of 117 out of 319 patients with invasive macroadenoma (36.7%) underwent MRI scans at other hospitals, with four patients (5.6%) in the preoperative medical therapy group and 113 patients (45.6%) in the primary surgery group. Consequently, the latter patients did not undergo further MRI evaluation or Knosp grading.

Remission rate after surgery

The patients were followed-up for at least 3 months following surgery (3–53 months, mean follow-up time:

Fig. 1 Flow diagram of patient recruitment and selection for the study

11.1 ± 10.9 months). GH levels were controlled in 46 out of 81 (56.8%) of patients treated with SSAs compared with 143 out of 277 (51.6%) patients who underwent surgery directly (*P* = 0.41). In contrast to the latter observation, 32 out of 79 (40.5%) of SSA- pretreated patients exhibited normalized IGF-1 level compared with 83 of 255 (32.6%) patients who underwent surgery (*P* = 0.19). This classification was conducted according to the biochemical remission criteria mentioned in the Chinese guideline.

In patients with microadenomas, the remission rate of GH in the preoperative medical therapy group was significantly higher compared with that of the primary surgery group (100% vs. 62.1%, *P* = 0.037), while the remission rate of IGF-1 was higher in the preoperative medical therapy group (60% vs. 35.7%, *P* = 0.267).

In patients with macroadenomas, the preoperative medical therapy did not improve the curative effect of surgery and there was no significant difference in the GH (50.7% vs. 50.4%, *P* = 0.96) or IGF-1 (37.7% vs. 32.2%, *P* = 0.39) remission rates between the two groups (Table 2).

Remission rate of macroadenoma according to Knosp grade

CS invasion is considered one of the most significant preoperative predictor of remission in the surgical treatment of pituitary GH adenomas. The remission rate for GH and IGF-1 decreased significantly with higher Knosp grade in both groups. The biochemical remission rates in the primary surgery group did not reveal a significant difference compared with those of the preoperative

Table 1 Patient characteristics at baseline

	Preoperative medical therapy (*n* = 81)	Primary surgery (*n* = 277)	*P*
M/F	41/40	125/152	0.38
Age of onset (y)	34.8 ± 11.4	34.6 ± 11.7	0.86
Age of diagnosis (y)	40.3 ± 11.9	40.1 ± 12.1	0.89
Mean basal GH (μg/L)	44.47 ± 16.13	48.17 ± 17.52	0.68
Mean IGF-1 (μg/L)	841.27 ± 313.26	889.50 ± 306.21	0.31
Microadenoma (%)	10 (12.3)	29 (10.5)	0.63
Macroadenoma (%)	71 (87.7)	248 (89.5)	0.63
[a]Tumor invasion (Knosp)	67	135	0.161
Knosp 0 (%)	21 (31.3)	49 (36.3)	
Knosp 1 (%)	6 (9.0)	12 (8.9)	
Knosp 2 (%)	19 (28.4)	42 (31.1)	
Knosp 3 (%)	14 (20.9)	29 (21.5)	
Knosp 4 (%)	7 (10.4)	3 (2.2)	

[a]Classified according to magnetic resonance imaging performed at Peking Union Medical College Hospital (China)

Table 2 Surgical remission rates of patients with acromegaly

		Preoperative medical thera
Remission rate for GH	Total (%)	46/81 (56.8)
	Microadenoma (%)	10/10 (100)
	Macroadenoma (%)	36/71 (50.7)
Remission rate for IGF-1	Total (%)	32/79 (40.5)
	Microadenoma (%)	6/10 (60)
	Macroadenoma (%)	26/69 (37.7)

medical therapy group in patients with Knosp grade 0 tumors (Table 3), but in patients with invasive macroadenoma (Knosp grade 1–3), the GH and IGF-1 remission rates were significantly higher in the preoperative medical therapy group compared with those in the primary surgery group (Table 3). No significant differences between the two groups were noted for Knosp grade 4 macroadenomas (Table 3). As a result, the patients with invasive macroadenomas (Knosp grade 1–3) may benefit from medical therapy prior to surgery (Table 3).

Remission rate of macroadenoma according to preoperative SSA therapy duration

The duration of the preoperative SSA therapy in some of the patients was >3–6 months, as recommended in previous studies [12]. To investigate the effects of the duration of the preoperative medical therapy on the surgical remission rate, the patients with macroadenoma were divided into two subgroups: ≤6 months (median time, 3 months) and >6 months (median time, 12 months). Comparison of the latter subgroups with the primary surgery group (Table 3) showed no significant differences in the mean GH and IGF-1 levels at diagnosis, but the IGF-1 remission rates in the patients who received >6 months of preoperative SSA treatment were significantly greater compared with those of the patients who underwent surgery directly and/or those who received ≤6 months of preoperative SSA treatment (Table 4). With regard to the GH, levels no significant difference in remission was noted between the two groups (Table 4). Among the patients with Knosp grade 1–3 disease, a significant difference was noted for

the remission ra
groups as regard
ferences noted in
not statistically si

Discussion

The present stud
fects of preopera
tive rate of pati
pituitary tumor
proach at our h
to the biochemi
the Chinese diag
romegaly [17, 1
62.1%) and IGF-
patients with mi
SSAs treatment v
patients who un
treatment did no
remission rate in
subgroup analysi
creased the post
the patients with
addition, the surg
rate were further
operative SSA tre

It has been re
present with acr
exhibit inadequat
and that the use
prove the clinica

Table 4 Surgica

Mean basal GH at	
Mean IGF-1 at diag	
Mean SSAs therap	
Remission rate for	
Knosp grade 0	
Knosp grade 1–	
Knosp grade 4	
Remission rate for	
Knosp grade 0	
Knosp grade 1–	
Knosp grade 4	

use of drug th
been limited t
with SSAs ca
those with inv
tions associate
plications of a
those who de
has been sugg
facilitated by S
addressing pre
cure rates are
the preoperati
tive GH (100%
mission rates
the results we
not for the IC
medical treatm
remission rate

The success
tients harbori
tive therapeut
[21, 29]. In on
(especially CS
tors of persis
and GH levels
ate with surge
tumors comp
tumor charac
ation) [38, 39
operative GH
Knosp grade
directly were
postoperative
markedly with
chemical remi
Knosp grade 4

The medica
IGF-1 levels e

Table 3 Surgical remission rates of patients with macroadenoma according to the Knos

		Preoperative medical thera
Remission rate for GH	Total (%)	38/67 (56.7)
	Knosp grade 0 (%)	15/21 (71.4)
	Knosp grade 1–3 (%)	22/39 (56.4)
	Knosp grade 4 (%)	1/7 (14.3)
Remission rate for IGF-1[a]	Total (%)	25/65 (38.5)
	Knosp grade 0 (%)	8/21 (38.1)
	Knosp grade 1–3 (%)	16/37 (43.2)
	Knosp grade 4 (%)	1/7 (14.3)

[a]IGF-1 results were not available for all patients

patients and the remission rates [19, 20]. Surgery was conducted via the endonasal transsphenoidal approach for the treatment of pituitary tumors [4, 10, 11].

Indicators and measurements

The patients were followed-up for at least 3 months following surgery. Postoperative remission was determined according to the Chinese biochemical remission criteria for acromegaly (2013) [17, 18]: random serum GH <2.5 μg/L, glucose GH inhibition test that exhibited GH levels lower than 1 μg/L, and/or IGF-1 levels that were decreased to normal levels according to the age and the sex of the patients. An oral glucose tolerance test (OGTT) has been proposed as an alternative method to assess remission in acromegaly [21, 22], but several studies have supported the use of GH and IGF-1 biomarkers in assessing remission in acromegaly [23–26]. The disease was evaluated at diagnosis, at 3 months following surgery, and at the last visit (≥3 months following surgery).

GH and IGF-1 levels were measured from fasting venous blood samples using a chemiluminescence method (IMMULITE2000 Growth Hormone (hGH) and IMMULITE2000 IGF-I, Siemens Healthcare Diagnostics, USA). For the glucose GH inhibition test, the patients were asked to ingest 75 g glucose in the morning without food, and the venous blood was obtained prior to and at 30, 60, 90, and 120 min following glucose ingestion.

Tumor invasiveness classification by MRI

A total of 202 patients with macroadenoma (67 in the preoperative medical therapy group and 135 in the primary surgery group) underwent sellar MRI scans at the Peking Union Medical College Hospital during at diagnosis. None of the patients had received any treatment (including drug therapy or surgery). Tumor invasion was evaluated by the doctors in the Radiology Department according to the Knosp criteria. The patients with invasive macroadenoma were grouped as the Knosp 1–3 and Knosp 4 subgroups. This selection was carried out because of the limited number of Knosp 4 patients, while both Knosp 1 and 2 tumors demonstrate considerably low percentage of invasion [27, 28].

The Knosp grading system comprises five categories [19, 20]: (0) no invasion with all of the lesion medial to the cavernous carotid artery (CCA); (1) invasion extending to, but not beyond, the medial aspect of the CCA; (2) invasion extending to, but not beyond, the lateral aspect of the CCA; (3) invasion past the lateral aspect of the CCA, but not completely filling the cavernous sinus (CS); and (4) completely filling the CS both medial and lateral to the CCA. Invasive macroadenoma was defined as macroadenoma with CS extension (Knosp ≥1).

Statistical analysis

Statistical analysis was carried out using the SPSS 16.0 software package (IBM, Armonk, NY, USA). Continuous data were expressed as mean ± standard deviation (SD). The chi-square test and Fisher's exact test were used to compare remission rates. Two-sided P-values <0.05 were considered statistically significant.

Results

Characteristics of the patients

A total of 520 patients were screened and 358 patients were eligible and met the study criteria (Fig. 1). Among these patients, the male (n = 166) to female (n = 192) ratio was 1:1.16, the mean age at disease onset was 34.7 years (range, 15–70 years), and the mean age at disease diagnosis was 40.3 years (range, 18–71 years). The Knosp grade system was used as an alternative stratification method.

The preoperative medical therapy group included 81 patients, 10 of which were diagnosed with microadenoma (adenoma diameter ≤ 1 cm), while 71 were diagnosed with macroadenoma (adenoma diameter > 1 cm). The preoperative drug treatment lasted 3–36 months, and the median treatment duration was 4 months. Only one patient had taken drug therapy for 36 months prior to surgery, with octreotide LAR 20 mg.

A total of 29 out of 277 patients who underwent initial surgery were diagnosed with microadenoma while the remaining 248 were diagnosed with macroadenoma. The patient characteristics at baseline are shown in Table 1.

Age at disease onset, disease duration, baseline biochemical parameters, and percentage of patients with macroadenoma were not significantly different between the two groups.

Among the patients with macroadenoma, 67 were in the preoperative medical therapy group, among which 21, 6, 19, 14, and 7 exhibited Knosp disease of grade 0, 1, 2, 3, and 4, respectively. This corresponded to an estimated percentage of 31.3%, 9.0%, 28.4%, 20.9%, and 10.4%, respectively. A total of 135 of the patients with macroadenoma were included in the primary surgery group. Among those patients 49, 12, 42, 29, and 3 corresponding to 36.3%, 8.9%, 31.1%, 21.5%, and 2.2%, respectively, exhibited disease Knosp grade 0, 1, 2, 3, and 4, respectively (Table 1).

A total of 117 out of 319 patients with invasive macroadenoma (36.7%) underwent MRI scans at other hospitals, with four patients (5.6%) in the preoperative medical therapy group and 113 patients (45.6%) in the primary surgery group. Consequently, the latter patients did not undergo further MRI evaluation or Knosp grading.

Remission rate after surgery

The patients were followed-up for at least 3 months following surgery (3–53 months, mean follow-up time:

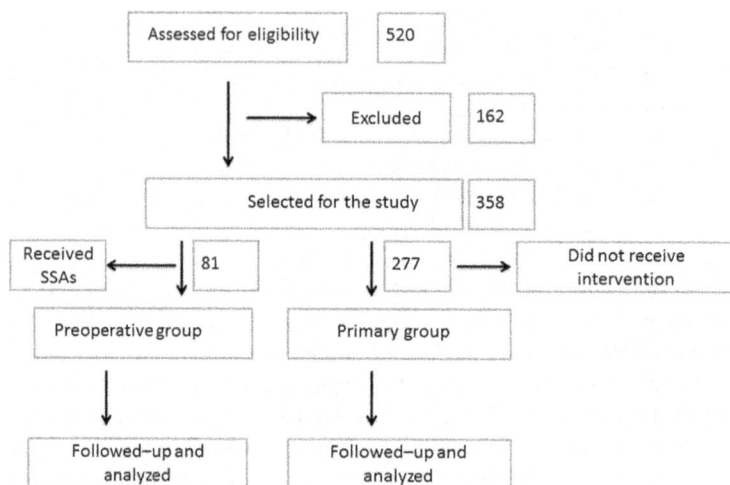

Fig. 1 Flow diagram of patient recruitment and selection for the study

11.1 ± 10.9 months). GH levels were controlled in 46 out of 81 (56.8%) of patients treated with SSAs compared with 143 out of 277 (51.6%) patients who underwent surgery directly (*P* = 0.41). In contrast to the latter observation, 32 out of 79 (40.5%) of SSA- pretreated patients exhibited normalized IGF-1 level compared with 83 of 255 (32.6%) patients who underwent surgery (*P* = 0.19). This classification was conducted according to the biochemical remission criteria mentioned in the Chinese guideline.

In patients with microadenomas, the remission rate of GH in the preoperative medical therapy group was significantly higher compared with that of the primary surgery group (100% vs. 62.1%, *P* = 0.037), while the remission rate of IGF-1 was higher in the preoperative medical therapy group (60% vs. 35.7%, *P* = 0.267).

In patients with macroadenomas, the preoperative medical therapy did not improve the curative effect of surgery and there was no significant difference in the GH (50.7% vs. 50.4%, *P* = 0.96) or IGF-1 (37.7% vs. 32.2%, *P* = 0.39) remission rates between the two groups (Table 2).

Remission rate of macroadenoma according to Knosp grade

CS invasion is considered one of the most significant preoperative predictor of remission in the surgical treatment of pituitary GH adenomas. The remission rate for GH and IGF-1 decreased significantly with higher Knosp grade in both groups. The biochemical remission rates in the primary surgery group did not reveal a significant difference compared with those of the preoperative

Table 1 Patient characteristics at baseline

	Preoperative medical therapy (*n* = 81)	Primary surgery (*n* = 277)	*P*
M/F	41/40	125/152	0.38
Age of onset (y)	34.8 ± 11.4	34.6 ± 11.7	0.86
Age of diagnosis (y)	40.3 ± 11.9	40.1 ± 12.1	0.89
Mean basal GH (μg/L)	44.47 ± 16.13	48.17 ± 17.52	0.68
Mean IGF-1 (μg/L)	841.27 ± 313.26	889.50 ± 306.21	0.31
Microadenoma (%)	10 (12.3)	29 (10.5)	0.63
Macroadenoma (%)	71 (87.7)	248 (89.5)	0.63
[a]Tumor invasion (Knosp)	67	135	0.161
Knosp 0 (%)	21 (31.3)	49 (36.3)	
Knosp 1 (%)	6 (9.0)	12 (8.9)	
Knosp 2 (%)	19 (28.4)	42 (31.1)	
Knosp 3 (%)	14 (20.9)	29 (21.5)	
Knosp 4 (%)	7 (10.4)	3 (2.2)	

[a]Classified according to magnetic resonance imaging performed at Peking Union Medical College Hospital (China)

Table 2 Surgical remission rates of patients with acromegaly

		Preoperative medical therapy	Primary surgery	P
Remission rate for GH	Total (%)	46/81 (56.8)	143/277 (51.6)	0.41
	Microadenoma (%)	10/10 (100)	18/29 (62.1)	0.037
	Macroadenoma (%)	36/71 (50.7)	125/248 (50.4)	0.96
Remission rate for IGF-1	Total (%)	32/79 (40.5)	83/255 (32.6)	0.19
	Microadenoma (%)	6/10 (60)	10/28 (35.7)	0.267
	Macroadenoma (%)	26/69 (37.7)	73/227 (32.2)	0.39

medical therapy group in patients with Knosp grade 0 tumors (Table 3), but in patients with invasive macroadenoma (Knosp grade 1–3), the GH and IGF-1 remission rates were significantly higher in the preoperative medical therapy group compared with those in the primary surgery group (Table 3). No significant differences between the two groups were noted for Knosp grade 4 macroadenomas (Table 3). As a result, the patients with invasive macroadenomas (Knosp grade 1–3) may benefit from medical therapy prior to surgery (Table 3).

Remission rate of macroadenoma according to preoperative SSA therapy duration

The duration of the preoperative SSA therapy in some of the patients was >3–6 months, as recommended in previous studies [12]. To investigate the effects of the duration of the preoperative medical therapy on the surgical remission rate, the patients with macroadenoma were divided into two subgroups: ≤6 months (median time, 3 months) and >6 months (median time, 12 months). Comparison of the latter subgroups with the primary surgery group (Table 3) showed no significant differences in the mean GH and IGF-1 levels at diagnosis, but the IGF-1 remission rates in the patients who received >6 months of preoperative SSA treatment were significantly greater compared with those of the patients who underwent surgery directly and/or those who received ≤6 months of preoperative SSA treatment (Table 4). With regard to the GH, levels no significant difference in remission was noted between the two groups (Table 4). Among the patients with Knosp grade 1–3 disease, a significant difference was noted for

the remission rate of the IGF-1 levels between the two groups as regards the Knosp grade 1–3, whereas the differences noted in the cases of Knosp 0 and 4 grades were not statistically significant (Table 4).

Discussion

The present study was a retrospective analysis of the effects of preoperative SSA treatment on the surgical curative rate of patients with acromegaly who underwent pituitary tumor resection via the transsphenoidal approach at our hospital from 2009 and 2014. According to the biochemical remission criteria recommended by the Chinese diagnostic and treatment guidelines for acromegaly [17, 18], the postoperative GH (100% vs. 62.1%) and IGF-1 (60% vs. 35.7%) remission rates in the patients with microadenoma who received preoperative SSAs treatment were higher compared with those in the patients who underwent surgery directly. Preoperative treatment did not increase the postoperative biochemical remission rate in the patients with macroadenoma. The subgroup analysis indicated that preoperative SSAs increased the postoperative biochemical remission rate in the patients with macroadenoma of Knosp grades ≥1. In addition, the surgical efficacy and biochemical remission rate were further improved by the administration of preoperative SSA treatment for a time period >6 months.

It has been reported that a majority of patients that present with acromegaly due to GH-secreting tumors exhibit inadequately controlled disease following surgery and that the use of SSAs is encouraged in order to improve the clinical symptoms [21, 29–31]. Although the

Table 3 Surgical remission rates of patients with macroadenoma according to the Knosp grade

		Preoperative medical therapy	Primary surgery	P
Remission rate for GH	Total (%)	38/67 (56.7)	68/135 (50.4)	0.10
	Knosp grade 0 (%)	15/21 (71.4)	37/49 (75.5)	0.72
	Knosp grade 1–3 (%)	22/39 (56.4)	31/83 (37.3)	0.048
	Knosp grade 4 (%)	1/7 (14.3)	0/3 (0)	~1.00
Remission rate for IGF-1[a]	Total (%)	25/65 (38.5)	42/125 (33.6)	0.51
	Knosp grade 0 (%)	8/21 (38.1)	29/48 (60.4)	0.09
	Knosp grade 1–3 (%)	16/37 (43.2)	13/74 (17.6)	0.004
	Knosp grade 4 (%)	1/7 (14.3)	0/3 (0)	~1.00

[a]IGF-1 results were not available for all patients

Table 4 Surgical remission rates in patients with macroadenoma according to preoperative SSA therapy duration

	SSAs ≤6 months (n = 49)	SSAs >6 months (n = 18)	P
Mean basal GH at diagnosis (µg/L)	46.11 ± 16.40	35.96 ± 14.69	0.383
Mean IGF-1 at diagnosis (µg/L)	874.9 ± 309.7	789.3 ± 257.1	0.702
Mean SSAs therapy duration (month)	3.6 ± 0.98	18.1 ± 11.0	<0.001
Remission rate for GH	25/49 (51.0)	13/18 (72.2)	0.121
Knosp grade 0 (%)	10/15 (66.7)	5/6 (83.3)	0.623
Knosp grade 1–3 (%)	15/28 (53.6)	7/11 (63.6)	0.725
Knosp grade 4 (%)	0/6 (0)	1/1 (100)	0.143
Remission rate for IGF-1	14/47 (29.8)	11/18 (61.1)	0.020
Knosp grade 0 (%)	4/15 (26.7)	4/6 (66.7)	0.146
Knosp grade 1–3 (%)	10/26 (38.5)	6/11 (54.5)	0.018
Knosp grade 4 (%)	0/6 (0)	1/1 (100)	0.143

use of drug therapy in pituitary tumors has traditionally been limited to the adjuvant setting, first-line treatment with SSAs can be used in selected patients, including those with invasive tumors, those at risk of complications associated with anesthesia, those with severe complications of acromegaly, those who refuse surgery, and those who desire to retain intact pituitary function. It has been suggested that tumor removal during surgery is facilitated by SSA pretreatment [27, 28]. Previous studies addressing preoperative SSAs and subsequent surgical cure rates are conflicting [32–37]. In the present study, the preoperative SSA treatment increased the postoperative GH (100% vs. 62.1%) and IGF-1 (60% vs. 35.7%) remission rates in patients with microadenoma, although the results were significantly different for the GH and not for the IGF-1 levels. In addition, the preoperative medical treatment did not increase the overall surgical remission rates in patients with macroadenoma.

The success rates of TSS decline substantially in patients harboring large and invasive tumors and alternative therapeutic modalities are required when TSS fails [21, 29]. In one study, male sex and parasellar extension (especially CS invasion) were the most powerful predictors of persistent disease [30, 31]. Knosp grade (0–2) and GH levels (<45 ng/mL) have been shown to correlate with surgery remission in patients with GH-secreting tumors compared with preoperative demographics and tumor characteristics (which did not exhibit an association) [38, 39]. The present study showed that the postoperative GH and IGF-1 remission rates in patients with Knosp grade 0 macroadenoma who underwent surgery directly were 75.5% and 60.4%, respectively, but that the postoperative GH and IGF-1 remission rates decreased markedly with increasing CS invasion. No cases of biochemical remission were noted among the patients with Knosp grade 4 tumors.

The medical treatment with SSAs reduced the GH and IGF-1 levels effectively and decreased the tumor size to some extent. Based on these observations, the involvement of the preoperative SSAs treatment in the increase of the surgical recovery rate in patients with invasive macroadenoma was investigated. The subgroup analysis indicated that in the Knosp grade 0 subgroup, the preoperative SSA treatment did not increase the surgical efficacy. In contrast to this finding, the postoperative GH and IGF-1 remission rates in the patients who received preoperative SSAs treatment and exhibited invasive macroadenoma (Knosp grade ≥ 1) were significantly greater compared with those in the patients who underwent surgery directly. The overall postoperative remission rate among the patients with Knosp grade 4 macroadenoma was very low, possibly due to the limited number of cases included in the present study. As a consequence, this group was not included in the analysis. In the subsequent analysis, the preoperative SSAs treatment significantly increased the surgical curative rates in the remaining patients with invasive macroadenoma (Knosp grades 1–3). The aforementioned findings indicate that the preoperative SSAs treatment provides beneficial effects in invasive macroadenoma patients with tumors that do not progress with complete CS invasion.

A review of published studies evaluating SSAs as first-line therapy has reported that octreotide LAR therapy for a period of 6–24 months conferred significant (20–30%) tumor volume reduction in 73–85% of patients, with an overall mean reduction in tumor volume of 35–68% [40]. In a prospective, multicenter study of 98 patients treated with octreotide LAR at a dose of 10–30 mg every 4 weeks, a reduction in tumor volume exceeding 20% tumor was reported in 63% and 75% of patients following 24 and 48 weeks of treatment, respectively. Furthermore, it has been shown that tumor shrinkage increases with time, with the largest decreases in tumor volume generally occurring in the first year of treatment [41]. To date, the studies that have addressed the effects of preoperative SSA treatment on the surgical outcomes have adopted a

3–6-month regimen. The novelty of the present study is focused on the effects of the preoperative SSAs duration on the postoperative biochemical remission rate, which have not yet been reported. In addition, the patients were divided into two subgroups according to the preoperative SSAs treatment duration (≤6 months and >6 months). In the present study, for IGF-1, the difference between the ≤6 and >6 months groups was significant (61.1% vs. 29.8%). Further subgroup analysis showed that treatment for ≤6 and >6 months had differential effects on IGF-1 in patients with Knosp 1–3 disease (54.5% vs. 38.5%). Considering that the patients with Knosp 1–3 disease and who directly underwent surgery only have a 17.6% remission rate, extension of pre-operative SSA treatment could be especially helpful. On the other hand, no effect of pre-operative treatment duration (≤6 vs. >6 months) was observed for GH despite that differences were observed for pre-operative treatment (regardless of duration) vs. direct surgery for Knosp grade 1–3 subjects.

It is important to highlight that the current study was focused on acromegalic patients and did not examine the possibility of potentially deranged pituitary axis, of co-existing conditions such as central adrenal insufficiency, and of impaired patterns of other hormones including prolactin. The selection of the subjects was based solely on the diagnosis of acromegaly. The diagnosis of acromegaly was confirmed by biochemical tests and MRI or CT scans that indicated the presence of the pituitary tumor in the sellar area. This diagnosis excluded the manifestation of further pituitary-associated hormonal conditions and symptoms.

The present study is limited by its retrospective nature, i.e. selection bias and information bias [42]. The lack of control, the lack of randomization, the single center, and the inclusion of additional clinicopathological parameters during SSA treatment in the statistical analysis of the study are all disadvantages that can be improved in a future study. In addition, the decrease in tumor invasion was not investigated in the patients who received preoperative drug therapy for >6 months. Furthermore, the postoperative GH and IGF-1 levels in some patients were not consistent [42] and the decrease in the IGF-1 levels following the operation was relatively slow, indicating that the IGF-1 remission rate was significantly lower than the GH remission rate in the present study. Nevertheless, similar retrospective analysis of acromegaly patients who received 3–6 months of pre-operative SSAs showed that this time duration is optimal [17, 18, 43]. The numbers of patients were different between the two groups because many patients were from different parts of the country and referred to our center only for second opinion and/or treatments, and many patients had no medical insurance and could not afford SSAs. Finally, the improvements in the complications prior to and following the treatment were not investigated. Further prospective controlled studies are required to elucidate whether individualized preoperative SSAs treatment can improve the surgical efficacy and provide evidence of the benefit of preoperative SSAs treatment in invasive macroadenoma patients.

Conclusions

Currently, there is no consensus regarding the potential of preoperative SSAs treatment to improve the surgical remission rate in patients with acromegaly. Preoperative SSAs aiming to improve the surgical remission rate are not recommended by the Clinical Practice Guidelines of the Endocrine Society, the European Society of Endocrinology, and the Chinese Diagnostic and Treatment Guidelines for Acromegaly. Nevertheless, the present study suggests that preoperative SSAs improve the surgical remission rate in patients with invasive macroadenoma (Knosp grades 1–3) and that longer preoperative SSA treatment (>6 months) improves the surgical results in specific cases. Consequently, the data suggest that the increase in the preoperative SSAs treatment duration, according to the disease conditions of the patients, has the potential to increase the surgical curative rate and improve the outcomes.

Abbreviations

CCA: Cavernous carotid artery; CS: Cavernous sinus; GH: Growth hormone; IGF-1: Insulin-like growth factor 1; LAR: Long acting repeatable; MRI: Magnetic Resonance imaging; OGTT: Oral glucose tolerance test; SSAs: Somatostatin analogs; TSS: Transsphenoidal surgery

Acknowledgements

The authors appreciate the contribution of the multidisciplinary team, including an endocrinologist, neurosurgeon, radiologist, pathologist and radiotherapist.

Funding

This study was supported by the National Key Program of Clinical Science (WBYZ2011).

Authors' contributions

LD conceived and coordinated the study, designed, performed and analyzed the experiments, wrote the paper. HZ, BX, and FG carried out the data collection, data analysis, and revised the paper. All authors reviewed the results and approved the final version of the manuscript.

Competing interests

The authors declare that they have no competing interests.

Author details

[1]Key Laboratory of Endocrinology, Ministry of Health; Department of Endocrinology, Peking Union Medical College Hospital, Peking Union Medical College and Chinese Academy of Medical Sciences, Beijing 100730, China. [2]Department of Neurosurgery, Peking Union Medical College Hospital, Peking Union Medical College and Chinese Academy of Medical Sciences, Beijing 100730, China.

References

1. DH S, Liao KM, Chen HW, Chang TC. Long-term primary medical therapy with somatostatin analogs in acromegaly. J Formos Med Assoc. 2006;105:664–9.
2. Melmed S. Medical progress: acromegaly. N Engl J Med. 2006;355:2558–73.
3. Ribeiro-Oliveira A, Jr., Barkan A. The changing face of acromegaly–advances in diagnosis and treatment. Nat Rev Endocrinol 2012;8:605–611.
4. Nomikos P, Buchfelder M, Fahlbusch R. The outcome of surgery in 668 patients with acromegaly using current criteria of biochemical 'cure. Eur J Endocrinol. 2005;152:379–87.
5. Sheppard MC. Primary medical therapy for acromegaly. Clin Endocrinol. 2003;58:387–99.
6. Colao A, Cappabianca P, Caron P, De Menis E, Farrall AJ, Gadelha MR, et al. Octreotide LAR vs. surgery in newly diagnosed patients with acromegaly: a randomized, open-label, multicentre study. Clin Endocrinol. 2009;70:757–68.
7. Luque-Ramirez M, Portoles GR, Varela C, Albero R, Halperin I, Moreiro J, et al. The efficacy of octreotide LAR as firstline therapy for patients with newly diagnosed acromegaly is independent of tumor extension: predictive factors of tumor and biochemical response. Horm Metab Res. 2010;42:38–44.
8. Carlsen SM, Svartberg J, Schreiner T, Aanderud S, Johannesen O, Skeie S, et al. Six-month preoperative octreotide treatment in unselected, de novo patients with acromegaly: effect on biochemistry, tumour volume, and postoperative cure. Clin Endocrinol. 2011;74:736–43.
9. Annamalai AK, Webb A, Kandasamy N, Elkhawad M, Moir S, Khan F, et al. A comprehensive study of clinical, biochemical, radiological, vascular, cardiac, and sleep parameters in an unselected cohort of patients with acromegaly undergoing presurgical somatostatin receptor ligand therapy. J Clin Endocrinol Metab. 2013;98:1040–50.
10. Katznelson L, Laws ER, Jr., Melmed S, Molitch ME, Murad MH, Utz A, et al. Acromegaly: an endocrine society clinical practice guideline. J Clin Endocrinol Metab 2014;99:3933–3951.
11. Newman CB, Melmed S, George A, Torigian D, Duhaney M, Snyder P, et al. Octreotide as primary therapy for acromegaly. J Clin Endocrinol Metab. 1998;83:3034–40.
12. Jacob JJ, Bevan JS. Should all patients with acromegaly receive somatostatin analogue therapy before surgery and, if so, for how long? Clin Endocrinol. 2014;81:812–7.
13. Fougner SL, Bollerslev J, Svartberg J, Oksnes M, Cooper J, Carlsen SM. Preoperative octreotide treatment of acromegaly: long-term results of a randomised controlled trial. Eur J Endocrinol. 2014;171:229–35.
14. Mao ZG, Zhu YH, Tang HL, Wang DY, Zhou J, He DS, et al. Preoperative lanreotide treatment in acromegalic patients with macroadenomas increases short-term postoperative cure rates: a prospective, randomised trial. Eur J Endocrinol. 2010;162:661–6.
15. Shen M, Shou X, Wang Y, Zhang Z, Wu J, Mao Y, et al. Effect of presurgical long-acting octreotide treatment in acromegaly patients with invasive pituitary macroadenomas: a prospective randomized study. Endocr J. 2010;57:1035–44.
16. Li ZQ, Quan Z, Tian HL, Cheng M. Preoperative lanreotide treatment improves outcome in patients with acromegaly resulting from invasive pituitary macroadenoma. J Int Med Res. 2012;40:517–24.
17. Helseth R, Carlsen SM, Bollerslev J, Svartberg J, Oksnes M, Skeie S, et al. Preoperative octreotide therapy and surgery in acromegaly: associations between glucose homeostasis and treatment response. Endocrine. 2016;51:298–307.
18. Yao Y, Wang RZ. The comment of guidelines for clinical diagnosis and treatment of acromegaly - 2013 update. Zhonghua Yi Xue Za Zhi. 2013;93:2101–2.
19. Knosp E, Steiner E, Kitz K, Matula C. Pituitary adenomas with invasion of the cavernous sinus space: a magnetic resonance imaging classification compared with surgical findings. Neurosurgery. 1993;33:610–7. discussion 7-8
20. Salvatori R, Woodmansee WW, Molitch M, Gordon MB, Lomax KG. Lanreotide extended-release aqueous-gel formulation, injected by patient, partner or healthcare provider in patients with acromegaly in the United States: 1-year data from the SODA registry. Pituitary. 2014;17:13–21.

21. Capatina C, Wass JA. 60 YEARS OF NEUROENDOCRINOLOGY: acromegaly. J Endocrinol. 2015;226:T141–60.
22. Yildirim AE, Sahinoglu M, Divanlioglu D, Alagoz F, Gurcay AG, Daglioglu E, et al. Endoscopic endonasal transsphenoidal treatment for acromegaly: 2010 consensus criteria for remission and predictors of outcomes. Turk Neurosurg. 2014;24:906–12.
23. Evran M, Sert M, Tetiker T. Clinical experiences and success rates of acromegaly treatment: the single center results of 62 patients. BMC Endocr Disord. 2014;14:97.
24. Wang YY, Higham C, Kearney T, Davis JR, Trainer P, Gnanalingham KK. Acromegaly surgery in Manchester revisited–the impact of reducing surgeon numbers and the 2010 consensus guidelines for disease remission. Clin Endocrinol. 2012;76:399–406.
25. Patt H, Jalali R, Yerawar C, Khare S, Gupta T, Goel A, et al. High-precision conformal fractionated radiotherapy is effective in achieving remission in patients with acromegaly after failed Transsphenoidal surgery. Endocr Pract. 2016;22:162–72.
26. Schofl C, Franz H, Grussendorf M, Honegger J, Jaursch-Hancke C, Mayr B, et al. Long-term outcome in patients with acromegaly: analysis of 1344 patients from the German acromegaly register. Eur J Endocrinol. 2013;168:39–47.
27. Abe T, Ludecke DK. Effects of preoperative octreotide treatment on different subtypes of 90 GH-secreting pituitary adenomas and outcome in one surgical centre. Eur J Endocrinol 2001;145:137–145.
28. Micko AS, Wohrer A, Wolfsberger S, Knosp E. Invasion of the cavernous sinus space in pituitary adenomas: endoscopic verification and its correlation with an MRI-based classification. J Neurosurg. 2015;122:803–11.
29. Jane JA, Jr., Starke RM, Elzoghby MA, Reames DL, Payne SC, Thorner MO, et al. Endoscopic transsphenoidal surgery for acromegaly: remission using modern criteria, complications, and predictors of outcome. J Clin Endocrinol Metab 2011;96:2732–2740.
30. van Bunderen CC, van Varsseveld NC, Baayen JC, van Furth WR, Aliaga ES, Hazewinkel MJ, et al. Predictors of endoscopic transsphenoidal surgery outcome in acromegaly: patient and tumor characteristics evaluated by magnetic resonance imaging. Pituitary. 2013;16:158–67.
31. Zhang L, Wu X, Yan Y, Qian J, Lu Y, Luo C. Preoperative somatostatin analogs treatment in acromegalic patients with macroadenomas. A meta-analysis. Brain and Development. 2015;37:181–90.
32. Kowalska A, Walczyk A, Palyga I, Gasior-Perczak D, Gadawska-Juszczyk K, Szymonek M, et al. The delayed risk stratification system in the risk of differentiated thyroid cancer recurrence. PLoS One. 2016;11:e0153242.
33. Pita-Gutierrez F, Pertega-Diaz S, Pita-Fernandez S, Pena L, Lugo G, Sangiao-Alvarellos S, et al. Place of preoperative treatment of acromegaly with somatostatin analog on surgical outcome: a systematic review and meta-analysis. PLoS One. 2013;8:e61523.
34. Maiza JC, Vezzosi D, Matta M, Donadille F, Loubes-Lacroix F, Cournot M, et al. Long-term (up to 18 years) effects on GH/IGF-1 hypersecretion and tumour size of primary somatostatin analogue (SSTa) therapy in patients with GH-secreting pituitary adenoma responsive to SSTa. Clin Endocrinol. 2007;67:282–9.
35. Nunes VS, Correa JM, Puga ME, Silva EM, Boguszewski CL. Preoperative somatostatin analogues versus direct transsphenoidal surgery for newly-diagnosed acromegaly patients: a systematic review and meta-analysis using the GRADE system. Pituitary. 2015;18:500–8.
36. Plockinger U, Quabbe HJ. Presurgical octreotide treatment in acromegaly: no improvement of final growth hormone (GH) concentration and pituitary function. A long-term case-control study. Acta Neurochir. 2005;147:485–93. discussion 93
37. Vilar L, Vilar CF, Lyra R, Lyra R, Naves LA. Acromegaly: clinical features at diagnosis. Pituitary. 2016;
38. Colao A, Pivonello R, Auriemma RS, Briganti F, Galdiero M, Tortora F, et al. Predictors of tumor shrinkage after primary therapy with somatostatin analogs in acromegaly: a prospective study in 99 patients. J Clin Endocrinol Metab. 2006;91:2112–8.
39. Starke RM, Raper DM, Payne SC, Vance ML, Oldfield EH, Jane JA, Jr. Endoscopic vs microsurgical transsphenoidal surgery for acromegaly: outcomes in a concurrent series of patients using modern criteria for remission. J Clin Endocrinol Metab 2013;98:3190–3198.
40. Colao A, Auriemma RS, Pivonello R. The effects of somatostatin analogue therapy on pituitary tumor volume in patients with acromegaly. Pituitary. 2016;19:210–21.

21

Utility of serum IGF-1 for diagnosis of growth hormone deficiency following traumatic brain injury and sport-related concussion

Kirstie Lithgow[1]* (iD), Alex Chin[2], Chantel T. Debert[3] and Gregory A. Kline[1]

Abstract

Background: Growth hormone deficiency (GHD) is a potential consequence of traumatic brain injury (TBI), including sport-related concussion (SRC). GH stimulation testing is required for definitive diagnosis; however, this is resource intensive and can be associated with adverse symptoms or risks. Measurement of serum IGF-1 is more practical and accessible, and pituitary tumour patients with hypopituitarism and low serum IGF-1 have been shown to have a high probability of GHD. We aimed to evaluate IGF-1 measurement for diagnosing GHD in our local TBI population.

Methods: We conducted a retrospective chart review of patients evaluated for GHD at the TBI clinic and referred for GH stimulation testing with insulin tolerance test (ITT) or glucagon stimulation test (GST) since December 2013. We obtained demographics, TBI severity, IGF-1, data pertaining to pituitary function, and GH stimulation results. IGF-1 values were used to calculate z-scores per age and gender specific reference ranges. Receiver operator curve analysis was performed to evaluate diagnostic threshold of IGF-1 z-score for determining GHD by GST or ITT.

Results: Sixty four patient charts were reviewed. 48 patients had mild, six had moderate, eight had severe TBI, and two had non-traumatic brain injuries. 47 patients underwent ITT or GST. 27 were confirmed to have GHD (peak hGH < 5 μg/L). IGF-1 level was within the age and gender specific reference range for all patients with confirmed GHD following GH stimulation testing. Only one patient had a baseline IGF-1 level below the age and gender specific reference range; this patient had a normal response to GH stimulation testing. ROC analysis showed IGF-1 z-score AUC f, confirming lack of diagnostic utility.

Conclusion: Baseline IGF-1 is not a useful predictor of GHD in our local TBI population, and therefore has no value as a screening tool. TBI patients undergoing pituitary evaluation will require a dynamic test of GH reserve.

Background

Growth hormone deficiency (GHD) is an increasingly recognized potential consequence following traumatic brain injury (TBI) [1, 2] Patients with GHD may present with impaired concentration, memory loss, low energy, depression, anxiety, social isolation, and poor quality of life [1, 3]. Due to the subtle and non-specific nature of these symptoms, as well as the potential overlap with neurologic and psychiatric sequelae of TBI, biochemical testing is crucial in making the diagnosis of GHD [2, 4]. GH stimulation testing is required for definitive diagnosis of GHD; the insulin tolerance test (ITT) is considered the reference standard and the glucagon stimulation test (GST) is an acceptable alternative, however, this testing is time consuming, resource intensive, and can be associated with adverse side effects [5]. Measurement of serum IGF-1, as a potential marker of GH activity, is comparatively more practical and accessible, and hypopituitary patients with low serum IGF-1 values have been shown to have a high probability of GHD [6]. Previous authors showed that in a population comprised

---
* Correspondence: kclithgo@ucalgary.ca
[1]Division of Endocrinology, Department of Medicine, Cumming School of Medicine, University of Calgary, 1820 Richmond Rd SW, Calgary, AB T2T 5C7, Canada
Full list of author information is available at the end of the article

of patients with moderate and severe TBIs, an IGF-1 greater than 175 ng/mL had high negative predictive value for true GHD according to a stimulation test with peak GH response of < 3 µg/L, and was therefore helpful in deciding which patients should undergo dynamic testing [7]. However, the IGF-1 method changed from a manual to an automated method during this study, and these findings have not been validated in a population that includes patients with mild, moderate, and severe traumatic brain injuries or sports-related concussion (SRC). The latter point is especially relevant considering patients with mild TBI also have significant risk of neuroendocrine dysfunction [8]. Our primary objective was to evaluate the performance of IGF-1 as a screening tool for GHD in a patient population that includes mild (including SRC), moderate, and severe TBI.

Methods

The procedures followed in this study were in accordance with the ethical standards of the Conjoint Health Research Ethics Board at the University of Calgary, Calgary, Alberta, Canada. We conducted a retrospective review of the electronic medical record of patients referred to endocrinology from the Calgary Brain Injury Program from December 2013–2016 for evaluation of hypopituitarism/GHD with either an ITT or GST. From each patient chart, we collected demographic information including age, sex, weight, and the number of months from injury to endocrinology assessment. We also collected data pertaining to the nature of the TBI including severity (mild, moderate, or severe) and whether the TBI had been classified as a SRC. Severity of injury was classified based on the Mayo Clinic Classification which includes initial GCS, length of loss of consciousness or length of post-traumatic amnesia to retrospectively determine TBI severity [9]. Baseline IGF-1 values were recorded, as well as all biochemical data pertaining to pituitary function. IGF-1 values were used to calculate a z-score for each patient per age and gender specific reference ranges. ITT and GST were performed in a dedicated endocrine testing unit with trained endocrine nurses according previously published standard protocols [10]. The choice of ITT or GST was made according to the availability of sufficient nursing staff as two nurses are required to perform the ITT. A successful insulin hypoglycemic test was determined by the achievement of a nadir blood glucose of < 2.5 mmol/L and all tests achieved this standard. Peak GH response following dynamic GH testing with ITT or GST was used to define the presence or absence of GHD where a peak hGH < 5.0 µg/L was considered abnormal and peak < 3.0 µg/L considered severe GHD. Using the dynamic test as the reference standard, the sensitivity and specificity of IGF-1 levels and IGF-1 Z-score to detect GHD was determined.

Assays

Insulin-like growth factor-1 (IGF-1) method

Serum IGF-1 was measured by a one-step immunometric (sandwich) chemiluminescent immunoassay using the Diasorin Liaison XL platform (DiaSorin, Stillwater, MN, USA). IGF-1 is separated from binding proteins and is captured by a murine monoclonal antibody coated onto solid-phase magnetic particles and a secondary murine monoclonal antibody conjugated with an isoluminol derivative to form an immune complex. After incubation, the unbound material is removed with a wash cycle and starter reagents are added to induce a flash chemiluminescence reaction which is measured by a photomultiplier and is directly proportional to the IGF-1 concentration (ug/L) in the serum. During the period of the study, the assay exhibited imprecision levels of < 8.4%. Age- and gender-specific reference intervals (95th percentile) were adapted according to the manufacturer's instructions for use. This assay is referenced to the 1st WHO International Standard for Insulin-like Growth Factor-I NIBSC code: 02/254.

Growth hormone method

Growth hormone was measured by a one-step immunometric chemiluminescent immunoassay using the Siemens Immulite 2000 XPi platform (Siemens Healthcare Diagnostics, Tarrytown, NY, USA). Growth hormone is captured by a murine monoclonal antibody coated onto the solid phase bead a rabbit polyclonal antibody conjugated with alkaline phosphatase. After incubation, unbound material is removed by a centrifugal wash and chemiluminescent substrate is added to produce a signal which is directly proportional to the growth hormone concentration (ug/L). During the period of the study, the assay exhibited imprecision levels of < 3.9%. Reference intervals (95th percentile) were adapted according to the manufacturer's instructions for use. This assay is referenced to WHO NIBSC 2nd International Standard 98/574.

Statistics

Standard descriptive statistics were used to define demographic variables. Group medians were compared using the Mann-Whitney U test. Statistical significance was set at $p = 0.05$. Receiver operator curve analysis was performed to evaluate diagnostic threshold of IGF-1 z-score for determining GHD by GST or ITT. All statistical calculations were performed using SPSS software version 24 [11].

Results

Sixty four patient charts were retrieved. Baseline demographics according to diagnostic GH status are presented in Table 1. There were 48 mild, 6 moderate,

Table 1 Baseline Demographics

	All patients $n = 62$	GH deficient $n = 29$	Non-GH deficient $n = 18$
Age (median, IQR)	43 (21.8)	46 (17)	39 (18) $p = 0.216$
Gender	M: $n = 29$	M: $n = 15$	M: $n = 7$
	F: $n = 33$	F: $n = 14$	F: $n = 11$
Weight (median, IQR)	78.1 kg (32.3)	83 kg (34.0)	74.2 kg (23.6) $p = 0.220$
#months to endo referral (median, IQR)	20 (16)	24 (13)	15 (20) $p = 0.317$
TBI Severity	Mild $n = 48$	Mild $n = 22$	Mild $n = 17$
	Mod $n = 6$	Mod $n = 1$	Mod $n = 1$
	Severe $n = 8$	Severe $n = 6$	
Documented Sport Concussion	$n = 15$	$n = 7$	$n = 5$
	Hockey n = 4	Hockey n = 3	Basketball $n = 1$
	Cycling $n = 2$	Cycling $n = 2$	Dirt biking $n = 1$
	Basketball $n = 2$	Basketball $n = 1$	Football $n = 1$
	Soccer $n = 2$	Football $n = 1$	Equestrian $n = 1$
	Football $n = 2$		Soccer $n = 1$
	Dirt biking $n = 1$		
	Wrestling $n = 1$		
	Equestrian $n = 1$		
Documented pituitary deficits	$n = 4$	$n = 2$	$n = 1$
	$n = 1$ secondary hypothyroidism	$n = 1$ secondary hypothyroidism	$n = 1$ secondary hypogonadism and hypothyroidism
	$n = 2$ secondary hypogonadism	$n = 1$ secondary hypogonadism	
	$n = 1$ secondary hypothyroidism and secondary hypogonadism		
IGF-1 Z score (median, IQR)	−0.193 (2.07)	−0.214 (1.52)	−0.060 (1.24) $p = 0.979$
Peak GH during stim test (median, IQR)	3.8 μg/L (6.9)	1.3 μg/L (2.6)	9.7 μg/L (4.3) $p = < 0.001$

and 8 severe TBIs. Two were excluded from analysis due to having brain injuries of non-traumatic etiology. One patient passed away during the interval between assessment and dynamic testing. 14 patients did not receive GH stimulation testing after endocrinology assessment. Of these patients, six were not felt to have symptoms in keeping with GHD at the time of endocrinology assessment so were not referred on for testing. Five patients declined testing due to improvement in their symptoms at the time of endocrinology assessment, or unwillingness to undergo testing procedures. Three agreed to testing but were lost to follow-up before testing was performed. Of the 47 patients that underwent GH stimulation testing with ITT ($n = 24$, 51%) or GST ($n = 23$, 49%), 27 (57%) were confirmed to have GHD (based on a peak GH level of 5 μg/L or less), 18 (38%) had normal results to stimulation testing. Two patients (4%) patients had borderline results with a peak GH levels of 5.2 and 5.5 μg/L following GST and were classified as GHD at the discretion of the treating clinician, as therapy was offered to these patients due to symptomatology in keeping with growth hormone deficiency. Of the patients with confirmed GHD, 20 (43%) had severe GHD with peak GH < 3.0 μg/L or less.

There was a total of 15 TBIs classified as SRC; seven of which were ultimately proved to be GH deficient. Four patients had documented evidence of other pituitary deficits, which were either central hypothyroidism, central hypogonadism, or both. Of these four patients, one of them had sustained a SRC, though this individual was known to have a history of anabolic steroid use.

For each patient, IGF-1 status was correlated with GH status after stimulation testing (Table 2). Patients were labelled as having "low" IGF-1 if the value fell below the assay reference range for matched age and gender, and "normal" IGF-1 if value was within this reference range. Baseline IGF-1 level was not available for four patients in GH deficient group and two patients in the non- GH deficient group. All but one patient had normal IGF-1 levels, and the single patient with low IGF-1 level tested

Table 2 IGF-1 and GH status

	GH deficient	Non-GH deficient
IGF-1 low	0	1
IGF-1 normal	25	15
Median z-score	−0.214	− 0.060 $p = 0.979$

negative for growth hormone deficiency with a peak GH of 50.2 µg/L. Mean IGF-1 z-score was lower for patients in the non-GHD group, but this was non-significant ($p = 0.979$). IGF-1 Z-scores' ability to diagnose GHD were examined by ROC curve analysis, shown in Fig. 1. ROC analysis showed AUC of 0.495, $p = 0.959$, confirming lack of diagnostic utility.

Discussion

Our results demonstrate that baseline serum IGF-1 level had no value in predicting GH deficiency, emphasizing the need for dynamic testing in this population. These findings contradict those of Zgaljardic et al. [7] There are several differences between our respective studies that may account for this. Our study includes an older patient population, and the majority of our subjects (48/62) sustained mild TBI, while the previous paper only included patients with moderate and severe TBI. Because almost all of our patients had normal IGF-1 levels, we cannot exclude the possibility that a truly low IGF-1 level, if present, may have a high specificity for true GHD as has been seen in other hypopituitary states. However, in our data, the single patient with overtly low IGF-1 was not GH deficient and as a group, the non-GHD patients tended to have lower IGF-1 values than the GHD patients and so it may be that in TBI patients, IGF-1 measurements of any kind have very poor sensitivity or specificity for true GHD. Importantly, the IGF-1 assay used at our centre differs from that used by Zgaljardic et al.; significant variability amongst different commercial IGF-1 immunoassays has been highlighted previously [12]. Furthermore, the

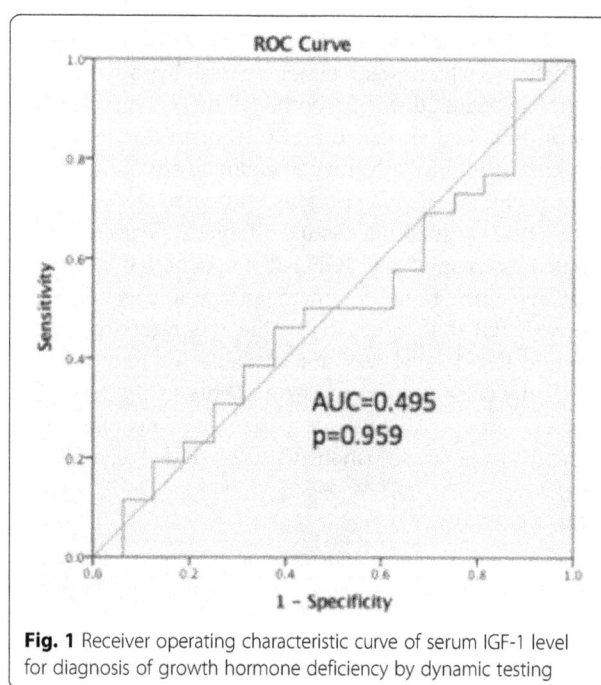

Fig. 1 Receiver operating characteristic curve of serum IGF-1 level for diagnosis of growth hormone deficiency by dynamic testing

different reference interval for each assay is a source of further complexity regarding the comparison of results between studies [13]. While reference intervals need to be method-specific, there is considerable variability in how reference ranges are derived for IGF-1 and may lead to different interpretations for the same patient [14]. Given this variability, it may require multicenter studies to validate robust reference ranges for specific IGF-1 methods to allow for better correlation between studies [12, 15]. Another factor can be due to the regulation of IGF-1 and its association with binding proteins, particularly with IGF binding proteins, whereby IGF-1 immunoassays have relied on displacement of IGF-1 from IGF binding proteins for proper measurement. Further advances in IGF-1 measurement by tandem mass spectrometry may be more specific and ensures the displacement of binding proteins by assay design. However, tandem mass spectrometry methods will similarly require proper validation of reference ranges as well as standardization [16]. In addition, the tandem mass spectrometry method may miss certain IGF-1 protein variants which have unknown functionality and will be unable to distinguish from wild type individuals [17]. Nevertheless, a repeat study that employs the use of a well-developed tandem mass spectrometry method for IGF-1 is warranted and will address the role of assay specificity in addition to variability in reference ranges. Taken together, the limitations in IGF-1 assay standardization and the results presented herein suggest the use of more specific dynamic testing of GH reserve.

Our findings add to a growing body of literature documenting pituitary dysfunction secondary to sport-related concussion. This can present with isolated or multiple pituitary hormone deficits, with GHD being the most common isolated deficit [18, 19]. While previous literature has implicated contact sports involving repetitive head trauma [4], our study includes two patients who developed growth hormone deficiency following an isolated concussion sustained while cycling. Therefore, even individuals who sustain a single concussion from non-contact sports appear to be susceptible to developing some degree of pituitary dysfunction.

Our study has several methodological limitations. Our results may not be generalizable to other institutions that use different IGF-1 assays, as we have outlined above. The referral process was not standardized; decisions about which patients are referred for endocrinology assessment reflect local practice patterns which may differ at other centres. For each patient, only a single dynamic test of GH reserve was performed, however, additional testing is not currently feasible due to cost and resource limitations. In the absence of other

Utility of serum IGF-1 for diagnosis of growth hormone deficiency following traumatic brain injury...

151

pituitary hormone deficits or obvious structural abnormalities in the pituitary, expert opinion suggests that two dynamic tests of GH reserve should be performed in order to confirm isolated GHD [20]. However, an FDA or Health Canada-approved GHRH method is not available in North America for GHRH stimulation testing, while insulin hypoglycemic testing may not be widely available at many centres and thus multi-modality testing may not be possible. In the absence of a "gold standard" diagnostic reference, it is also unknown as to whether the combination of dynamic GH stimulation tests truly improves diagnosis. In theory, diagnostic specificity may be improved but at an unknown loss of diagnostic sensitivity; this requires further study. We are unable to obtain BMI data from our EMR, which may have diagnostic implications as BMI can influence peak GH response, though the evidence on this matter is conflicting [7].

Conclusion

Our study has demonstrated the need for dynamic testing of GH reserve for patients with TBI who are suspected to have GHD at our centre. Individual measurement of IGF-1 levels and interpretation of the results according to method-specific reference ranges is ineffective to screen for GH deficiency in patients with TBI. Sport-related concussion, not just repetitive SRC of any nature appears to be a risk factor for subsequent GHD.

Abbreviations

GH: Growth hormone; GHD: Growth hormone deficiency; GST: glucagon stimulation test; hGH: human growth hormone; ITT: insulin tolerance test; SRC: sport-related concussion; TBI: traumatic brain injury

Acknowledgements

None

Funding

There is no funding source to disclose.

Authors' contributions

KL, CD, and GK were all responsible for study planning and design. KL was responsible for data collection, data analysis, and drafting the manuscript. AC assisted in data analysis and revised the lab methodology section of the manuscript. CD assisted with data analysis and statistics, reviewed all versions of the manuscript and provided minor revisions and editorial feedback. GK assisted with data analysis and statistics, reviewed all versions of the manuscript and provided major revisions and editorial feedback. All authors have given final approval of for work to be published, take responsibility for appropriate portions of the content, and agreed to be accountable for all aspects of the work.

Ethics approval and consent to participate

The authors declare that the procedures followed in this study were in accordance with the ethical approval s of the Conjoint Health Research Ethics Board at the University of Calgary, Calgary, Alberta, Canada (REB16–0355). Our study was granted waiver of consent by the Conjoint Health Research Ethics Board on the grounds that contacting all patients was thought to be unfeasible (due to the study's retrospective nature, we did not have up to date contact information for all participants) as well as the minimal risk of harm to participants given our study did not involve any direct interaction or procedures.

Competing interests

The authors declare that they have no competing interests.

Author details

[1]Division of Endocrinology, Department of Medicine, Cumming School of Medicine, University of Calgary, 1820 Richmond Rd SW, Calgary, AB T2T 5C7, Canada. [2]Clinical Biochemistry, Calgary Laboratory Services and Department of Pathology and Laboratory Medicine, Cumming School of Medicine, University of Calgary, 9, 3535 Research Road NW, Calgary, AB T2L 2K8, Canada. [3]Division of Physical Medicine and Rehabilitation, Department of Clinical Neurosciences Cumming School of Medicine, University of Calgary, 2500 University Dr. NW, Calgary, AB T2N 1N4, Canada.

References

1. Behan LA, Phillips J, Thompson CJ, Agha A. Neuroendocrine disorders after traumatic brain injury. J Neurol Neurosurg Psychiatry. 2008;79(7):753–9.
2. Brod M, Pohlman B, Højbjerre L, Adalsteinsson JE, Rasmussen MH. Impact of adult growth hormone deficiency on daily functioning and well-being. BMC Res Notes. 2014;7:813.
3. Hartman ML, Crowe BJ, Biller BM, Ho KK, Clemmons DR, Chipman JJ, Board HA, Group USHS. Which patients do not require a GH stimulation test for the diagnosis of adult GH deficiency? J Clin Endocrinol Metab. 2002;87(2):477–85.
4. Dubourg J, Messerer M. Sports-related chronic repetitive head trauma as a cause of pituitary dysfunction. Neurosurg Focus. 2011;31(5):E2.
5. Molitch ME, Clemmons DR, Malozowski S, Merriam GR, Vance ML, Society E. Evaluation and treatment of adult growth hormone deficiency: an Endocrine Society clinical practice guideline. J Clin Endocrinol Metab. 2011;96(6):1587–609.
6. Lissett CA, Jönsson P, Monson JP, Shalet SM, Board KI. Determinants of IGF-I status in a large cohort of growth hormone-deficient (GHD) subjects: the role of timing of onset of GHD. Clin Endocrinol. 2003;59(6):773–8.
7. Zgaljardic DJ, Guttikonda S, Grady JJ, Gilkison CR, Mossberg KA, High WM, Masel BE, Urban RJ. Serum IGF-1 concentrations in a sample of patients with traumatic brain injury as a diagnostic marker of growth hormone secretory response to glucagon stimulation testing. Clin Endocrinol. 2011;74(3):365–9.
8. Tanriverdi F, Kelestimur F. Pituitary dysfunction following traumatic brain injury: clinical perspectives. Neuropsychiatr Dis Treat. 2015;11:1835–43.
9. Malec JF, Brown AW, Leibson CL, Flaada JT, Mandrekar JN, Diehl NN, Perkins PK. The mayo classification system for traumatic brain injury severity. J Neurotrauma. 2007;24(9):1417–24.
10. Berg C, Meinel T, Lahner H, Yuece A, Mann K, Petersenn S. Diagnostic utility of the glucagon stimulation test in comparison to the insulin tolerance test in patients following pituitary surgery. Eur J Endocrinol. 2010;162(3):477–82.
11. IBM SPSS Statistics for Windows, version 24.0 (IBM Corp., Armonk, N.Y., USA.
12. Chanson P, Arnoux A, Mavromati M, Brailly-Tabard S, Massart C, Young J, Piketty ML, Souberbielle JC, Investigators V. Reference values for IGF-I serum concentrations: comparison of six immunoassays. J Clin Endocrinol Metab. 2016;101(9):3450–8.

13. Ranke MB, Osterziel KJ, Schweizer R, Schuett B, Weber K, Röbbel P, Vornwald A, Blumenstock G, Elmlinger MW. Reference levels of insulin-like growth factor I in the serum of healthy adults: comparison of four immunoassays. Clin Chem Lab Med. 2003;41(10):1329–34.

14. Pokrajac A, Wark G, Ellis AR, Wear J, Wieringa GE, Trainer PJ. Variation in GH and IGF-I assays limits the applicability of international consensus criteria to local practice. Clin Endocrinol. 2007;67(1):65–70.

15. Bidlingmaier M, Friedrich N, Emeny RT, Spranger J, Wolthers OD, Roswall J, Körner A, Obermayer-Pietsch B, Hübener C, Dahlgren J, et al. Reference intervals for insulin-like growth factor-1 (igf-i) from birth to senescence: results from a multicenter study using a new automated chemiluminescence IGF-I immunoassay conforming to recent international recommendations. J Clin Endocrinol Metab. 2014;99(5):1712–21.

16. Cox HD, Lopes F, Woldemariam GA, Becker JO, Parkin MC, Thomas A, Butch AW, Cowan DA, Thevis M, Bowers LD, et al. Interlaboratory agreement of insulin-like growth factor 1 concentrations measured by mass spectrometry. Clin Chem. 2014;60(3):541–8.

17. Hines J, Milosevic D, Ketha H, Taylor R, Algeciras-Schimnich A, Grebe SK, Singh RJ. Detection of IGF-1 protein variants by use of LC-MS with high-resolution accurate mass in routine clinical analysis. Clin Chem. 2015;61(7):990–1.

18. Popovic V. GH deficiency as the most common pituitary defect after TBI: clinical implications. Pituitary. 2005;8(3–4):239–43.

19. Langelier DM, Kline GA, Debert CT. Neuroendocrine dysfunction in a young athlete with concussion: a case report. Clin J Sport Med. 2017;

20. Glynn N, Agha A. Diagnosing growth hormone deficiency in adults. Int J Endocrinol. 2012;2012:972617.

22

The association between biochemical control and cardiovascular risk factors in acromegaly

John D. Carmichael[1], Michael S. Broder[2], Dasha Cherepanov[2*], Eunice Chang[2], Adam Mamelak[1], Qayyim Said[3], Maureen P. Neary[3] and Vivien Bonert[1]

Abstract

Background: The study aim was to estimate the proportion of acromegaly patients with various comorbidities and to determine if biochemical control was associated with reduced proportion of cardiovascular risk factors.

Methods: Data were from a single-center acromegaly registry. Study patients were followed for ≥12 months after initial treatment. Study period was from first to last insulin-like growth factor-I and growth hormone tests.

Results: Of 121 patients, 55% were female. Mean age at diagnosis was 42.4 (SD: 15.0). Mean study period was 8.8 (SD: 7.2) years. Macroadenomas were observed in 93 of 106 patients (87.7%), and microadenomas in 13 (12.3%). Initial treatment was surgery in 104 patients (86%), pharmacotherapy in 16 (13.2%), and radiation therapy in 1 (0.8%). Of 120 patients, 79 (65.8%) achieved control during the study period. New onset comorbidities (reported 6 months after study start) were uncommon (<10%). Comorbidities were typically more prevalent in uncontrolled versus controlled patients—24 (58.5%) vs. 33 (41.8%) had hypertension, 17 (41.5%) vs. 20 (25.3%) had diabetes, 11 (26.8%) vs. 16 (20.3%) had sleep apnea, and 3 (7.3%) vs. 3 (3.8%) had cardiomyopathy—except for colon polyps or cancer (19.5% vs. 20.3%), left ventricular hypertrophy (9.8% vs. 11.4%), and visual defects (14.6% vs. 17.7%).

Conclusions: A greater number of comorbidities were observed in biochemically uncontrolled patients with acromegaly compared to their controlled counterparts in this single-center registry. About a third of the patients remained uncontrolled after a mean of >8 years of treatment, demonstrating the difficulty of achieving control in some patients.

Keywords: Chart review, Patient registry, Acromegaly, Biochemical control, Comorbidities

Background

Acromegaly results from excessive growth hormone (GH) production, usually caused by a benign pituitary adenoma. GH has direct metabolic effects and also stimulates hepatic insulin-like growth factor-I (IGF-1) production. IGF-1 in turn facilitates somatic growth and metabolic function [1]. The disease affects between 40 and 130 individuals per million persons, or approximately 20,000 people in the US [2], and recent studies indicate incidence of pituitary tumors in the US is increasing [3]. Although untreated acromegaly has

clinically significant consequences, most signs and symptoms appear slowly, often resulting in delayed diagnosis. Most acromegaly patients are diagnosed at an average age of about 40 years [2, 4]. Diagnosis is made clinically on the basis of typical signs and symptoms and confirmed with laboratory assessment of GH and/or IGF-1 levels.

The primary goal of therapy is to normalize GH and IGF-1 levels, as these values have been shown to correspond to a reduction in mortality similar to that of an unaffected population [5, 6]. Initial treatment is generally transsphenoidal surgical resection of the adenoma, but about half of the patients require additional treatment [7]. Current guidelines recommend somatostatin receptor ligands (SRLs) (octreotide and lanreotide) or GH-receptor

* Correspondence: dasha@pharllc.com
[2]Partnership for Health Analytic Research, LLC, 280 S. Beverly Dr., Suite 404, Beverly Hills, CA 90212, USA
Full list of author information is available at the end of the article

antagonist pegvisomant for initial medical therapy in patients with moderate-to-severe signs and symptoms of GH excess. In patients with very mild signs and symptoms, guidelines suggest an initial trial of the dopamine agonist cabergoline [7, 8].

In addition to direct effects from the tumor mass, untreated patients with acromegaly may develop diabetes mellitus, hypertension, cardiomyopathy, sleep apnea, and colon polyps at rates much higher than the non-acromegaly population [9]. The risk of developing these comorbid conditions generally increases with the length and severity of biochemical abnormalities. Successful treatment appears to reduce myocardial thickness [10] and improve sleep apnea [11], but a link between biochemical control and hypertension, diabetes, and other key outcomes has not been established. We sought, using medical records from a single referral center, to estimate the proportion of acromegaly patients with various comorbid conditions, and to determine if biochemical disease control was associated with reduced rate of cardiovascular risk factors.

Methods

This was a prospective cohort study of an acromegaly registry established at the Cedars-Sinai Medical Center Pituitary Center (CSMC-PC), with retrospective chart data at CSMC-PC for some patients dating as far back as 1985. Consenting patients had data abstracted from medical records and entered in a database. This registry contains data on demographics, medical and surgical therapy, symptoms, laboratory values, cardiology and colonoscopy results, pathology, radiology, surgical information, and visual field data. The database is updated periodically. The current study focused on acromegaly patients treated at the center from 1985 through June 2013. Registry participants followed for at least 12 months after initial treatment were eligible for inclusion in the current study. The first and last values for IGF-1 and GH tests for each patient were used to define the study start and end dates. The study was approved by the CSMC Institutional Review Board.

Baseline measures, determined in the 6 months following the first recorded biochemical test, included patient demographics (age, sex, and race/ethnicity), tumor size, and presence of hormonal abnormalities (prolactin elevation [hyperprolactinemia], adrenal insufficiency [use of adrenal replacement], gonadal insufficiency [use of sex steroid replacement], and hypothyroidism [use of thyroid replacement]). Adrenal insufficiency was diagnosed with standard cortrosyn (ACTH) stimulation testing with a cutoff point of 18 mcg/dl. Treatments for acromegaly, including surgery, radiation, and pharmacotherapy, were recorded, as were the dates of those treatments. Patients receiving presurgical pharmacotherapy of short duration

were reported simply as having had surgery, unless pharmacotherapy was continued after the procedure. The presence of comorbid conditions, including hypertension (i.e., diagnosis of hypertension or use of hypertensive medication), diabetes (i.e., diagnosis of diabetes or HbA1c ≥6.5% or use of antihyperglycemic medication), left ventricular hypertrophy (LVH), cardiomyopathy, congestive heart failure (CHF), sleep apnea, colon polyps, colon cancer, and visual field defects (i.e., diagnosis of any visual acuity impairment or visual field cut), was recorded, as was the use of antihypertensive and antihyperglycemic medications. All comorbidities were diagnosed by specialists in their respective fields, using standard diagnostic methods. All GH and IGF-1 values were recorded. The primary predictor variable was biochemical control at study end, defined as a last IGF-1 less than or equal to the upper limit of normal for patient's age and gender [12, 13]. Considering the possiblity of discordance between values of GH and IGF-I in different treatment scenarios, to maintain a robust definition of control we opted to rely solely on IGF-I for this analysis [13]. The primary and secondary outcomes of interest were the proportion of patients with new onset (noted any time after the first 6 months of observation) comorbidities and the proportion with a comorbidity of interest at any time during the study period.

Descriptive statistics, including means, standard deviations (SD), medians, and percentages, were estimated for all study measures as applicable, and reported separately for patients who did and did not achieve biochemical control. For the primary analysis, presence of existing and new onset comorbidities were examined in patients, stratified on the basis of whether or not they had attained biochemical control. All data transformations and statistical analyses were performed using SAS® version 9.4 (SAS Institute, Cary, NC).

Results

A total of 121 acromegaly patients met the inclusion criteria, provided written consent, and were included in the study. The mean (SD) patient age at the time of this study was 55.4 (16.7) years, and the mean age at diagnosis was 42.4 (15.0). Overall, 67 (55%) patients were female. Race/ethnicity was reported as Caucasians for 88 (72.7%) patients, Asian for 16 (13.2%), and Hispanic for 12 (9.9%); 5 (4.1%) patients were of other race/ethnicity. The mean (SD) time from first to last recorded biochemical value (study period) was 8.8 (7.2) years, and the median (25th to 75th percentile) was 5.8 (3.2-13.7) years. For 106 patients, data were available on initial tumor size. Macroadenomas were observed in 93 patients (87.7%) and microadenomas in 13 patients (12.3%) in this cohort. On presentation, 20 (16.5%) patients had gonadal insufficiency, 19 (15.7%) had hypothyroidism, 18

(14.9%) had adrenal insufficiency, and 1 (0.8%) had elevated prolactin (Table 1).

Initial treatment was surgery, observed in 104 patients (86%), which included 13 patients with short duration pre-surgical pharmacologic therapy. Initial treatment was pharmacologic in 16 patients (13.2%), and radiation therapy in the 1 remaining patient. For patients treated with primary medical therapy, somatostatin analogues

Table 1 Baseline characteristics of 121 acromegaly patients

		All N = 121
Age, year	Mean	55.4
	(SD)	(16.7)
Age[a] at diagnosis, year	n	109
	Mean	42.4
	(SD)	(15.0)
Female	n	67
	(%)	(55.4)
Race/ethnicity		
Caucasian	n	88
	(%)	(72.7)
Asian	n	16
	(%)	(13.2)
Hispanic	n	12
	(%)	(9.9)
Other	n	5
	(%)	(4.1)
Years of follow-up	Mean	8.8
	(SD)	(7.2)
	25th percentile	3.2
	Median	5.8
	75th percentile	13.7
Tumor size[b]	n	106
Macroadenoma	n	93
	(%)	(87.7)
Microadenoma	n	13
	(%)	(12.3)
Additional Hormonal Abnormalities		
Gonadal insufficiency	n	20
	(%)	(16.5)
Hypothyroidism	n	19
	(%)	(15.7)
Adrenal insufficiency	n	18
	(%)	(14.9)
Prolactin elevation	n	1
	(%)	(0.8)

[a]109 patients had information about age at diagnosis
[b]106 patients had tumor size information

were the most common initial pharmacologic treatment, observed in 11 patients (9.1%), followed by dopamine agonists in 5 patients (4.1%) (Table 2). By the end of a median of 5.8 years of follow-up, 92 (76%) patients had been treated with multiple modalities. Of 104 initially surgically treated patients, 78 (75%) required second line treatment: 67 had pharmacotherapy, 7 a subsequent surgery, and 4 received radiotherapy as second line treatment.

Of the 121 subjects, 1 had no IGF-1 values reported, and consequently was dropped from the main analysis. Among the remaining 120, 79 (65.8%) had achieved biochemical control during the period of observation (mean 8.8 years, median 6.1 years) and 41 (34.2%) had not. The mean IGF-1 level at study start was 260% of upper limit of normal (ULN) in patients who were eventually controlled and 242% of ULN in those not controlled. The mean last IGF-1 was 67.7% of ULN in controlled and 177.8% in uncontrolled patients (Table 3).

New onset comorbidities (those first reported after the initial six months of the study period) were uncommon. There were 6 (7.6%) new cases of hypertension and 3 (3.8%) of diabetes in controlled patients compared to 3 (7.3%) and 4 (9.8%) in uncontrolled patients. There were 7 (8.9%) cases of LVH in controlled compared to 2 (4.9%) in uncontrolled patients. No new cases of cardiomyopathy were observed during the study period. There was 1 case of colon polyp or cancer in each group (1.3% controlled vs. 2.4% uncontrolled), 6 (7.6%) cases of visual field defects in controlled and 2 (4.9%) cases in uncontrolled patients, with visual field defects present in all at presentation, and not worsening during therapy (Table 4).

Considering comorbidities identified at any time during care, rather than new onset comorbidities, in the controlled group, 33 (41.8%) had hypertension compared to 24 (58.5%) in the uncontrolled group. Diabetes was observed in 20 (25.3%) of controlled compared to 17

Table 2 Initial treatment

		All N = 121
Pituitary surgery[a]	n	104[b]
	(%)	(86.0)
Radiation	n	1
	(%)	(0.8)
Pharmacotherapy	n	16
	(%)	(13.2)
Somatostatin analogues	n	11
	(%)	(9.1)
Dopamine agonists	n	5
	(%)	(4.1)

[a]Includes patients with pre-surgical medication (≤6 months medication prior to surgery)
[b]13 had presurgical medication

Table 3 Change from initial to last IGF-1 over the study period

		Controlled N = 79; 65.8%	Uncontrolled N = 41; 34.2%	All N = 120
Baseline IGF-1 (% of UNL)	Mean	260.3	241.6	253.9
Last IGF-1 (% of UNL)	Mean	67.7	177.8	105.3
Difference (last test value minus the baseline value)	Mean	192.6	−63.8	−148.6

IGF-1 insulin-like growth factor I, *ULN* upper limit of normal

(41.5%) of uncontrolled patients. LVH and cardiomyopathy were identified in 9 (11.4%) and 3 (3.8%) of controlled patients compared to 4 (9.8%) and 3 (7.3%) of uncontrolled patients. Sleep apnea was present in 16 (20.3%) of controlled and 11 (26.8%) of uncontrolled patients. Colon polyps or cancer were present in 16 (20.3%) of controlled and 8 (19.5%) of uncontrolled patients. Visual field defects were observed in 14 (17.7%) of controlled and 6 (14.6%) of uncontrolled patients (Table 5).

Discussion

In a large sample of acromegaly patients treated at a single US referral center, we demonstrated a greater number of cardiovascular and other comorbidities in biochemically uncontrolled patients with acromegaly compared to their controlled counterparts. We also observed that despite the use of multiple treatment modalities by experienced clinicians, about a third of the patients presenting to a tertiary referral center remained biochemically uncontrolled after a mean of more than eight years of treatment, demonstrating the difficulty of achieving biochemical control in some patients. Finally, we identified a higher prevalence

of hypertension, diabetes, and sleep apnea than has been reported in other acromegaly registries [14, 15].

Cardiovascular disease in general, and LVH in particular, are a significant cause of mortality in acromegaly [1, 5]. The biochemical basis of cardiac remodeling and subsequent LVH in acromegaly is not fully established but appears to result, at least in part, as a direct effect of elevated levels of GH and IGF-1 on cardiac cells [16]. Treatment of these biochemical abnormalities improves LVH. A review of 15 studies, most less than 1 year in duration, showed consistent reduction in LVH after biochemical control of the disease [9], and subsequent studies have had similar results [10]. Factors other than a direct hormonal effect on cardiac muscle may influence development of cardiac disease. Colao et al. [17] reported that hypertension and diabetes also correlate with the presence of cardiomyopathy.

Hypertension (47.5%) and diabetes (30.8%) were the most commonly observed comorbidities during the study period, and both were more common in uncontrolled patients than in controlled patients. LVH was reported in 10.8%, and CHF in 5% of patients. Hypertension was more

Table 4 New onset comorbid conditions[a], stratified by last observed biochemical control

		Controlled N = 79; 65.8%	Uncontrolled N = 41; 34.2%	All N = 120
Cardiovascular				
Hypertension	n	6	3	9
	(%)	(7.6)	(7.3)	(7.5)
Diabetes mellitus	n	3	4	7
	(%)	(3.8)	(9.8)	(5.8)
Left ventricular hypertrophy	n	7	2	9
	(%)	(8.9)	(4.9)	(7.5)
Cardiomyopathy or heart failure	n	0	0	0
	(%)	(0.0)	(0.0)	(0.0)
Other				
Sleep apnea	n	0	0	0
	(%)	(0.0)	(0.0)	(0.0)
Colonic polyps or colon cancer	n	1	1	2
	(%)	(1.3)	(2.4)	(1.7)
Visual field defects	n	6	2	8
	(%)	(7.6)	(4.9)	(6.7)

[a]New onset comorbidities were defined as evidence of condition during the study period, excluding the first 6 months comprising the baseline period

Table 5 Comorbid conditions, stratified by last observed biochemical control

		Controlled N = 79; 65.8%	Uncontrolled N = 41; 34.2%	All N =120
Cardiovascular				
Hypertension	n	33	24	57
	(%)	(41.8)	(58.5)	(47.5)
Diabetes mellitus	n	20	17	37
	(%)	(25.3)	(41.5)	(30.8)
Left ventricular hypertrophy	n	9	4	13
	(%)	(11.4)	(9.8)	(10.8)
Cardiomyopathy or heart failure	n	3	3	6
	(%)	(3.8)	(7.3)	(5.0)
Other				
Sleep apnea	n	16	11	27
	(%)	(20.3)	(26.8)	(22.5)
Colonic polyps or colon cancer	n	16	8	24
	(%)	(20.3)	(19.5)	(20.0)
Visual field defects	n	14	6	20
	(%)	(17.7)	(14.6)	(16.7)

commonly encountered in the current study than has been reported in several European registries, and somewhat higher than a commonly cited figure of 40% [18]. For example, in a Belgian acromegaly registry of 418 patients, Bex et al. [14] reported that 39.4% of reported cases had hypertension. From a Spanish registry of more than 1000 patients, Mestron et al. [15] reported 39.1% with hypertension. Diabetes was less common (25.3%) in the Belgian study and slightly more common (36.5%) in the Spanish study [14, 15]. Hypertension and diabetes are associated with mortality in the non-acromegaly population, although the current literature is inconsistent with regard to the impact of biochemical acromegaly control on reduction in these risk factors [9]. We observed higher prevalence of both conditions in uncontrolled compared to controlled patients. New onset of major comorbidities was uncommonly encountered, regardless of biochemical control status. Hypertension (7.5%), left ventricular hypertrophy (7.5%), visual field defects (6.7%), and diabetes (5.8%) were the most frequently observed new-onset comorbidities; all other comorbidities of interest occurred were uncommon (<2%).

Despite the availability of multiple therapies, including newer pharmacologic treatments, reducing serum IGF-1 levels to within the normal range remains challenging in some patients. Overall, IGF-1 dropped substantially: from 254% of ULN at study start to 105% of ULN at study end. Achieving this reduction required the use of multiple therapeutic modalities, and even with these treatments, 34% of patients did not attain biochemical control at the end of the study. However, even among uncontrolled patients, IGF-1 values fell from 242% to 178% of ULN, suggesting that continued treatment over time is likely to provide some biochemical improvement. It is unclear with this analysis if this improvement imparts benefit in terms of comorbidities, in patients not meeting a definition of biochemical control. Nonadherence may have reduced the number of patients who were in control at the end of the study. It is unclear from the current data the extent to which patients were adherent to therapy.

This study has several limitations. Firstly, despite the relatively large sample size for a study of acromegaly, small numbers moderate the power of statistical comparisons. Secondly, the results reflect care at a single institution over more than two decades. Practices have changed significantly over that time, and the results, therefore, may not be representative of what would be experienced were the study to be repeated today. Thirdly, some patients were treated elsewhere before referral to CSMC-PC. This is a study of population of patients with complex acromegaly, referred for specialized tertiary or quaternary care. Data entered in the registry reflects care from a variety of providers both within and outside CSMC and documentation may not have been optimal. Finally, this is not a randomized-placebo controlled study, where the study design would have required strict medication titration protocol and oversight until control was attained. This is a registry where there could have been treatment interruption (e.g., insurance coverage) and unsupervised or possibly sub-optimal dose titration that may have had impact attainment of control.

Conclusion

Overall, a greater number of comorbidities were observed in biochemically uncontrolled patients with acromegaly compared to their controlled counterparts in this single-center registry. This study indicates that about a third of the patients remained uncontrolled after a mean of >8 years of treatment, demonstrating the difficulty of achieving control in some patients.

Abbreviations
CHF: Congestive heart failure; CSMC-PC: Cedars-Sinai Medical Center Pituitary Center; GH: Growth hormone; IGF-1: Insulin-like growth factor-I; LVH: Left ventricular hypertrophy; SD: Standard deviations; SRLs: Somatostatin receptor ligands; ULN: Upper limit of normal

Acknowledgements
Not applicable.

Funding
This study was funded by Novartis Pharmaceuticals Corporation. The funder reviewed the manuscript.

Authors' contributions
JDC, MSB, DC, EC, AM, QS, MPN, and VB all met the ICMJE criteria for authorship. JDC, MSB, DC, EC, AM, QS, MPN, and VB were involved in the design of the study, interpretation of results, and writing of the manuscript. Additionally, JDC, AM, and VB participated in data acquisition and EC conducted the statistical analyses. All authors read and approved the final manuscript.

Competing interests
Maureen P. Neary and Qayyim Said are employees of Novartis Pharmaceuticals Corporation. Michael S. Broder, Eunice Chang, and Dasha Cherepanov are employees of the Partnership for Health Analytic Research, LLC, a health services research company paid by Novartis to conduct this research.

Author details
[1]Cedars-Sinai Medical Center, 8700 Beverly Blvd, Los Angeles, CA 90048, USA. [2]Partnership for Health Analytic Research, LLC, 280 S. Beverly Dr., Suite 404, Beverly Hills, CA 90212, USA. [3]Novartis Pharmaceuticals Corporation, One Health Plaza, East Hanover, NJ 07936-1080, USA.

References
1. Melmed S. Medical progress: Acromegaly. N Engl J Med. 2006;355(24):2558–73. Review. Erratum in: N Engl J Med. 2007 Feb 22;356(8):879.
2. Chanson P, Salenave S. Acromegaly. Orphanet J Rare Dis. 2008;3:17.
3. Gittleman H, Ostrom QT, Farah PD, Ondracek A, Chen Y, Wolinsky Y, Kruchko C, Singer J, Kshettry VR, Laws ER, Sloan AE, Selman WR, Barnholtz-Sloan JS. Descriptive epidemiology of pituitary tumors in the United States, 2004–2009. J Neurosurg. 2014;121(3):527–35.
4. Chanson P, Salenave S, Kamenicky P, Cazabat L, Young J. Pituitary tumours: acromegaly. Best Pract Res Clin Endocrinol Metab. 2009;23(5):555–74.
5. Colao A, Auriemma RS, Pivonello R, Galdiero M, Lombardi G. Medical consequences of acromegaly: what are the effects of biochemical control? Rev Endocr Metab Disord. 2008;9(1):21–31. Review.
6. Swearingen B, Barker 2nd FG, Katznelson L, Biller BM, Grinspoon S, Klibanski A, Moayeri N, Black PM, Zervas NT. Long-term mortality after transsphenoidal surgery and adjunctive therapy for acromegaly. J Clin Endocrinol Metab. 1998;83(10):3419–26.
7. Katznelson L, Laws Jr ER, Melmed S, Molitch ME, Murad MH, Utz A, Wass JA. Endocrine Society.. Acromegaly: an endocrine society clinical practice guideline. J Clin Endocrinol Metab. 2014;99(11):3933–51.
8. Melmed S, Casanueva F, Cavagnini F, Chanson P, Frohman LA, Gaillard R, Ghigo E, Ho K, Jaquet P, Kleinberg D, Lamberts S, Laws E, Lombardi G, Sheppard MC, Thorner M, Vance ML, Wass JA, Giustina A. Consensus statement: medical management of acromegaly. Eur J Endocrinol. 2005;153(6):737–40.
9. Colao A, Ferone D, Marzullo P, Lombardi G. Systemic complications of acromegaly: epidemiology, pathogenesis, and management. Endocr Rev. 2004;25(1):102–52. Review.
10. De Marinis L, Bianchi A, Mazziotti G, Mettimano M, Milardi D, Fusco A, Cimino V, Maira G, Pontecorvi A, Giustina A. The long-term cardiovascular outcome of different GH-lowering treatments in acromegaly. Pituitary. 2008;11(1):13–20.
11. Herrmann BL, Wessendorf TE, Ajaj W, Kahlke S, Teschler H, Mann K. Effects of octreotide on sleep apnoea and tongue volume (magnetic resonance imaging) in patients with acromegaly. Eur J Endocrinol. 2004;151(3):309–15.
12. Puder JJ, Nilavar S, Post KD, Freda PU. Relationship between disease-related morbidity and biochemical markers of activity in patients with acromegaly. J Clin Endocrinol Metab. 2005;90(4):1972–8.
13. Carmichael JD, Bonert VS, Mirocha JM, Melmed S. The utility of oral glucose tolerance testing for diagnosis and assessment of treatment outcomes in 166 patients with acromegaly. J Clin Endocrinol Metab. 2009;94(2):523–7.
14. Bex M, Abs R, T'Sjoen G, Mockel J, Velkeniers B, Muermans K, Maiter D. AcroBel–the Belgian registry on acromegaly: a survey of the 'real-life' outcome in 418 acromegalic subjects. Eur J Endocrinol. 2007;157(4):399–409.
15. Mestron A, Webb SM, Astorga R, Benito P, Catala M, Gaztambide S, Gomez JM, Halperin I, Lucas-Morante T, Moreno B, Obiols G, de Pablos P, Paramo C, Pico A, Torres E, Varela C, Vazquez JA, Zamora J, Albareda M, Gilabert M. Epidemiology, clinical characteristics, outcome, morbidity and mortality in acromegaly based on the Spanish Acromegaly Registry (Registro Espanol de Acromegalia, REA). Eur J Endocrinol. 2004;151(4):439–46.
16. Saccà L, Cittadini A, Fazio S. Growth hormone and the heart. Endocr Rev. 1994;15(5):555–73. Review.
17. Colao A, Baldelli R, Marzullo P, Ferretti E, Ferone D, Gargiulo P, Petretta M, Tamburrano G, Lombardi G, Liuzzi A. Systemic hypertension and impaired glucose tolerance are independently correlated to the severity of the acromegalic cardiomyopathy. J Clin Endocrinol Metab. 2000;85(1):193–9.
18. Melmed S, Casanueva FF, Klibanski A, Bronstein MD, Chanson P, Lamberts SW, Strasburger CJ, Wass JA, Giustina A. A consensus on the diagnosis and treatment of acromegaly complications. Pituitary. 2013;16(3):294–302.

23

Clinical Management of Malignant Insulinoma: a single Institution's experience over three decades

Jie Yu, Fan Ping, Huabing Zhang, Wei Li, Tao Yuan, Yong Fu, Kai Feng, Weibo Xia, Lingling Xu[*] and Yuxiu Li[*]

Abstract

Background: Malignant insulinoma is extremely rare and accounts for only 10% of total insulinoma cases. The goal of this study is to retrospectively analyze clinical data from 15 patients with malignant insulinoma treated at Peking Union Medical College Hospital (PUMCH) from 1984 to April 2017.

Methods: "Malignant insulinoma" was used as the keywords in the PUMCH medical record retrieval system to search and obtain patients' clinical information. We identified subjects diagnosed with malignant insulinoma based on clinical or surgical pathological signs and subsequently analyzed their clinical data.

Results: Eight males and seven females with a median age at diagnosis of 40 years (38–54 years) were included. Eight patients (53%) had developed metastases at diagnosis, while the others (46.67%) developed metastases during the follow-up visits. The major sites of metastasis were the liver (86.7%), local tissues and blood vessels (33%) and abdominal lymph nodes (13%). All patients displayed neuroglycopenic (100%) and/or autonomic (60%) symptoms, mostly during fasting periods (73.3%), with an average blood glucose level of 1.66 ± 0.51 mmol/L. A total of 93% of the patients had one primary pancreatic lesion, 53% had a lesion in the head of the pancreas, and 47% had a lesion in the tail of the pancreas, with diameters ranging between 0.9 and 6.0 cm. Most liver metastases were multiple lesions. Selective celiac arteriography yielded 100% sensitivity for both primary pancreatic lesions and liver metastases. Most patients received synthetical treatments, including surgery, chemoembolization, and octreotide.

Conclusions: Malignant insulinomas have a similar diagnostic process to that of benign insulinomas but require far more comprehensive therapies to alleviate hypoglycemic symptoms and extend patients' survival.

Keywords: Malignant insulinoma, Metastasis, Hyperinsulinism, Hypoglycemia, Diagnosis, Therapeutics

Background

Insulinoma is a type of functional pancreatic neuroendocrine tumor (pNET) that originates from islet beta cells, which excessively secrete insulin and cause hypoglycemia. Insulinoma is the most common functional pNET, with a prevalence of approximately one to four cases per million people [1]. Four features of insulinoma are associated with four "90%" parameters: 90% are benign, 90% are solitary, 90% occur in the pancreas, and 90% are less than 2 cm in diameter [1]. Malignant insulinoma is extremely rare and accounts for only about 10% of all insulinoma cases [2]. Malignant insulinoma refers to cases exhibiting local invasion or distal metastasis, which is the only biological property that differentiates malignant cases from benign cases. Clinical manifestations, biochemical traits, and pathology cannot be used as direct evidence for identification. Benign insulinomas are typically treated surgically, whereas malignant insulinomas often require comprehensive approaches to maximize patient survival. In this study, we analyzed the clinical data of 15 cases of malignant insulinoma treated at the Peking Union Medical College Hospital (PUMCH) from 1984 to April 2017.

* Correspondence: llxuwsh@163.com; liyuxiu@medmail.com.cn
Department of Endocrinology, Chinese Academy of Medical Sciences and Peking Union Medical College, Peking Union Medical College Hospital, Beijing, China

Methods

Study subjects

"Malignant insulinoma" was used as the keywords to search the PUMCH medical record retrieval system for patients with a discharge diagnosis of malignant insulinoma and their related clinical data from 1984 to April 2017. The search yielded 25 patients. Among these patients, the medical records of three patients were unavailable, two patients were later diagnosed with benign insulinoma, two patients were diagnosed with recurrent insulinoma, two patients were diagnosed with multiple insulinomas, and one patient had no clear diagnosis; therefore, 15 patients diagnosed with malignant insulinoma based on clinical and/or pathological evidence were included in this study. The clinical diagnostic criteria for malignant insulinoma included the following: i) hypoglycemic symptoms and the Whipple triad; ii) endogenous hyperinsulinemic hypoglycemia symptoms, with a blood glucose level < 3 mmol/L, insulin level > 3 μIU/mL, and C-peptide level > 0.6 ng/mL; and iii) pancreatic tumors with local infiltration or distant metastases based on evidence from one or several imaging methods. In addition, the pathological diagnostic criteria included a clinical diagnosis with surgical or puncture specimens indicative of a pNET [3].

Study methods

Retrieval of clinical information

We retrospectively analyzed the detailed clinical information of the 15 patients, including 1) general information, such as gender, age at disease onset, age at diagnosis, family history, and the presence of multiple endocrine neoplasia; 2) clinical signs, such as the time of hypoglycemia onset and neuroglycopenic and autonomic symptoms at hypoglycemia onset; and 3) qualitative and localization diagnostic information; the qualitative diagnosis included the blood glucose, insulin, and C-peptide levels at hypoglycemia onset, and localization methods included abdominal ultrasound, abdominal enhanced computed tomography (CT), pancreatic volume perfusion CT, octreotide imaging, and selective celiac arteriography; 4) treatments, including surgery, interventional approaches, chemotherapy, and somatostatin analogues; 5) tumor characteristics, including the number, size, distribution, and location and metastasis information; and 6) pathological information. Most patients did not have detailed histological information, and we could not perform tumor staging or analyze the Ki-67 index. Moreover, we divided the 15 patients into two groups according to the timing of metastasis diagnosis: metastasis upon diagnosis or metastasis during the follow-up. Then, some clinical characteristics were compared between the groups. All follow-up visits were performed by phone calls in which the patients or their family members stated the disease conditions.

Biochemical assays

Glucose detection The glucose oxidase assay was performed to determine the serum glucose level. The serum insulin and C-peptide levels were examined using radioimmunoassays (DPC, America) prior to 1991 and chemiluminescence assays (ADVIA Centaur XP, Siemens) after 1991. All tests were performed in the Clinical Laboratory of the PUMCH.

Data analysis

Continuous data are expressed as the mean ± standard deviation when they were normally distributed or as the median (interquartile range) when they were not normally distributed. A t test was performed to compare the means of the continuous data with a normal distribution, whereas the Mann-Whitney U test was used for continuous data with a non-normal distribution. Statistical analyses were performed using IBM SPSS Statistics Version 22.0 (Chicago, IL, USA). A two-tailed $P < 0.05$ was considered significant.

Results

Basic characteristics

The 15 patients included eight males and seven females with a median age at diagnosis of 40 (38–54) years. Eight patients (53%), including four males and four females, had metastases upon diagnosis, whereas the seven remaining patients, including four males and three females, developed hepatic metastases 2 to 25 years after the insulinoma diagnosis. The most common site of metastasis was the liver (86.7%), followed by local tissues and blood vessels (33%) and abdominal lymph nodes (13%). Two patients (13%, Nos. 9 and 15) experienced hepatic metastases and pancreatic local recurrence during the follow-up visits (Table 1).

Clinical manifestations

All 15 subjects showed symptoms of hypoglycemia manifesting as neuroglycopenic symptoms (100%) and/or autonomic symptoms (60%). The most common neuroglycopenic symptoms included confusion (80%), coma (46.7%), behavioral changes (46.7%), and seizure (40%). The most common autonomic symptoms included sweating (53.3%), weakness (40%), palpitations (33.3%), and hunger (20%). Symptoms other than hypoglycemia were rare, and only one patient (No. 1) developed repeated back pain at disease onset, while one patient (No. 12) presented with discomfort under the xiphoid process and in the right abdomen at the time of liver metastasis diagnosis at a follow-up visit.

Hypoglycemia most often occurred during periods of fasting (73.3%), followed by before lunch or before dinner (46.7%), whereas hypoglycemia was rare after meals

Table 1 Clinical characteristics of the 15 patients with malignant insulinoma

No.[c]	Gender	Age at diagnosis	Hypoglycemia time	GLU (mmol/L)	INS (µIU/mL)	C-P (ng/mL)	Number and diameter (cm) of primary lesions	Location of primary lesions[a]	Local infiltration	Sites and numbers of metastases	Treatment after metastasis occurrence	Prognosis	Follow-up duration (years)[b]
1	F	54	Fasting, before meals	1.4	32.05	5.6	1, 5×5	Head	Yes	Multiple liver metastases	TACE for 1 course	N.A.	Loss to follow-up
2	F	63	Fasting	1.3	81.41	3.9	1, 1.8×1.4	Neck	No	Multiple pulmonary metastases, bone metastases?	Automatic discharge	No symptoms of hypoglycemia	Survival (7 years)
3	M	46	Fasting	1.6	62.52	5.2	1, 5.8×4.3	Tail	Yes	Multiple liver and lymph nodes metastases	Somatostatin analogues for 9 courses	Alleviation of hypoglycemia	Loss to follow-up
4	M	51	Before meals	1.0	N.A.[d]	N.A.	3, 3×4	Tail	Yes	Multiple liver metastases	Distal pancreatectomy	No remission	Loss to follow-up
5	M	26	Fasting	2.2	121.8	N.A.	1, 1.5	Head	No	Multiple intracranial metastases	Pancreatic lesion enucleation	Blood glucose increased, still in a coma	Loss to follow-up
6	F	30	Before meals	1.0	300	7.9	1, 0.9	Body	No	Multiple liver and lymph nodes metastases	Enucleation with partial hepatectomy, Sandostatin LAR for 2 courses	No hypoglycemia	Survival (0.8 years)
7	M	55	Fasting	1.9	148	N.A.	1, 6	Tail	Yes	Multiple liver metastases	Exploratory laparotomy, TACE for 1 course	N.A.	Loss to follow-up
8	F	39	Fasting, after meals and exercise	1.9	15.2	2.9	1, N.A.	Head	No	Multiple liver metastases	pancreatic surgery (unspecified)	No hypoglycemia	Survival (14 years)
9	M	72	Fasting, before meals	2.3	29.48	2.7	1, 1.5	Head	No	Solitary liver metastases	Surgical resection of liver metastases	No remission	Survival (4 years)
10	F	39	Before meals	1.5	42.2	2.5	1, 1.2	Head	No	Multiple liver metastases	Exploratory laparotomy, absolute ethanol injection ablation for 3 courses, TACE for 10 courses	Temporary remission	Survival (13 years)
11	M	40	Fasting	2.9	5.2	0.6	1, 0.8×1	Head	No	Multiple liver metastases	Sandostatin LAR for 2 courses	No remission	Loss to follow-up
12	F	50	Fasting, before meals, after exercise	1.9	300	21.61	1, N.A.	N.A.	No	Multiple liver metastases	Liver interventional therapy for 4 courses, liver surgery (unspecified)	No hypoglycemia	Survival (6 years)
13	M	38	Fasting, after exercise	2.1	N.A.	N.A.	1, 1	Tail	No	Solitary liver metastases	Surgical resection of liver metastases	No hypoglycemia	Loss to follow-up
14	M	36	Fasting	0.9	17	3.7	1, N.A.	Neck	No	Multiple liver metastases	Exploratory laparotomy, TACE for 1 courses	N.A.	Loss to follow-up
15	F	38	Fasting, before meals	1.6	71.8	7.3	1, 6×4	Tail	No	Multiple liver metastases	TACE for 4 courses	3 years of remission	Loss to follow-up

[a]Location of primary lesions: final determination was based on preoperative mapping and intraoperative positioning
[b]Survival duration: the period between metastasis occurrence and follow-up visits
[c]Case Nos. 1–8 had developed metastasis upon diagnosis, whereas case Nos. 9–15 developed metastasis during the follow-up visits
[d]N.A., data not available

(6.7%). The average blood glucose level upon symptom onset was 1.66 ± 0.51 mmol/L.

Patient No. 11 additionally presented with asymptomatic primary hyperparathyroidism and was clinically diagnosed with multiple endocrine neoplasia type 1 (MEN1). Patient No. 8 additionally presented with left adrenal nonfunctional adenoma and was clinically suspected of having MEN1. Neither of the two cases had a family history of MEN1 or received the MEN1 gene test.

Biochemical analysis and lesion localization

All patients denied previous use of sulfonylureas or insulin. Eleven patients had documented blood glucose, insulin, and C-peptide levels (Table 1), which were all consistent with the criteria for endogenous hyperinsulinemic hypoglycemia. A comparison between the patients with metastases upon diagnosis and their counterparts who developed metastases during the follow-up revealed that the former group appeared to have lower glucose levels but higher insulin and C-peptide levels than the latter group, although the differences were not significant (Table 2). Ten patients had histological confirmation of a pancreatic primary lesion or liver metastatic lesion through surgical or puncture biopsy pathology.

All patients except for one had a solitary pancreatic primary lesion. The maximal diameters of the primary lesions ranged between 0.9 and 6.0 cm, 53% of the lesions were located in the head and neck, and 47% of the lesions were located in the body and tail. The most common metastatic site was the liver (86.7%), and almost all cases of liver metastasis (84.6%) involved multiple hepatic metastases. Among the eight patients with metastasis at diagnosis, tumors were evenly distributed in the head, body, and tail of the pancreas; however, among the seven patients who developed metastasis during the follow-up visits, 50% of the tumors were in the head of the pancreas (Table 1).

Spearman analysis was performed to test the associations between the tumor size and insulin, C-peptide, and glucose levels. We have found a positive correlation between tumor size with both insulin and C-peptide levels($r = 0.183$, $P = 0.613$; and $r = 0.268$, $P = 0.493$, respectively), but a negative correlation between tumor size and glucose levels ($r = -0.182$, $P = 0.572$), although none of the differences reached significance due to the small sample size.

Sensitivity of localization tests

Of the 10 patients with a histologically confirmed pancreatic primary lesion or liver metastatic lesion, 6 patients received selective celiac arteriography 7 times, and the sensitivity for both primary pancreatic lesions and liver metastases was 100%. Next, we used celiac arterial angiography or pathological confirmation as the gold standard to analyze the sensitivity of other preoperative noninvasive localization examinations, as shown in Table 3.

Treatment and efficacy

Of the eight patients with metastases at diagnosis, four patients underwent surgery, three of whom displayed total or partial remission of hypoglycemia (75%) (Table 1). Among the other four patients who did not undergo surgery, one rejected any treatment, two underwent transcatheter arterial (chemo) embolization (TAE/ TACE) but were later lost to follow-up, and one patient (Patient No. 3) received somatostatin analogues (five treatments of Sandostatin LAR and four treatments of Somatuline), which alleviated hypoglycemic symptoms.

Of the seven patients who showed no metastases at diagnosis, five patients underwent enucleation, one patient (Patient No. 13) underwent distal pancreatectomy and splenectomy, and one patient (Patient No. 11) underwent complete pancreatectomy; all patients achieved complete remission of hypoglycemia. During the follow-up, two of these patients displayed a single liver metastasis, and resection of the liver lesion relieved hypoglycemia in only one of these patients (50%). Of the other 5 patients who displayed multiple liver metastases, one underwent surgery combined with TAE/ TACE, which resulted in complete remission of hypoglycemia, one patient received somatostatin analogues, and three patients received only TAE/ TACE, resulting in only temporary remission or no remission (Table 1).

Because the availability of diazoxide was limited in hospitals and pharmacies in mainland China, only one patient (Patient No. 10) received diazoxide in a short period of time, but the drug was discontinued due to poor performance.

Follow-up visits

Of the 15 patients, six completed the follow-up visits, with a duration ranging from nine months to 29 years. All six of these subjects survived. The period from metastasis occurrence to follow-up ranged from nine months to 14

Table 2 Blood glucose, insulin, and C-peptide concentrations with hypoglycemia

	Metastasis identified upon diagnosis	Metastasis occurred during follow-up	P value
Glucose (median, quartile, mmol/L)	1.5 (1.1–1.9)	1.9 (1.5–2.3)	0.23
Insulin (median, quartile, μIU/mL)	81.41 (32.05–148.00)	35.84 (14.05–128.85)	0.28
C-peptide (median, quartile, ng/mL)	5.20 (3.40–6.75)	3.20 (2.03–10.88)	0.36

Table 3 Sensitivity of preoperative noninvasive localization tests

	Primary lesions		Liver metastases	
	Cases examined	Sensitivity	Cases examined	Sensitivity
Abdominal ultrasound	10	50%	6	85.7%
Abdominal enhanced CT	7	50%	6	83.3%
Pancreatic volume perfusion CT	2	50%	2	100%
Octreotide imaging	1	0	2	0

years, with a median of 6.5 years. Among these patients, five (83.3%) were females with a median diagnostic age of 42.5 (30–47) years. Three patients had metastases at diagnosis, whereas the other three showed metastases during the follow-up visits. All patients had a single primary pancreatic lesion with a maximal diameter of 0.9–1.8 cm. Four patients had multiple liver metastases, and one patient had multiple pulmonary metastases and suspected bone metastases, while the other one patient successively developed a single hepatic metastasis and pancreatic recurrence in situ. Five patients underwent cytoreductive surgery and/or combined with TAE/ TACE and/or somatostatin treatment. Currently, four patients have no hypoglycemic symptoms, and two patients need extra meals every day (Table 1).

Discussion

Insulinoma is the most common functional pancreatic neuroendocrine tumor (pNET), and malignant insulinoma is very rare, with a prevalence of only one case per million people [4], accounting for 7–10% of all cases of insulinoma [1, 5]. In this study, we retrospectively analyzed the clinical data of 15 cases of malignant insulinoma treated at the PUMCH from 1984 to April 2017. The numbers of males and females were similar, and the median age at diagnosis was 40 (38–54) years. More than 50% of the patients exhibited metastases at diagnosis, with the liver as the most common metastatic site. The main clinical manifestations were hypoglycemia-related symptoms. Unlike patients with benign insulinoma, those with the malignant type exhibit pronounced neuroglycopenic symptoms. Selective celiac arteriography yielded 100% positive rates for both pancreatic primary lesions and liver metastases. Almost all patients had solitary lesions of different sizes in the pancreas, which were evenly distributed in the pancreas. The therapeutic approaches included surgery, TAE/ TACE, and somatostatin analogue administration.

Malignant insulinoma has a reported onset age of 50–60 years, which is older than the ages of the patients in our report, and no gender preference [2]. Affected patients mostly exhibit neuroglycopenic symptoms, resulting from higher insulin and proinsulin secretion, which is consistent with our study. Although, the severity of hypoglycemia symptoms is reportedly not proportional to the tumor

burden, we found a positive correlation between tumor size and insulin and C-peptide level [2, 6].

Liver metastasis upon disease onset is the most common manifestation of malignant insulinoma. Rarely, malignancy is diagnosed at the time of recurrence, which occurs for only 2% of insulinomas overall [2]. The most common metastatic sites of malignant insulinoma are the abdomen, including the retroperitoneal lymph nodes and liver, while bone, lung or other metastasis sites are rare [1, 2, 7]. In our study, more than 80% of the patients displayed liver metastasis, more than 30% of the patients showed invasion into local blood vessels or neighboring tissues, only one patient had brain metastasis, and one patient showed lung metastasis and suspected bone metastasis, which are consistent with previous studies.

Among noninvasive localization methods for insulinoma, abdominal ultrasound had a relatively low sensitivity of 9–64% [8], CT and magnetic resonance imaging (MRI) yielded a sensitivity of 56–70% and 63–86% separately [9, 10]. As for invasive approaches, sensitivity of endoscopic ultrasonography (EUS) was 86.6–92.3% [9], and arteriography had a sensitivity of approximately 70% [11]. In our previous study, we separately analyzed the sensitivity for primary pancreatic lesions and liver metastases, and found that arteriography had the best performance and all of abdominal ultrasound, enhanced CT and volume perfusion CT (VPCT) had considerable higher sensitivities for detecting liver metastases versus pancreatic lesions. As for somatostatin receptor imaging, it was reported to generate a positive rate of 30–50% [2, 12], and Jin et al. reported that it had an 85.7% sensitivity for malignant insulinoma, which was higher than for benign insulinoma (37.9%) [13]. In our study, because of only few cases detected, the results were all negative. Alternatively, if we used a clinical diagnosis of malignant insulinoma as the criterion, it produced a sensitivity of 80% (4/5) for pancreatic primary lesions and 50% (3/6) for liver metastases, which is consistent with previous results [13].

A comprehensive approach is needed to treat malignant insulinoma, which includes medication, surgery, and interventional therapy. For patients with advanced or metastatic lesions, cytoreductive surgery is conducive to control hormone secretion [2], although whether it can extend survival remains controversial. TAE/TACE is often used to manage liver metastases and has an effectiveness rate greater than

50% [3]. Therapy using somatostatin analogues has an objective remission rate (ORR) of less than 10% and a disease control rate (DCR) between 35 and 40% [3]. In our study, 7 patients underwent cytoreductive surgery when they developed metastases, 71.4% of whom displayed increased blood glucose levels and showed complete or partial remission of hypoglycemia. Therefore, surgery is an effective approach to control symptoms for patients with malignant insulinoma, although the curative outcome may differ from one patient to another. TAE/TACE and somatostatin treatment approaches generated remission rates lower than those reported in a previous study [14], and the discrepancy may be due to the small study population and high loss to follow-up rate.

Lepage et al. studied 81 patients with malignant insulinomas and found that they had a five-year survival rate of 55.6% [15]. A report from the Mayo Clinic following 13 cases of malignant insulinoma found that these patients had a 10-year survival rate of 29% [16]. No consensus has been reached regarding this discrepancy, although Ki67 was proposed to affect total survival [4]. Hirshberg et al. compared survivors of a long course of disease and patients with a poor prognosis and discovered that the two groups were almost indistinguishable in terms of their pathomorphology, insulin levels, and proinsulin levels and that neither liver metastasis nor lymph node metastasis was a factor that contributed to a poor prognosis [7]. Our study had relatively limited follow-up data and did not calculate time-dependent survival. However, one patient survived for 14 years from the discovery of metastasis, indicating that malignant insulinoma did not necessarily mean a poor prognosis and that patients may still have a long survival period [7].

Strengths and limitations

This study has some strengths and limitations. The strengths include the long observation period analyzed and the comprehensive patient analysis. The main study limitations are those associated with the retrospective nature of the study, the small patient number, and the long enrollment period spanning over decades (1984–2017), which implies a lack of uniformity in the diagnostic criteria, imaging resources, and treatment options, as well as an absence of detailed histological information and a small number of patients who were followed up. Therefore, we could not perform tumor staging and grading, and analyze the survival rate.

Conclusion

Malignant insulinoma is extremely rare. More than 50% of the patients had already developed metastases upon diagnosis, with the liver as the most common site. The main clinical manifestations are hypoglycemia-related symptoms. Unlike benign insulinoma, the malignant type causes prominent neuroglycopenic symptoms. Regarding the localization examination, selective celiac arteriography generated positive rates of 100% for both pancreatic primary lesions and liver metastases. Some malignant insulinoma tumors were initially diagnosed as solitary benign pancreatic tumors, indicating that the two types of tumor were difficult to distinguish clinically. However, patients with malignant insulinoma may develop metastasis during follow-up visits. Therefore, long-term follow-up visits are critical for patients with insulinoma.

Abbreviations

ASVS: arterial calcium stimulation with hepatic venous sampling; CT: computed tomography; DCR: disease control rate; EUS: endoscopic ultrasonography; MEN1: type 1 multiple endocrine neoplasia; MRI: magnetic resonance imaging; ORR: objective remission rate; pNET: pancreatic neuroendocrine tumor; PUMCH: Peking Union Medical College Hospital; TAE/TACE: transcatheter arterial (chemo) embolization; VPCT: volume perfusion CT

Acknowledgements

The authors would like to thank all the participants in this study.

Funding

No funding was received for this study.

Authors' contributions

JY: data acquisition, analysis and interpretation of the data, and drafting of the manuscript; FP, HBZ, WL, TY, YF, KF, and WBX: data acquisition and analysis and interpretation of the data. LLX and YXL: study concept and design, critical revision of the manuscript for important intellectual content, and study supervision. All authors read and approved the final manuscript

Competing interests

The authors declare that they have no competing interests.
All authors have read and approved the manuscript for publication.

References

1. Okabayashi T, Shima Y, Sumiyoshi T, Kozuki A, Ito S, Ogawa Y, Kobayashi M, Hanazaki K. Diagnosis and management of insulinoma. World J Gastroenterol. 2013;19:829–37.
2. Baudin E, Caron P, Lombard-Bohas C, Tabarin A, Mitry E, Reznick Y, Taieb D, Pattou F, Goudet P, Vezzosi D, et al. Malignant insulinoma: recommendations for characterisation and treatment. Ann Endocrinol (Paris). 2013;74:523–33.
3. Xu J, Liang H, Qin S. L W: expert consensus on gastrointestinal pancreatic neuroendocrine tumors in China (2016 version). Chin Clin Oncol. 2016;21:927–46.
4. Giuroiu I, Reidy-Lagunes D. Metastatic insulinoma: current molecular and cytotoxic therapeutic approaches for metastatic well-differentiated panNETs. J Natl Compr Cancer Netw. 2015;13:139–44.
5. Iglesias P, Lafuente C, Martin AM, Lopez GA, Castro JC, Diez JJ. Insulinoma: a multicenter, retrospective analysis of three decades of experience (1983-2014). Endocrinol Nutr. 2015;62:306–13.
6. Wang L, Zhao Y, Chen G, Liao Q. The diagnosis and treatment of malignant insulinoma. J Hepatobiliary Surg. 2004:88–90.
7. Hirshberg B, Cochran C, Skarulis MC, Libutti SK, Alexander HR, Wood BJ, Chang R, Kleiner DE, Gorden P. Malignant insulinoma: spectrum of unusual clinical features. Cancer-Am Cancer Soc. 2005;104:264–72.
8. ON T, PL C. KC C: the management of insulinoma. Br J Surg. 2006;93:264–75.
9. Goh BKP, Ooi LLPJ, Cheow P, Tan Y, Ong H, Chung YA, Chow PKH, Wong W, Soo K. Accurate preoperative localization of Insulinomas avoids the need for blind resection and reoperation: analysis of a single institution experience with 17 surgically treated tumors over 19 years. J Gastrointest Surg. 2009;13:1071–7.

10. Zhu L, Xue H, Sun Z, Li P, Qian T, Xing X, Li N, Zhao Y, Wu W, Jin Z. Prospective comparison of biphasic contrast-enhanced CT, volume perfusion CT, and 3 tesla MRI with diffusion-weighted imaging for insulinoma detection. J Magn Reson Imaging. 2017;46:1648–55.

11. Jackson JE. Angiography and arterial stimulation venous sampling in the localization of pancreatic neuroendocrine tumours. Best Pract Res Cl En. 2005;19:229–39.

12. Zhang T, Zhao Y, Cong L, Liao Q, Dai M, Guo J. Noninvasive examinations for localization of insulinoma. Chinese Journal of Surgery. 2009;47:1365–7.

13. Jing H, Li F, Du Y, Long M, Xing X, Zhao Y, Niu N, Ma Y, Liu Y, Ba J, et al. Clinical evaluation of detecting insulinoma with 99mTc-HYNIC-TOC imaging. Chinese Journal of Medicine. 2012:35–7.

14. Li X, Jin Z, Yang N, Liu W, Pan J. Transcatheter arterial chemoperfusion or chemoembolizaiton for treatment of liver metastasis from malignant insulinoma. Journal of Interventional Radiology. 2008:803–6.

15. Lepage C, Ciccolallo L, De Angelis R, Bouvier AM, Faivre J, Gatta G. European disparities in malignant digestive endocrine tumours survival. Int J Cancer. 2010;126:2928–34.

16. Service FJ, MM MM, O'Brien PC, Ballard DJ. Functioning insulinoma--incidence, recurrence, and long-term survival of patients: a 60-year study. Mayo Clin Proc. 1991;66:711–9.

24

Efficacy of combined treatment with pasireotide, pegvisomant and cabergoline in an acromegalic patient resistant to other treatments

A. Ciresi, S. Radellini, V. Guarnotta and C. Giordano[*] ⓘ

Abstract

Background: The approach to acromegalic patients with persistent acromegaly after surgery and inadequate response to first-generation somatostatin receptor ligands (SRLs) should be strictly tailored. Current options include new pituitary surgery and/or radiosurgery, or alternative medical treatment with SRLs high dose regimens, pegvisomant (PEG) as monotherapy, or combined therapy with the addition of PEG or cabergoline to SRLs. A new pharmacological approach includes pasireotide, a second-generation SRL approved for patients who do not adequately respond to surgery and/or for whom surgery is not an option. No reports on efficacy and safety of combined therapy with pasireotide and pegvisomant (PEG) in acromegaly are available.

Case presentation: Here we report the case of a 41-year-old acromegalic man with a mixed GH/PRL pituitary adenoma post-surgical resistant to first-generation SRLs both alone and in combination with cabergoline and PEG who achieved biochemical and tumor control with the combined triple treatment with pasireotide, PEG and cabergoline without adverse events and with a good compliance to treatment.

Conclusions: Twelve months of therapy with pasireotide, PEG and cabergoline proved to be safe and effective in this particular patient and the clinical improvement of disease resulted in an improved compliance to treatment.

Keywords: Pasireotide, Pegvisomant, Acromegaly, Cotreatment, Resistant

Background

In acromegaly, medical therapy is recommended in patients with persistent or recurrent disease following surgery. The medical treatment includes long-acting somatostatin receptor ligands (SRLs), dopamine agonists (usually cabergoline) and the GH receptor antagonist [pegvisomant (PEG)] [1]. The first-generation SRLs have high affinity for somatostatin receptors (SSTR)2 and weak to moderate affinity for SSTR3 and SSTR5 [2].

The percentage of achievement of biochemical control widely varies in the different studies. Actually, without the use of stringent inclusion criteria required for clinical trials, in unselected treatment-naïve acromegalic patients a biochemical control can be achieved in a percentage which is far lower than those reported in the past [3], while real life studies indicate a biochemical control rate around 40% [4].

Resistance to SRLs may be defined as a failure to achieve biochemical control criteria (GH < 1.0 μg/L and a normal age-adjusted IGF-1) and tumor volume increase or absence of > 20% decrease after at least 12 months of treatment [5].

The approach to patients with persistent acromegaly after surgery and inadequate response to first-generation SRLs should be strictly tailored [6]. Current options include new pituitary surgery (in a patient with persistent disease and residual intrasellar adenoma following initial surgery), use of either a SRLs or PEG (as the initial adjuvant medical therapy in a patient with significant disease without local mass effects), a trial of a dopamine agonist, usually cabergoline (as the initial adjuvant medical

* Correspondence: carla.giordano@unipa.it
Section of Endocrinology, Diabetology and Metabolic Diseases, Biomedical Department of Internal and Specialist Medicine (DIBIMIS), University of Palermo, Piazza delle Cliniche 2, 90127 Palermo, Italy

Efficacy of combined treatment with pasireotide, pegvisomant and cabergoline in an acromegalic...

167

therapy in a patient with modest elevations of serum IGF-1 and mild signs and symptoms of GH excess), the combined therapy with the addition of PEG or cabergoline (in a patient with inadequate response to SRLs) or, finally, the use of radiation therapy (in the setting of residual tumor mass following surgery if medical therapy is unavailable, unsuccessful or not tolerated) [1].

The switch to treatment with PEG as monotherapy or in association with SRLs represents nowadays a valid therapeutic strategy to achieve full disease control in acromegalic patients resistant or poorly responders to SRLs [1, 7].

PEG has been shown to control acromegaly in 60–90% of patients across several clinical trials. If in the real life the rate of disease control was lower, not exceeding 65–70%, an appropriate PEG dose titration up to the maximum allowed dosage was shown to normalize IGF-1 levels in up to 90% of cases even in the real life setting [3, 8, 9].

A new pharmacological approach includes pasireotide, a second-generation SRL approved for patients who do not adequately respond to surgery and/or for whom surgery is not an option [10].

Unlike first-generation SRLs which primarily exert their effects through binding to SSTR2, pasireotide binds with high affinity to SSTR5 [11].

Pasireotide has proven to be superior to first-generation SRLs both as first line medical treatment in naïve patients [12] and in patients classified as resistant [13].

To our knowledge, although the outcomes of combined therapy with the addition of PEG to first-generation SRLs are widely known, there are no reports available on the efficacy and safety of combined therapy with pasireotide and PEG. Here we report our experience with this new combined treatment in an acromegalic patient.

This study was carried out in accordance with the recommendations of Endocrine Society Clinical Practice Guidelines and at the time of hospitalization a written informed consent was obtained from the patient for publication of this case report and any accompanying images, in accordance with the Declaration of Helsinki.

Case presentation

A 41-year-old man with clinically evident acromegaly was referred to our department on his own initiative due to the physical changes over the years that had been noticed by the new wife by looking at past pictures. He stated that 1 year before had undergone surgery for carpal tunnel syndrome and for some months he reported snoring, profuse sweating, joint aches and occasional headache. He denied to have hypertension, galactorrhea, signs and symptoms of diabetes mellitus.

At clinical examination, the patient showed a clear acromegalic phenotype, with prominence of the brow, enlargement of the nose, thickening of the lips, prognathism, macroglossia, increased interdental spacing, acral enlargement, evident thyroid goiter. He showed blood pressure values into normal range, normal cardiac and respiratory exam, a mild splenomegaly.

Initial testing revealed IGF-1 1369 µg/l (normal: 109-204), basal-GH 31 µg/l with GH-nadir during an oral glucose tolerance test (OGTT) 16 µg/l, prolactin 2386 ng/ml (normal: < 15.2 ng/ml), total testosterone 0.88 µg/l (normal: 2.4-9.3 µg/l) with normal gonadotropins, parathyroid hormone 52 pg/ml (normal: 15-65 pg/ml), normal adrenal and thyroid function. The patient showed normal glucose tolerance (fasting glucose 4.78 mmol/l), with mild hyperinsulinism (OGTT-peak 230.6 µU/ml), glycosylate hemoglobin (HbA1c) 5.9%) and normal lipid profile. Magnetic resonance imaging (MRI) revealed a large hyperintense mass of 28,512 mm^3 (largest diameter 33 mm) with supra- and latero-sellar extension (with bilateral, mostly left, involvement of the cavernous sinus). Campimetry showed monolateral inferior quadrantanopsia.

The patient refused surgery as a first line treatment and started treatment with cabergoline (0.5-1.0 mg/weekly) and lanreotide-autogel 90 mg/monthly.

After 3 and 6 months he showed, respectively, IGF-1 1049-908 µg/l, basal-GH 35.6-44 µg/l; prolactin 1526-959 ng/ml. No side effects were reported, except for a quite significant increase in fasting glucose (6.44 mmol/l) and HbA1c (6.5%). At 6 months MRI revealed a volumetric tumor reduction (23,500 mm^3) with depression of the superior profile. Treatment was modified by increasing cabergoline to 1.5 mg/weekly and lanreotide to 120 mg/monthly for 6 months. A further, very small, decrease in hormonal levels was obtained, but without reaching the target, as follows: IGF-1850 µg/l, basal-GH 32 µg/l, prolactin 589 ng/ml. MRI showed an almost unchanged tumor mass. Fasting glucose (6.22 mmol/l) and HbA1c (6.5%) did not significantly change.

The patient was persuaded to undergo transsphenoidal adenomectomy, without complications, in july 2012. Histologically, the tumor was classified as GH/PRL and sparsely-granulated type, with a Ki-67 labeling index < 1%.

Despite a significant debulking of tumor, surgery was not curative but it probably led to a better biochemical response to subsequent medical treatment. The early random-GH after 1 month was 47 µg/L and the evaluation at 3 months confirmed persistent disease, with IGF-1631 µg/l, random-GH 15.2 µg/L, nadir-GH 11.5 µg/L. PRL was 251.9 ng/ml, total testosterone slightly increased (1.85 µg/l) and glucose metabolism back in the norm (fasting glucose 5.17 mmol/l, HbA1c 6.0%, insulin OGTT-peak 132.6 µU/ml). MRI revealed a residual tumor with left extension and campimetry was normal.

The patient started adjuvant therapy with octreotide-LAR and cabergoline, with the dosage progressively increased (maximum doses octreotide 40 mg/monthly and cabergoline 2.25 mg/weekly). This treatment did not result in hormonal normalization, as shown by random-GH 10.9 µg/L, IGF-1549 µg/l, PRL 76 ng/ml.

In august 2013 PEG was added to octreotide with a 3-times-a-week schedule as follows: 60 mg/weekly for 4 months, 90 mg/weekly for other 4 months and 120 mg/weekly for just 3 months (cabergoline dose unchanged). A dose-responsive IGF-1 reduction (437, 410 and 305 µg/l, respectively) was observed as the PEG dose gradually increased, although IGF-1 and PRL (72 ng/ml) remained above the norm. No significant change in tumor volume was seen and the glucose metabolism slightly improved (last HbA1c 5.8%). However, PEG was stopped by the patient due to lack of clinical improvement and poor compliance of patient to PEG treatment in the following weeks.

In july 2014, as there was still no commercial use of pasireotide, we had the opportunity to use it as compassionate treatment. We replaced octreotide with pasireotide-LAR 40 mg/monthly (cabergoline dose unchanged). After

6 months random-GH was 12.07 µg/L, IGF-1613 µg/L and PRL 41.2 ng/ml, with increased fasting glucose (6.17 mmol/l) and HbA1c (6.4%). MRI showed a decrease in tumor volume (15,525 mm^3) and a heterogeneous signal intensity, with predominant hyperintensity, on both T1 and T2-weighted images compatible with presence of necrotic areas.

Pasireotide was increased to 60 mg/monthly for 4 months without significant biochemical benefits: random-GH 10.9 µg/L, IGF-1518.9 µg/L.

In june 2015, after obtaining informed consent from the patient who refused surgery, PEG was added to pasireotide with a 6-times-a-week schedule, with a starting daily dose of 10 mg (60 mg/weekly), gradually increased to 15 (90 mg/weekly) up to 20 mg (120 mg/weekly) after 3 and 6 months (cabergoline dose unchanged). After 3 months of PEG-10 mg, 3 months of PEG-15 mg and 6 months of PEG-20 mg, IGF-1 was 344-234-172 µg/L and PRL 30-28.5-19 ng/ml, respectively. Fasting glucose was 6.5-5.06-5.39 mmol/l, while HbA1c

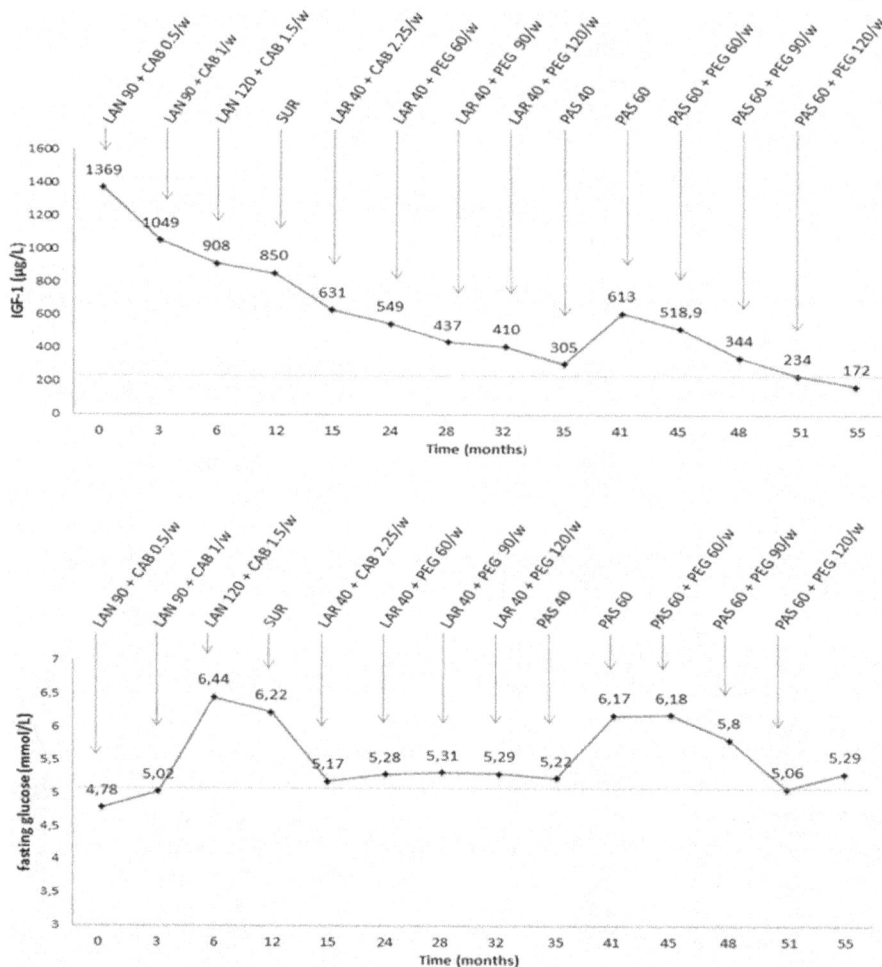

Fig. 1 IGF-1 (top) and fasting glucose (bottom) levels during the entire clinical follow-up of the patient. *LAN: lanreotide autogel; CAB: cabergoline; SUR: surgery (transsphenoidal adenomectomy); LAR: octreotide LAR; PEG: pegvisomant; PAS: pasireotide; w: weekly. All drugs doses are expressed in mg*

changed from 6.4 to 6.8-5.9-5.5%. After 12 months, MRI revealed an unchanged tumor volume. Clinically, an improvement in tiredness and joint pain was reported. The patient's compliance was satisfactory throughout the whole period of treatment and no side effects were reported. To date, the patient is continuing the treatment with the latest available IGF-1174 μg/L and PRL 9.5 ng/ml.

IGF-1 and fasting glucose levels during the entire clinical follow-up of the patient are presented in the Fig. 1.

MR coronal images at diagnosis and during the follow-up of the patient are presented in the Fig. 2.

Discussion

We describe for the first time the effectiveness of combined treatment with pasireotide and PEG in a patient with post-surgical active disease resistant to combined treatment with first-generation SRLs and PEG.

It is widely accepted that the post-surgical management of acromegalic patients with residual disease should be tailored. In patients with active disease the use of SRL as initial adjuvant medical therapy is suggested, with the subsequent addition of PEG or cabergoline (this latter in case of mild disease activity) to SRL in patients with inadequate response to an SRL [1].

According to these guidelines, following surgery we first started octreotide LAR up to the maximum monthly dosage. The poor response to octreotide as an adjuvant therapy was probably expected because of the biochemical resistance already shown to lanreotide before surgery. Indeed, octreotide and lanreotide seem to be equally effective in the biochemical control of acromegaly [14].

However, surgical debulking may significantly improve subsequent response to medical therapy, particularly in cases of highly active disease [15] as in this case, but when at least 75% of the tumor is removed [16], while here the debulking was much lower.

This patient had many determinants of a poor response, such as age, tumor volume, high baseline hormonal levels and sparsely granulated adenoma [17] and these parameters probably should have led us to anticipate other therapeutic decisions.

In addition, low tissue SSTR2 expression as a determinant of poor response to SRLs can not be excluded. Indeed, the expression of an adequate amount of SSTR2 is a requisite for response to treatment [18]. Unfortunately the characterization of SSTR subtypes was not performed in this case. However, since pasireotide monotherapy was not more effective than SRLs in decreasing IGF-1 levels, the better outcome can not be attributed only to this factor.

The switch to PEG as a monotherapy or in association with SRLs represents a valid strategy in resistant patients [1, 9]. Despite an initial optimal compliance to treatment, in our patient the addition of PEG to octreotide was able to reduce IGF-1 by just 20%, while the combined therapy with pasireotide resulted in a progressive decline in IGF-1 already after 3 months up to complete control, using the same weekly dose as already used in the first attempt at combination with octreotide.

Probably, both the different binding to SSTR [11] and the different behavior on post-SSTR intracellular cascade had a fundamental role. Indeed, pasireotide modulates

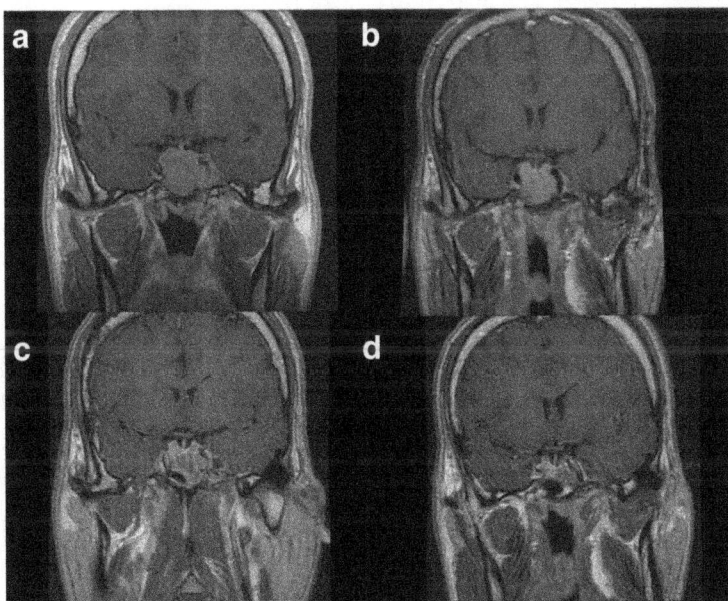

Fig. 2 Sellar MR coronal images at diagnosis (**a**), after 6 months of lanreotide autogel (**b**), 3 months after surgery (**c**) and 6 months after pasireotide treatment (**d**)

SSTR trafficking differently than octreotide, resulting in quicker recycling of SSTRs, particularly SSTR2, and may counteract SSTR2-desensitization [10].

In addition, we could speculate that, despite the same weekly dose, the 6-times-a-week schedule of PEG administration, compared to the 3-times-a-week schedule, may have been more effective in IGF-1 reduction. The patient surprisingly showed better compliance probably because of the associated clinical improvement. Consequently, the better outcome can be attributed to a better dosing schedule and association with pasireotide rather than with a better compliance to pegvisomant treatment.

Of course, it is worth noting that this combined treatment, which must be practiced for the rest of life, is very expensive and the health economics issue and the cost-effectiveness of different treatments are important considerations in management decisions in acromegaly. For these reasons, in the near future we will again try to offer to the patient other therapeutic options, such as new surgery or radiotherapy, which at present the patient refused.

Similarly, we carefully informed the patient of the possible expected adverse events of current therapy, the main of which being the latent negative effect of pasireotide on glucose metabolism [19]. Indeed, the highest binding affinity of pasireotide for SSTR5 has an important role in mediating insulin secretion. Conversely, glucagon secretion is mainly mediated by SSTR2, and this may account for the more modest suppressive effect of pasireotide on glucagon secretion, which can lead to a deterioration of glucose metabolism. Although this effect to date seems to be well balanced by the favorable effect on glycemic profile of PEG, a close monitoring of glucose homeostasis will be necessary during the entire course of the follow-up.

Conclusions

In conclusion, 12 months of therapy with pasireotide and PEG proved to be safe and effective in achieving biochemical and tumor control and clinical improvement of acromegaly resulted in improved compliance. This combined treatment may represent a valid therapeutic strategy to achieve full disease control in acromegalic patients resistant or poorly responders to first-generation SRLs. However, although in this particular patient the combined treatment was safe and effective, we are well aware that this is only one case and that we can not generalize safety issues based only in one patient. Clinical trials involving several patients and with longer periods of follow-up are needed to confirm these findings.

Abbreviations
HbA1c: Glycosylate hemoglobin; MRI: Magnetic resonance imaging; OGTT: Oral glucose tolerance test; PEG: Pegvisomant; SRLs: Somatostatin receptor ligands; SSTR: Somatostatin receptors

Acknowledgements
Not applicable

Funding
This research did not receive any specific grant from any funding agency in the public, commercial or not-for-profit sector.

Authors' contributions
A.C. and C.G. had full control of the study design, data analysis and interpretation, and preparation of article. All authors (A.C., S.R., V.G., C.G.) were involved in planning the analysis and drafting the article. The final draft article was approved by all the authors.

Competing interests
All authors declare that there is no conflict of interest that could be perceived as prejudicing the impartiality of the research reported.

References
1. Katznelson L, Laws ER Jr, Melmed S, Molitch ME, Murad MH, Utz A, et al. Acromegaly: an endocrine society clinical practice guideline. J Clin Endocrinol Metab. 2014;99(11):3933–351. https://doi.org/10.1210/jc.2014-2700.
2. Ben-Shlomo A, Melmed S. Somatostatin agonists for treatment of acromegaly. Mol Cell Endocrinol. 2008;286(1-2):192–8. https://doi.org/10.1016/j.mce.2007.11.024.
3. Giustina A, Chanson P, Kleinberg D, Bronstein MD, Clemmons DR, Klibanski A, et al. Expert consensus document: a consensus on the medical treatment of acromegaly. Nat Rev Endocrinol. 2014;10(4):243–8. https://doi.org/10.1038/nrendo.2014.21.
4. Colao A, Auriemma RS, Pivonello R, Kasuki L, Gadelha MR. Interpreting biochemical control response rates with first-generation somatostatin analogues in acromegaly. Pituitary. 2016;19(3):235–47. https://doi.org/10.1007/s11102-015-0684-z.
5. Colao A, Auriemma RS, Lombardi G, Pivonello R. Resistance to somatostatin analogs in acromegaly. Endocr Rev. 2011;32(2):247–71. https://doi.org/10.1210/er.2010-0002.
6. Katznelson L. Approach to the patient with persistent acromegaly after pituitary surgery. J Clin Endocrinol Metab. 2010;95(9):4114–23. https://doi.org/10.1210/jc.2010-0670.
7. Jørgensen JO, Feldt-Rasmussen U, Frystyk J, Chen JW, Kristensen LØ, Hagen C, et al. Cotreatment of acromegaly with a somatostatin analog and a growth hormone receptor antagonist. J Clin Endocrinol Metab. 2005;90(10):5627–31. https://doi.org/10.1210/jc.2005-0531.
8. Neggers SJ, Franck SE, de Rooij FW, Dallenga AH, Poublon RM, Feelders RA, et al. Long-term efficacy and safety of pegvisomant in combination with long-acting somatostatin analogs in acromegaly. J Clin Endocrinol Metab. 2014;99(10):3644–52. https://doi.org/10.1210/jc.2014-2032.
9. Giustina A, Arnaldi G, Bogazzi F, Cannavò S, Colao A, De Marinis L, et al. Pegvisomant in acromegaly: an update. J Endocrinol Investig. 2017;40(6):577–89. https://doi.org/10.1007/s40618-017-0614-1.
10. Cuevas-Ramos D, Fleseriu M. Pasireotide: a novel treatment for patients with acromegaly. Drug Des Devel Ther. 2016;10:227–39. https://doi.org/10.2147/DDDT.S77999.
11. Bruns C, Lewis I, Briner U, Meno-Tetang G, Weckbecker G. SOM230: a novel somatostatin peptidomimetic with broad somatotropin release inhibiting factor (SRIF) receptor binding and a unique antisecretory profile. Eur J Endocrinol 2002; 146(5): 707-716. PMID: 11980628.
12. Colao A, Bronstein MD, Freda P, Gu F, Shen CC, Gadelha M, et al. Pasireotide versus octreotide in acromegaly: a head-to-head superiority study. J Clin Endocrinol Metab. 2014;99(3):791–9. https://doi.org/10.1210/jc.2013-2480.

Efficacy of combined treatment with pasireotide, pegvisomant and cabergoline in an acromegalic...

171

13. Gadelha MR, Bronstein MD, Brue T, Coculescu M, Fleseriu M, Guitelman M, et al. Pasireotide versus continued treatment with octreotide or lanreotide in patients with inadequately controlled acromegaly (PAOLA): a randomised, phase 3 trial. Lancet Diabetes Endocrinol. 2014;2(11):875–84. https://doi.org/10.1016/S2213-8587(14)70169-X.

14. Tutuncu Y, Berker D, Isik S, Ozuguz U, Akbaba G, Kucukler FK, et al. Comparison of octreotide LAR and lanreotide autogel as post-operative medical treatment in acromegaly. Pituitary. 2012;15(3):398–404. https://doi.org/10.1007/s11102-011-0335-y.

15. Karavitaki N, Turner HE, Adams CB, Cudlip S, Byrne JV, Fazal-Sanderson V, et al. Surgical debulking of pituitary macroadenomas causing acromegaly improves control by lanreotide. Clin Endocrinol. 2008;68(6):970–5. https://doi.org/10.1111/j.1365-2265.2007.03139.x.

16. Colao A, Attanasio R, Pivonello R, Cappabianca P, Cavallo ML, Lasio G, et al. Partial surgical removal of growth hormone-secreting pituitary tumors enhances the response to somatostatin analogs in acromegaly. J Clin Endocrinol Metab. 2006;91(1):85–92. https://doi.org/10.1210/jc.2005-1208.

17. Bhayana S, Booth GL, Asa SL, Kovacs K, Ezzat S. The implication of somatotroph adenoma phenotype to somatostatin analog responsiveness in acromegaly. J Clin Endocrinol Metab. 2005;90(11):6290–5. https://doi.org/10.1210/jc.2005-0998.

18. Ferone D, de Herder WW, Pivonello R, Kros JM, van Koetsveld PM, de Jong T, et al. Correlation of in vitro and in vivo somatotropic adenoma responsiveness to somatostatin analogs and dopamine agonists with immunohistochemical evaluation of somatostatin and dopamine receptors and electron microscopy. J Clin Endocrinol Metab. 2008;93(4):1412–7. https://doi.org/10.1210/jc.2007-1358.

19. Pivonello R, Auriemma RS, Grasso LF, Pivonello C, Simeoli C, Patalano R, et al. Complications of acromegaly: cardiovascular, respiratory and metabolic comorbidities. Pituitary. 2017;20(1):46–62. https://doi.org/10.1007/s11102-017-0797-7.

25

A case of malignant insulinoma responsive to somatostatin analogs treatment

Mariasmeralda Caliri[1†], Valentina Verdiani[1†], Edoardo Mannucci[2], Vittorio Briganti[3], Luca Landoni[4], Alessandro Esposito[4], Giulia Burato[5], Carlo Maria Rotella[2], Massimo Mannelli[1] and Alessandro Peri[1*]

Abstract

Background: Insulinoma is a rare tumour representing 1–2% of all pancreatic neoplasms and it is malignant in only 10% of cases. Locoregional invasion or metastases define malignancy, whereas the dimension (> 2 cm), CK19 status, the tumor staging and grading (Ki67 > 2%), and the age of onset (> 50 years) can be considered elements of suspect.

Case presentation: We describe the case of a 68-year-old man presenting symptoms compatible with hypoglycemia. The symptoms regressed with food intake. These episodes initially occurred during physical activity, later also during fasting. The fasting test was performed and the laboratory results showed endogenous hyperinsulinemia compatible with insulinoma. The patient appeared responsive to somatostatin analogs and so he was treated with short acting octreotide, obtaining a good control of glycemia. Imaging investigations showed the presence of a lesion of the uncinate pancreatic process of about 4 cm with a high sst2 receptor density. The patient underwent exploratory laparotomy and duodenocephalopancreasectomy after one month.

The definitive histological examination revealed an insulinoma (T3N1MO, AGCC VII G1) with a low replicative index (Ki67: 2%).

Conclusions: This report describes a case of malignant insulinoma responsive to octreotide analogs administered pre-operatively in order to try to prevent hypoglycemia. The response to octreotide analogs is not predictable and should be initially assessed under strict clinical surveillance.

Keywords: Insulinoma, Hypoglycemia, Somatostatin analogs, Octreotide

Background

Insulinoma is a rare tumour representing 1–2% of all pancreatic neoplasms [1]. It is malignant in only 10% of cases [2]. The malignancy can be stated only in the presence of locoregional invasion into the surrounding soft tissue, lymph node or liver metastases [3]. The dimension > 2 cm, CK19 status, the tumor staging and grading (Ki67 > 2%), and the age of onset > 50 years can be considered indicators of malignancy [4–6]. However, in literature, there are some reports where about 40–50% of malignant insulinomas are < 2 cm [7]. Most of malignant insulinomas are sporadic (about 97%), even if a few cases

of association with MEN1 and 1 case of association with type-1 neurofibromatosis have been described [8].

In affected patients, the control of glycemia before surgical excision, or for a prolonged time if surgery is not feasible, may be very problematic. Admittedly, the description of new cases may be of help for clinicians, who have to deal with similar situations. We report a case of malignant insulinoma associated with local infiltration, neoplastic thrombosis and lymph node metastasis, in which medical treatment with octreotide effectively counteracted hypoglycemia before surgery. One peculiarity of this case is represented by the fact that short acting octreotide was used, in agreement with the surgeon, in order to avoid any possible pharmacological interference caused by long acting formulations at the time of surgery, which was performed shortly after the diagnosis.

* Correspondence: alessandro.peri@unifi.it

†Mariasmeralda Caliri and Valentina Verdiani contributed equally to this work.

[1]Endocrine Unit, Department of Experimental and Clinical Biomedical Sciences "Mario Serio", University of Florence, Careggi University Hospital, Florence, Italy

Full list of author information is available at the end of the article

Case presentation

A 68-year-old man presented a weight increase of 7 kg during the last year and symptoms compatible with hypoglycemia (objective vertigo, feeling of an empty head, sweating, palpitations). During some of these episodes low blood glucose levels (< 40 mg/dl) were documented by glucometer measurement. The symptoms regressed with food intake. These episodes initially occurred during physical activity and later also during fasting.

He had no family history of endocrine disease.

At admission, his body mass index was 28 kg/m^2. The rest of the physical examination was unremarkable. Biochemical assessment did not show any abnormality, and glucose level was 70 mg/dl (n.v. 65–110). Plasma cortisol at 8 a.m. was in the normal range (394.8 nmol/l, n.v. 138–685 nmol/l), anti-insulin antibodies were negative, chromogranin A was 69 ng/ml (n.v. 10–185), prolactin was 247 mU/l (n.v. 53–369), gastrin was 12.7 pg/ml (n.v. < 180), PTH was 6.4 pmol/l (n.v. 1–6.8) and serum calcium level was 8.8 mg/dl (n.v. 8.6–10.4).

The fasting test was performed, which was interrupted after 12 h due to the onset of symptomatic hypoglycemia (44 mg/dl, glucometer measurement). Plasma glucose level was 41 mg/dl, insulin level 16.3 U/L and C-peptide 1.27 nmol/l (Table 1). Per protocol, 1 mg of glucagon was injected intravenously after interruption of the fasting test and plasma glucose was measured (time 0′, 41 mg/dl; after 10 min 75 mg/dl, after 20 min 94 mg/dl and after 30 min 93 mg/dl). The patient's laboratory results showed endogenous hyperinsulinemia, according to published guidelines (fasting test: plasma glucose < 55 mg/dl, with insulin and C-peptide levels > 3 U/L and > 0.2 nmol/L, respectively; glucagone test: > 25 mg/dL increase of glucose levels after fasting) [9]. The short octreotide test (subcutaneous infusion of 100 mg of short-term octreotide at 7.00 a.m. after an overnight fast, and blood glucose, insulin and C-peptide hourly sampling for six hours) was performed to evaluate the efficacy of a possible treatment with somatostatin analogs, in order to counteract hypoglycemia [10]. No food was allowed during the test. The test showed an increase in plasma glucose above 100 mg/dl (Table 2), and the patient was considered to be responsive to somatostatin analogs [10].

Table 2 Short term octreotide test. The test was performed according to ref. [2]

	0′	1 h	2 h	3 h	4 h	5 h	6 h
Glycemia (basal 65–110 mg/dL)	54	61	116	134	133	130	122
Insulin level (basal 3–17 U/L)	16.8	2.5	3.1	4.3	4.5	5.2	6
C-peptide (basal 0.37–1.47 nmol/L)	1.39	0.56	0.49	0.51	0.54	0.56	0.59

Additional procedures included:

- MRI, which revealed a lesion of the uncinate pancreatic process of about 4 cm, which presented a brief contact with the upper mesenteric artery and a > 180° contact with the superior mesenteric vein with suspected infiltration (Fig. 1).
- Octreoscan, which showed a lesion located in the pancreatic site, with a high somatostatin receptor (sstR) density (Fig. 2).
- Abdominal CT scan with contrast, which revealed a polylobed lesion with sharp margins at the level of the uncinate pancreas process, in contact with the superior mesenteric vein and reaching the margins of the superior mesenteric artery. No signs of vessels infiltration were observed.

All these imaging procedures were indicative of the presence of an insulinoma as the cause of endogenous hyperinsulinemia.

Surgical treatment was scheduled. Before surgery, considering the response to the short octreotide test, the patient was treated with short acting octreotide (0.1 mcg twice a day), obtaining a good control of glycemia by glucometer measurement, disappearance of hypoglycemic symptoms and no recurrence of hypoglycemic episodes.

The patient underwent exploratory laparotomy and duodenocephalopancreasectomy after one month.

The postoperative course was complicated by the appearance of a pancreatic (grade B) [11] and a biliary fistula, whereby the patient was conservatively treated with fasting and parenteral nutritional intake and subsequenty via a naso-enteral tube. The control CT scan,

Table 1 Fasting test results. The test has been performed according to the Endocrine Society Clinical Pratice Guidelines on adult hypoglycemic disorders (ref [9])

	12 a.m.	2 a.m.	4 a.m.	8 a.m.	10 a.m.	12 p.m.
Glucometer measurement mg/dL	111	68	67	66	62	45
Glycemia (basal 65–110 mg/dL)		70		58		41
Insulin level (basal 3–17 U/L)		8.7		13.3		16.3
C-peptide (basal 0.37–1.47 nmol/L)		1.11		1.03		1.27

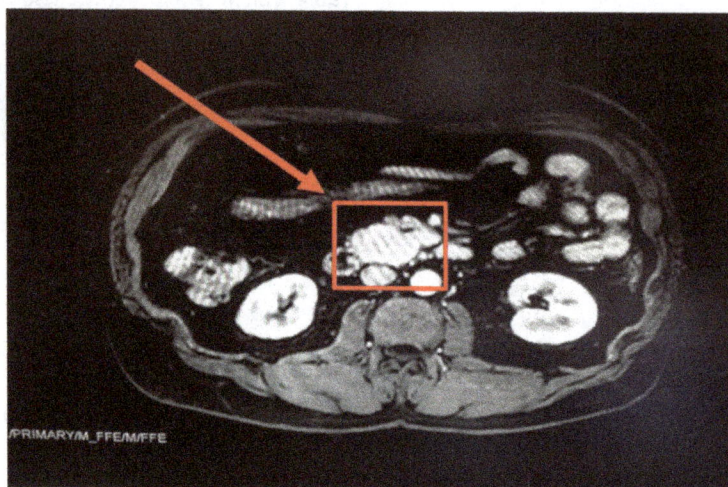

Fig. 1 Abdominal MRI showing a solid tumor with definite margins of the uncinate pancreatic process of 4x3x3.5 cm

performed a month later, did not reveal intra-abdominal spill and drainages were removed. Oral feeding was resumed one month after the operation.

The definitive histological examination revealed a neuroendocrine tumor with insulin receptors (insulinoma) of 3.5 cm infiltrating the duodenum, retroperitoneal adipose tissue, with widespread neoplastic thrombosis, and with metastasis in 3 pancreatic-duodenal lymph nodes among the 48 that had been surgically removed (T3N1MO, AjCC VIII edition G1), with a low replicative index (Ki67: 2%); radical resection (R0). Vascular and adipose tissue infiltration by the tumor, which are indicative of malignancy, were observed. Immunohistochemical staining was positive for insulin and synaptophysin (Fig. 3).

The most recent abdominal MRI, performed 6 months after surgery, did not reveal any recurrence of disease and currently the patient is in good conditions and with normal glycemic levels.

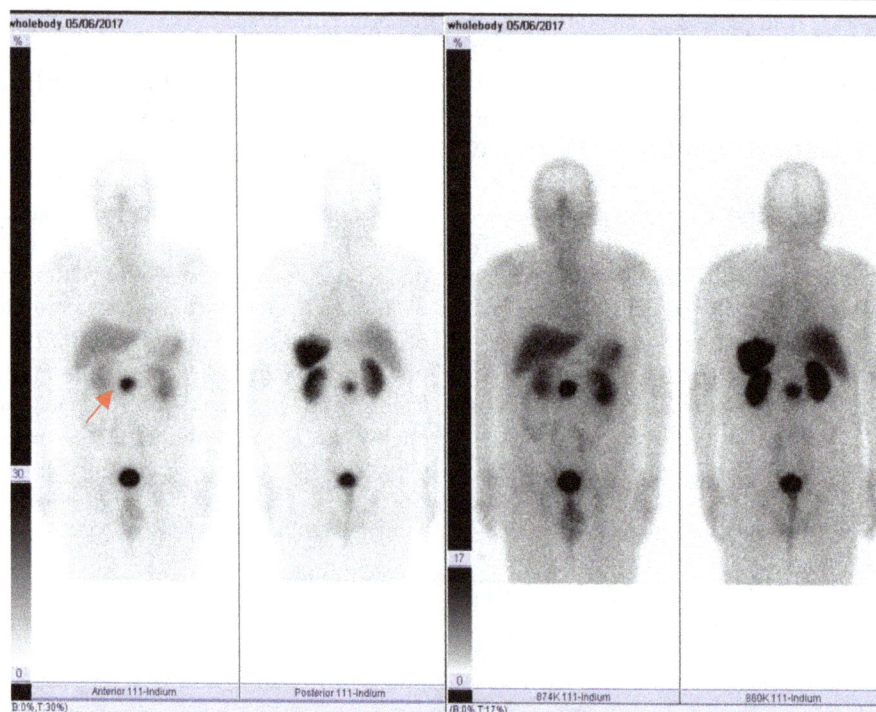

Fig. 2 Octreoscan showing a lesion localized in the pancreatic site, with high sstR density

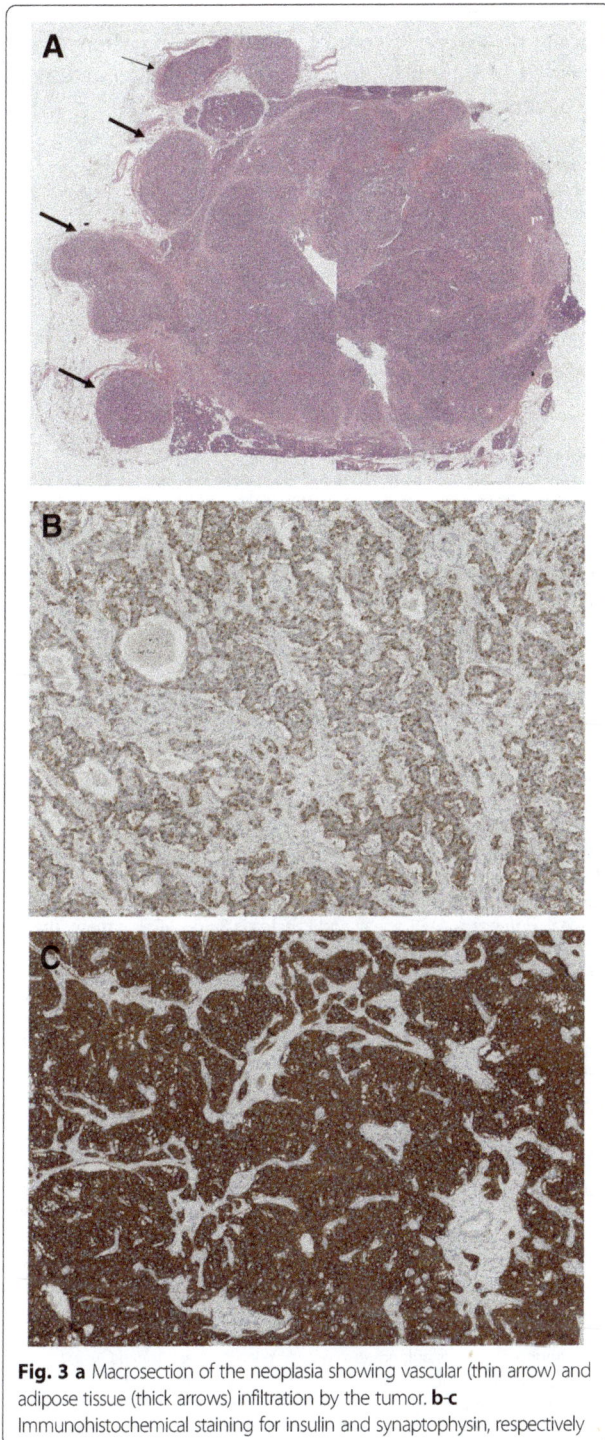

Fig. 3 a Macrosection of the neoplasia showing vascular (thin arrow) and adipose tissue (thick arrows) infiltration by the tumor. **b-c** Immunohistochemical staining for insulin and synaptophysin, respectively

Discussion and conclusions

Clinical hypoglycemia occurs when plasma glucose concentration is low enough to cause symptoms and/or signs, which include neurological alterations. The clinical feautures of hypoglycemia are non specific and it is not possible to establish a single plasma glucose concentration that definitively confirms clinical hypoglycemia.

Therefore, hypoglycemia is confirmed by the documentation of the Whipple's triad [12], e.g. symptoms and/or signs consistent with hypoglycemia, a low plasma glucose concentration, and resolution of clinical alterations after the plasma glucose concentration is increased [12, 13].

The most common cause of hypoglycemia is represented by insulin, insulin secretagogues, alcohol abuse and drugs of different classes [14]. Hypoglycemia may occur during sepsis and other critical illnesses, which include renal or hepatic failure. Hypoglycemia can be also secondary to cortisol deficiency [15]. It is therefore reasonable to assess plasma cortisol in the presence of hypoglycemia, although adrenocortical failure is not a common cause of hypoglycemia in adults in the absence of other clinical evidence. A low plasma cortisol concentration found in the presence of hypoglycemia is not per se indicative of adrenocortical insufficiency. In fact, recurrent hypoglycemia shifts glycemic thresholds for cortisol secretion [16].

Hypoglycemia may be caused by hyperinsulinism in the absence of prior gastric surgery or after Roux-en-Y gastric bypass for obesity [15]. It can also be associated to the presence of anti-insulin antibodies, such as in Hirata syndrome [17]. Finally, hyperinsulinemic hypoglycemia may be due to uncontrolled insulin release either from tumoral pancreatic beta-cells or from functionally defective beta-cells, as observed in nesidioblastosis, which is usually seen in newborns [18].

Although rare, insulinoma is the most common neuroendocrine tumor of the pancreas with an annual incidence of four in every 1 million persons. Malignancy is observed in only 10% of cases [2]. The clinical manifestation of insulinoma are variable and nonspecific and are related to the presence of hypoglycemia. The symptoms, which are often precipitated during physical exercise, become typically evident after fasting. The 72-h fasting test remains the gold standard for the diagnosis of insulinoma and includes the measurement of plasma glucose, insulin, C-peptide, at the time hypoglycemic symptoms appear [19]. We used this test for the diagnosis of primary hyperinsulinism in our case and the severe hypoglycemia with measurable insulin levels occurred after only 12 h unequivocally confirmed the hypothesis.

Non-invasive imaging procedures, such as CT and MRI, are used when a the biochemical diagnosis of primary hyperinsulinism has been made. Invasive modalities, such as endoscopic ultrasonography and arterial stimulation venous sampling, have frequently been shown to be superior to non-invasive localization techniques to preoperatively localize insulinomas [19]. Numerous studies have shown that the cell surface in neuroendocrine tumors (NETs) express sstR and have led to the development of new localization techniques. 11In-[DTPA-D-Phe1] octreotide scintigraphy (Octreoscan) can be used for the localization of primary tumours and their metastases in patients presenting with the clinical and biochemical features of NETs [20]. However only 20–50% of insulinoma can be dectected by octreoscan with planar imaging [10, 21, 22], although it has been described that the use of SPECT improves the detection of insulinomas by octreoscan scintigraphy [23]. GLP-1R imaging by ^{111}In-DOTA-exendin-4 administration is another non-invasive diagnostic approach that may succesfully localize small insulinomas pre- and intraoperatively [24]. Very recently, the ENETS guidelines recommend ^{68}Ga-DOTA-somatostatin analog PET/CT, because it is largely superior to somatostatin receptor scintigraphy, and facilitates the diagnosis of most types of NET lesions [25]. In our patient MRI showed the presence of a lesion of the uncinate pancreatic process of about 4 cm. Subsequent octreoscan revealed that the lesion expressed high levels of sstR.

Surgery is the first choice therapy for resectable insulinomas. A pharmacological approach can be useful both during the preoperative period, and for preventing hypoglycaemia in insulinomas with unknown localization. Diazoxide can prevent hypoglycemia by suppressing the release of insulin from insulinoma cells via opening ATP-sensitive potassium channels [26]. The use of this drug may be limited by side effects, such as hypotension, water retention with declining edema, hyperuricaemia, hypertriglyceridaemia, thrombocytopenia and neutropenia. Somatostatin analogs represent another possible medical strategy to suppress uncontrolled insulin secretion and control the symptoms of hypoglycemia in patients with insulinoma [27]. They can be used for instance in patients who are not eligible for surgery and when diazoxide is not applicable due to its inefficiency or adverse effects. In malignant insulinomas the use of somatostatin analogs may have an additional indication, due to the antiproliferative and moderate antineoplastic activity of these molecules [28–31].

It has to be said that the response to somatostatin analogs may differ according to the presence of various subtypes of sstR on insulinoma cells. Octreotide binds predominantly to sstR subtype 2. The absence of these receptors on insulinoma cells may aggravate hypoglycemia when a patient is treated with octreotide. This effect may be due to the inhibition of contra-insular hormones such as growth hormone and glucagon by somatostatin [32, 33]. The glycemic response to somatostatin analogs in any single patient is unpredictable and for this reason testing the drug while the patient is hospitalized is mandatory. In the case we described, a very good response was obtained with octreotide administration and the patient did not experience any new hypoglycemic episode before surgery.

In summary, we have described a rare case of malignant insulinoma in a patient with recurrent hypoglycemic episodes. The patient was successfully treated with short acting octreotide analogs before surgery, after testing its efficacy on glycemic control. No disease recurrence was observed at 6 month after surgery and the condition of the patient is currently very satisfactorily.

Abbreviations

CT scan: Computed Tomography scan; MEN-1: Multiple Endocrine neoplasia-1; MRI: Magnetic Resonance Imaging; PTH: Parathyroid hormone

Acknowledgements

N/A

Funding

N/A

Authors' contributions

MC and VV contributed to the patient's clinical care and preparation of the manuscript; VB contributed to octreoscan imaging and revision of the manuscript, LL and AE contributed to surgery and revision of the manuscript, GB contributed to histopathological assessment and revision of the manuscript, EM, CRM, MM and AP contributed to the patient's clinical care, revision and final approval of the manuscript of the manuscript.

Competing interests

The authors declare that they have no competing interests.

Author details

[1]Endocrine Unit, Department of Experimental and Clinical Biomedical Sciences "Mario Serio", University of Florence, Careggi University Hospital, Florence, Italy. [2]Diabetology Unit, Department of Experimental and Clinical Biomedical Sciences "Mario Serio", University of Florence, Careggi University Hospital, Florence, Italy. [3]Division of Nuclear Medicine, Careggi University Hospital, Florence, Italy. [4]General and Pancreatic Surgery Department, The Pancreas Institute-University of Verona Hospital Trust, Verona, Italy. [5]Department of Pathology and Diagnostics, University of Verona Hospital Trust, Verona, Italy.

References

1. Oberg K, Eriksson B. Endocrine tumours of the pancreas. Best Pract Res Clin Gastroenterol. 2005;19:753–81.
2. Hirshberg B, Cochran C, Skarulis MC, Libutti SK, Alexander HR, Wood BJ, et al. Malignant insulinoma: spectrum of unusual clinical features. Cancer. 2005; 104:264–72.
3. Grant CS. Insulinoma. Best Pract Res Clin Gastroenterol. 2005;19:783–98.
4. Jonkers YM, Claessen SM, Veltman JA, Geurts van Kessel A, Din-jens WN, Skogseid B, et al. Molecular parameters associated with insulinoma progression: chromosomal instability versus p53 and CK19 status. Cytogenet Genome Res. 2006;115:289–97.
5. Pape UF, Berndt U, Müller-Nordhorn J, Böhmig M, Roll S, Koch M, et al. Prognostic factors of long-term outcome in gastroenteropancreatic neuroendocrine tumours. Endocr Relat Cancer. 2008;15:1083–97.
6. Pape UF, Jann H, Müller-Nordhorn J, Bockelbrink A, Berndt U, Willich SN, et al. Prognostic relevance of a novel TNM classification system for upper gastroenteropancreatic neuroendocrine tumors. Cancer. 2008;113:256–65.
7. E B, Caron P, Lombard-Bohas C, Tabarin A, Mitry E, Reznick Y, et al. Malignant insulinoma: recommendations for characterisation and treatment. Ann Endocrinol. 2013;74:523–33.
8. Perren A, Wiesli P, Schmid S, Montani M, Schmitt A, Schmid C, et al. Pancreatic endocrine tumors are a rare manifestation of the neurofibromatosis type 1 phenotype: molecular analysis of a malignant insulinoma in a NF-1 patient. Am J Surg Pathol. 2006;30:1047–51.
9. Cryer PE, Axelrod L, Grossman AB, Heller SR, Montori VM, Seaquist ER, Service FJ, Endocrine Society. Evaluation and management of adult hypoglycemic disorders: an Endocrine Society clinical practice guideline. J Clin Endocrinol Metab. 2009;94:709–28.

10. Vezzosi D, Bennet A, Rochaix P, Courbon F, Selves J, Pradere B, et al. Octreotide in insulinoma patients: efficacy on hypoglycemia, relationships with octreosacan scintigraphy and immunostaining with anti-sst2A and anti-sst5 antibodies. Eur J Endocrinol. 2005;152:757–67.

11. Bassi C, Marchegiani G, Dervenis C, Sarr M, Abu Hilal M, Adham M, et al. The 2016 update of the international study group (ISGPS) definition and grading of postoperative pancreatic fistula: 11 years after. Surgery. 2017;161:584–91.

12. Whipple AO. The surgical therapy of hyperinsulinism. J Int Chir. 1938;3:237–76.

13. Cryer PE. Symptoms of hypoglycemia, thresholds for their occurrence, and hypoglycemia unawareness. Endocrinol Metab Clin N Am. 1999;28:495–500.

14. Murad MH, Coto-Yglesias F, Wang AT, Sheidaee N, Mullan RJ, Elamin MB, et al. Clinical review: drug-induced hypoglycemia: a systematic review. J Clin Endocrinol Metab. 2009;94:741–5.

15. Nieman LK, Chanco Turner M. Addison's disease. Clin Dermatol. 2006;276–80.

16. A M, Fanelli C, Veneman T, Perriello G, Calderone S, Platanisiotis D, et al. Reversibility of unawareness of hypoglycemia in patients with insulinomas. N Engl J Med. 1993;329:834–9.

17. Gullo D, Evans JL, Sortino G, Goldfine ID, Vigneri R. Insulin autoimmune syndrome (Hirata disease) in European Caucasians taking α-lipoic acid. Clin Endocrinol. 2014;81:204–9.

18. Raffel A, Raffel A, Krausch MM, Anlauf M, Wieben D, Braunstein S, Klöppel G, et al. Diffuse nesidioblastosis as a cause of hyperinsulinemic hypoglycemia in adults: a diagnostic and therapeutic challenge. Surgery. 2007;141:179–84.

19. Okabayashi T, Shima Y, Sumiyoshi T, Kozuki A, Ito S, Ogawa Y, et al. Diagnosis and management of insulinoma. World J Gastroenterol. 2013;19: 829–37.

20. Shi W, Johnston CF, Buchanan KD, Ferguson WR, Laird JD, Crothers JG, Mcilrath EM. Localization of neuroendocrine tumours with [111In] DTPAoctreotide scintigraphy (Octreoscan): a comparative study with CT and MR imaging. Q J Med. 1998;91:295–301.

21. Krenning EP, Kwekkeboom DJ, Bakker WH, Breeman WA, Kooij PP, Oei HY, et al. Somatostatin receptor scintigraphy with [111In-DTPA-D-Phe1]- and [123I-Tyr3]-octreotide: the Rotterdam experience with more than 1000 patients. Eur J Nucl Med. 1993;20:716–31.

22. de Herder WW, Kwekkeboom DJ, Valkema R, Feelders RA, van Aken MO, Lamberts SW, et al. Neuroendocrine tumors and somatostatin: imaging techniques. J Endocrinol Investig. 2005;28:132–6.

23. Schillaci O, Massa R, Scopinaro F. 111In-pentetreotide scintigraphy in the detection of insulinomas: importance of SPECT imaging. J Nucl Med. 2000; 41:459–62.

24. Christ E, Wild D, Forrer F, Brändle M, Sahli R, Clerici T, et al. Glucagon-like peptide-1 receptor imaging for localization of insulinomas. J Clin Endocrinol Metab. 2009;94:4398–444.

25. Sundin A, Arnold R, Baudin E, Cwikla JB, Eriksson B, Fanti S, et al. ENETS consensus guidelines for the standards of Care in Neuroendocrine Tumors: radiological, Nuclear Medicine & Hybrid Imaging. Neuroendocrinology. 2017; 105:212–44.

26. Gill GV, Rauf O, MacFarlane IA. Diazoxide treatment for insulinoma: a national UK survey. Postgrad Med J. 1997;73:640–1.

27. Matej A, Bujwid H, Wroński J. Glycemic control in patients with insulinoma. Hormones (Athens). 2016;15:489–99.

28. Romeo S, Milione M, Gatti A, Fallarino M, Corleto V, Morano S, Baroni MG. Complete clinical remission and disappearance of liver metastases after treatment with somatostatin analogue in a 40-year-old woman with a malignant insulinoma positive for somatostatin receptors type 2. Horm Res. 2006;65:120–5.

29. Usukura M, Yoneda T, Oda N, Yamamoto Y, Takata H, Hasatani K, Takeda Y. Medical treatment of benign insulinoma using octreotide LAR: a case report. Endocr J. 2007;54:95–101.

30. Jawiarczyk A, Bolanowski M, Syrycka J, Bednarek-Tupikowska G, Kałużny M, Kołodziejczyk A, Domosławski P. Effective therapy of insulinoma by using long-acting somatostatin analogue. A case report and literature review. Exp Clin Endocrinol Diabetes. 2012;120:68–72.

31. Baudin E, Caron P, Lombard-Bohas C, Tabarin A, Mitry E, Reznick Y, et al. Malignant insulinoma: recommendations for characterisation and treatment. Ann Endocrinol (Paris). 2013;74:523–33.

32. Stehouwer CDA, Lems WF, Fischer HRA, Hackeng WHL, Naafs MAB. Aggravation of hypoglycemia in insulinoma patients by the long-acting somatostatin analogue octreotide (Sandostatin). Acta Endocrinol. 1989;121: 34 40.

33. Appetecchia M, Baldelli R. Somatostatin analogues in the treatment of gastroenteropancreatic neuroendocrine tumours, current aspects and new perspectives. J Exp Clin Cancer Res. 2010;29:19.

26

Long-term treatment outcomes of acromegaly patients presenting biochemically-uncontrolled at a tertiary pituitary center

John D. Carmichael[1], Michael S. Broder[2], Dasha Cherepanov[2]* ⓘ, Eunice Chang[2], Adam Mamelak[1], Qayyim Said[3], Maureen P. Neary[4] and Vivien Bonert[1]

Abstract

Background: Acromegaly is a rare, slowly progressive disorder resulting from excessive growth hormone (GH) production by a pituitary somatotroph tumor. The objective of this study was to examine acromegaly treatment outcomes during long-term care at a specialized pituitary center in patients presenting with lack of biochemical control.

Methods: Data came from an acromegaly registry at the Cedars-Sinai Medical Center Pituitary Center (center). Acromegaly patients included in this study were those who presented biochemically-uncontrolled for care at the center. Biochemical control status, based on serum insulin-like growth factor-1 values, was determined at presentation and at study end. Patient characteristics and acromegaly treatments were reported before and after presentation by presenting treatment status and final biochemical control status. Data on long-term follow-up were recorded from 1985 through June 2013.

Results: Seventy-four patients presented uncontrolled: 40 untreated (54.1%) and 34 (45.9%) previously-treated. Mean (SD) age at diagnosis was 43.2 (14.7); 32 (43.2%) were female patients. Of 65 patients with tumor size information, 59 (90.8%) had macroadenomas. Prior treatments among the 34 previously-treated patients were pituitary surgery alone (47.1%), surgery and medication (41.2%), and medication alone (11.8%). Of the 40 patients without prior treatment, 82.5% achieved control by study end. Of the 34 with prior treatment, 50% achieved control by study end.

Conclusions: This observational study shows that treatment outcomes of biochemically-uncontrolled acromegaly patients improve with directed care, particularly for those that initially present untreated. Patients often require multiple modalities of treatment, many of which are offered with the highest quality at specialized pituitary centers. Despite specialized care, some patients were not able to achieve biochemical control with methods of treatment that were available at the time of their treatment, showing the need for additional treatment options.

Keywords: Patient registry, Acromegaly, Biochemical control, Insulin-like growth factor-1, Treatment

* Correspondence: dasha@pharllc.com
[2]Partnership for Health Analytic Research, LLC, 280 S. Beverly Dr., Suite 404, Beverly Hills, CA 90212, USA
Full list of author information is available at the end of the article

Background

Acromegaly is a rare, slowly progressive disorder resulting from excessive growth hormone (GH) production by a pituitary somatotroph tumor. GH produces direct metabolic effects and induces hepatic insulin-like growth factor (IGF)-1 production. IGF-1 in turn also contributes to somatic growth and metabolic dysfunction [1]. Acromegaly affects up to 130 individuals per million persons, or approximately 20,000 people in the US, and recent reports indicate that incidence of pituitary tumors is increasing [2, 3]. Because of the slow progression of symptoms, diagnosis may be delayed for many years, with most acromegaly patients diagnosed after age 40 [2, 4–7]. Diagnosis is made clinically on the basis of typical signs and symptoms confirmed with laboratory assessment of GH and/or IGF-1 levels.

Initial treatment is surgery to resect the adenoma, but at least half of the patients require additional treatment [8–10]. First-line pharmacologic treatment usually consists of one of the first generation somatostatin receptor ligands (SRLs) such as octreotide or lanreotide. The goal of treatment is to reduce GH and/or IGF-1 levels to normal. The efficacy of SRL therapy is highly variable, with an average biochemical response rate of approximately 55% across most large series; however, lower response rates of 17-54% have been observed in several recent prospective studies that included only drug naïve patients [11, 12]. If initial pharmacologic therapy fails to achieve biochemical control, strategies for attempting to improve control include switching to or adding a dopamine agonist or pegvisomant, a GH-receptor antagonist; performing further surgery; or proceeding to radiotherapy [8–10].

The need to better understand this rare and complex disease had resulted in initiation of a number of acromegaly registries worldwide (e.g., [13–21]), although only a few such observational center-specific studies have been conducted in the US. [22–26]. The objective of this study was to report treatment patterns and outcomes of acromegaly patients that presented biochemically-uncontrolled for care at a single US pituitary center, based on data from a US acromegaly registry.

Methods

Study design and data sources

This study included patients from an observational acromegaly registry at the Pituitary Center at Cedars-Sinai Medical Center (CSMC) (center). The patients were followed by that center over time, some as early as 1985, and the database was periodically updated, resulting in approximately 300 acromegaly patients in the registry. The data in the registry include demographics, past medical and surgical history, symptoms, laboratory values, medications, cardiology and colonoscopy results, pathology, radiology, and surgical and visual field information.

All data were abstracted from medical records into the registry database by center investigators. The study was approved by the CSMC Institutional Review Board.

Study population and follow-up

The current study focused on acromegaly patients who were followed for at least 12 months after initial treatment and those who were not biochemically-controlled on presentation at CSMC. Presenting biochemical control status was determined based on the initial IGF-1 on presentation to the center. IGF-1 ≤ 100% of upper limit of normal (ULN) was defined as "controlled" and >100% ULN as "uncontrolled" [27]. Although all GH and IGF-1 values were recorded in the study, considering the possiblity of discordance between values of GH and IGF-I in different treatment scenarios, to maintain a robust definition of control we opted to rely solely on IGF-I for this analysis [27].

The first visit at the center was defined as the index date, the baseline period was defined as any time before the index date, and the follow-up period was defined as the time from the index date until the last observed IGF-1 test. Patients with no IGF-1 within the first 90 days after the index date were excluded.

Study measures

Baseline measures included patient characteristics, coexisting hormonal abnormalities, initial acromegaly treatments, and other medication use. Patient characteristics included age at the index date, age at diagnosis, gender, race/ethnicity, presenting biochemical control status, any abnormal finding on the first magnetic resonance imaging (MRI) or computed tomography (CT) (invasion of cavernous sinus; compression of optic chiasm; and carotid artery encasement), and first reported tumor size (microadenoma [<1 cm] vs. macroadenoma [≥1 cm]). Coexisting hormonal abnormalities included hyperprolactinemia, adrenal insufficiency (i.e., use of adrenal replacement [steroids]), gonadal insufficiency (or use of sex steroid replacement), hypothyroidism (or use of thyroid replacement), and use of antihyperglycemic or antihypertensive medications.

We described each patient's treatment course both during the baseline period and during follow-up. An individual treatment course was defined as the period from the first date of treatment until a different treatment was instituted. If there were no subsequent treatments, the treatment course ended on the last date of the treatment. Each surgical procedure was counted as a different treatment course. Combination treatment was defined as two or more medications used in conjunction for >90 days. Short (<6 month) pre-surgical medical treatment was not

Table 1 Baseline patient characteristics by presenting status

	Presenting Uncontrolled Without Prior Treatment for Acromegaly n = 40 (54.1%)	Presenting Uncontrolled with Prior Treatment for Acromegaly n = 34 (45.9%)	All N = 74
Age at index date, year[a]			
mean	44.7	50.1	47.2
(SD)	(15.5)	(15.6)	(15.6)
Age at diagnosis, year[b]			
n	35	31	66
mean	43.8	42.5	43.2
(SD)	(15.5)	(14.0)	(14.7)
Female			
n	16	16	32
(%)	(40.0)	(47.1)	(43.2)
Race/ethnicity			
Caucasian			
n	30	25	55
(%)	(75.0)	(73.5)	(74.3)
Asian			
n	5	5	10
(%)	(12.5)	(14.7)	(13.5)
Hispanic			
n	4	4	8
(%)	(10.0)	(11.8)	(10.8)
Other			
n	1	0	1
(%)	(2.5)	(0.0)	(1.4)
Years of follow-up at center			
mean	5.1	8.5	6.7
(SD)	(4.4)	(5.7)	(5.3)
min - max	0.3–23.0	0.2–21.3	0.2–23.0
median	4.2	7.8	4.9
Tumor Size[c]			
n	36	29	65
Macroadenoma			
n	33	26	59
(%)	(91.7)	(89.7)	(90.8)
Microadenoma			
n	3	3	6
(%)	(8.3)	(10.3)	(9.2)
Abnormal finding on MRI or CT			
n	25	15	40
(%)	(62.5)	(44.1)	(54.1)

Table 1 Baseline patient characteristics by presenting status (Continued)

Hormonal Abnormalities			
Prolactin elevation			
n	0	1	1
(%)	(0.0)	(2.9)	(1.4)
Adrenal insufficiency			
n	4	3	7
(%)	(10.0)	(8.8)	(9.5)
Gonadal insufficiency			
n	5	4	9
(%)	(12.5)	(11.8)	(12.2)
Hypothyroidism			
n	4	6	10
(%)	(10.0)	(17.6)	(13.5)

[a]Index date was defined as the first visit the center;
[b]66 patients had information about age at diagnosis;
[c]65 patients had tumor size available in the patient medical record; percent among non-missing observations

counted as a treatment course, nor was subcutaneous octreotide SA for ≤30 days immediately preceding the use of octreotide LAR or lanreotide.

Finally, final biochemical control status was assessed for all study patients, based on the last observed IGF-1 test result at the center and the same definition as the one described above for presenting biochemical control status. The assays used at the center included: GH and IGF-I assays at Nichols Institute Reference Laboratories (San Juan Capistrano, CA) from 1986 to 1994; Esoterix Inc. (Calabasas, CA) from 1994 to 2005; the Nichols Advantage assay at Nichols Institute/Quest Diagnostics (San Juan Capistrano, CA) from 2005 to 2006; and the DPC Immulite 2000 assay (Diagnostic Products Corp., Los Angeles, CA) at Quest Diagnostics from 2006 to present [27]. All GH and IGF-I assays are two-site RIAs, and each was standardized against World Health Organization international standard preparations, with changes in reference preparations made over the years [27].

Analyses

Baseline characteristics and baseline treatment variables were presented descriptively for two separate acromegaly cohorts: those presenting uncontrolled and untreated versus those presenting uncontrolled and treated. The two cohorts were then further stratified into those that reached final biochemical control and those that did not, for description of treatment during care at the center. Descriptive statistics, including means, standard deviations (SD), medians, and percentages, were estimated for all study measures when applicable, and reported separately for each control status cohort and for all patients. All data transformations and statistical analyses were performed using SAS® version 9.4 (SAS Institute, Cary, NC).

Results

Of 300 acromegaly patients in the registry, 121 were followed for at least 12 months after initial treatment, and of these only 74 patients presented biochemically uncontrolled at the center and were included in the study. Of these, 40 patients presented untreated (54.1%), and 34 (45.9%) presented after having received at least one prior treatment. The mean (SD) age at diagnosis was 43.2 (14.7) years and was 47.2 (15.6) years at the time of this study. There were 32 (43.2%) female patients, 55 (74.3%) Caucasian patients, 10 (13.5%) Asian patients, 8 (10.8%) Hispanic patients, and one of other race/ethnicity. Median follow-up at the center was 4.9 years. For 65 of 74 patients, data on baseline tumor size was available: 59 (90.8%) patients had macroadenomas and 6 (9.2%) had microadenomas. Abnormal findings on MRI or CT were observed in 40 (54.1%) patients; 10 (13.5%) patients had hypothyroidism, 9 (12.2%) patients gonadal insufficiency, 7 (9.5%) had adrenal insufficiency, and 1 (1.4%) had elevated prolactin. These patient characteristics were distributed relatively similarly by presenting treatment status (Table 1).

In the cohort with prior treatment, the pre-presentation (baseline) treatment was pituitary surgery alone in 16 (47.1%) patients, surgery and medication in 14 (41.2%) patients, and medication alone in 4 (11.8%) patients. Medications for acromegaly included only somatostatin analogues and dopamine agonists. In addition, 11.8% used antihyperglycemics and 26.5% antihypertensives. In the untreated cohort, 12.5% used antihyperglycemics and 22.5% used antihypertensive medications (Table 2).

At the end of follow up, 33 (82.5%) of 40 patients without prior treatment achieved control and 7 remained uncontrolled (17.5%). Of 34 patients that presented uncontrolled but with prior treatment, 17 (50%) patients achieved control and 17 remained uncontrolled by study end. Patients that remained uncontrolled tended to be older on average than those that reached control, especially those who were uncontrolled and treated at baseline. Overall, a higher proportions of patients that remained uncontrolled had prolactin elevation (4.2% vs. 0%), adrenal insufficiency (16.7% vs. 6%), and hypothyroidism (20.8% vs. 10.0%) (Table 3).

Among the 33 initially uncontrolled and untreated patients that reached control by study end, most were managed with surgery and medication (51.5%) or surgery alone (42.4%) after presentation. Among the 17 initially uncontrolled but treated patients that reached control

by study end, most were managed with medication alone (58.8%) during care at the center (Table 4).

Discussion

This study describes the treatment patterns and outcomes of acromegaly patients that presented without biochemical control at a single major specialized pituitary center in the US. The study showed that of those patients that presented at the center biochemically-uncontrolled and previously untreated for acromegaly, a majority (82.5%) achieved biochemical control during care at the center by study end. However, only 50% of patients that presented as biochemically-uncontrolled

Table 2 Baseline treatment by presenting status

	Presenting Uncontrolled Without Prior Treatment for Acromegaly $n = 40$ (54.1%)	Presenting Uncontrolled with Prior Treatment for Acromegaly $n = 34$ (45.9%)	All $N = 74$
Treatment Patterns			
No treatment	40	0	40
	(100.0)	(0.0)	(54.1)
Surgery and medication	0	14	14
	(0.0)	(41.2)	(18.9)
Medication only	0	4	4
	(0.0)	(11.8)	(5.4)
Surgery only	0	16	16
	(0.0)	(47.1)	(21.6)
Pituitary surgery	0	30	30
	(0.0)	(88.2)	(40.5)
Pharmacologic treatment	0	18	18
	(0.0)	(52.9)	(24.3)
Somatostatin analogues	0	12	12
	(0.0)	(35.3)	(16.2)
Pasireotide	0	0	0
	(0.0)	(0.0)	(0.0)
Dopamine agonists	0	12	12
	(0.0)	(35.3)	(16.2)
Pegvisomant	0	0	0
	(0.0)	(0.0)	(0.0)
Antihyperglycemic medication	5	4	9
	(12.5)	(11.8)	(12.2)
Insulin	0	1	1
	(0.0)	(2.9)	(1.4)
Antihypertensive medication	9	9	18
	(22.5)	(26.5)	(24.3)

Somatostatin analogues include octreotide LAR, octreotide SA, and lanreotide; dopamine agonists include bromocriptine and cabergoline

Table 3 Patient characteristics by presenting status and final biochemical control status

Final Biochemical Control	Presenting Uncontrolled Without Prior Treatment for Acromegaly n = 40 (54.1%)		Presenting Uncontrolled with Prior Treatment for Acromegaly n = 34 (45.9%)		All N = 74
	Controlled n = 33 (82.5%)	Uncontrolled n = 7 (17.5%)	Controlled n = 17 (50.0%)	Uncontrolled n = 17 (50.0%)	
Age at index date, year[a]					
mean	44.5	45.6	46.8	53.4	47.2
(SD)	(15.9)	(14.5)	(12.9)	(17.7)	(15.6)
Age at diagnosis, year[b]					
N	30	5	16	15	66
mean	44.5	40.0	41.4	43.6	43.2
(SD)	(15.9)	(13.6)	(12.1)	(16.1)	(14.7)
Years of follow-up at center					
mean	5.0	5.3	8.7	8.3	6.7
(SD)	(4.7)	(2.7)	(6.3)	(5.3)	(5.3)
min-max	0.3-23.0	2.2-9.4	0.2-21.3	0.6-20.2	0.2-23.0
median	4.2	4.5	8.0	7.3	4.9
Tumor Size[c]					
n	31	5	15	14	65
Macroadenoma					
n	29	4	14	12	59
(%)	(93.5)	(80.0)	(93.3)	(85.7)	(90.8)
Microadenoma					
n	2	1	1	2	6
(%)	(6.5)	(20.0)	(6.7)	(14.3)	(9.2)
Abnormal finding on MRI or CT					
n	21	4	7	8	40
(%)	(63.6)	(57.1)	(41.2)	(47.1)	(54.1)
Hormonal Abnormalities					
Prolactin elevation					
n	0	0	0	1	1
(%)	(0.0)	(0.0)	(0.0)	(5.9)	(1.4)
Adrenal insufficiency					
n	2	2	1	2	7
(%)	(6.1)	(28.6)	(5.9)	(11.8)	(9.5)
Gonadal insufficiency					
n	4	1	4	0	9
(%)	(12.1)	(14.3)	(23.5)	(0.0)	(12.2)
Hypothyroidism					
n	3	1	2	4	10
(%)	(9.1)	(14.3)	(11.8)	(23.5)	(13.5)

[a]Index date was defined as the first visit at the center;
[b]35 patients had information about age at diagnosis in the presenting uncontrolled without prior treatment group; 31 patients had the information in the presenting uncontrolled with prior treatment group;
[c]36 patients had tumor size available in the patient medical record in the presenting uncontrolled without prior treatment group; 29 patients had the information in the presenting uncontrolled with prior treatment group

Table 4 Treatment during care at center by presenting status and final biochemical control status

Final Biochemical Control	Presenting Uncontrolled Without Prior Treatment for Acromegaly n = 40 (54.1%)		Presenting Uncontrolled With Prior Treatment for Acromegaly n = 34 (45.9%)		All N = 74
	Controlled n = 33 (82.5%)	Uncontrolled n = 7 (17.5%)	Controlled n = 17 (50.0%)	Uncontrolled n = 17 (50.0%)	
Treatment Patterns					
Surgery and medication	17	4	2	4	27
	(51.5)	(57.1)	(11.8)	(23.5)	(36.5)
Medication only	2	2	10	12	26
	(6.1)	(28.6)	(58.8)	(70.6)	(35.1)
Surgery only	14	1	3	1	19
	(42.4)	(14.3)	(17.6)	(5.9)	(25.7)
No treatment	0	0	2	0	2
	(0.0)	(0.0)	(11.8)	(0)	(2.7)
Pituitary surgery	31	5	5	5	46
	(93.9)	(71.4)	(29.4)	(29.4)	(62.2)
Pharmacologic treatment	19	6	12	16	53
	(57.6)	(85.7)	(70.6)	(94.1)	(71.6)
Somatostatin analogues	15	4	9	15	43
	(45.5)	(57.1)	(52.9)	(88.2)	(58.1)
Pasireotide	0	0	1	0	1
	(0.0)	(0.0)	(5.9)	(0.0)	(1.4)
Dopamine agonists	8	2	6	10	26
	(24.2)	(28.6)	(35.3)	(58.8)	(35.1)
Pegvisomant	5	1	2	4	12
	(15.2)	(14.3)	(11.8)	(23.5)	(16.2)

Somatostatin analogues include octreotide LAR, octreotide SA, and lanreotide; dopamine agonists include bromocriptine and cabergoline; dopamine agonists include bromocriptine and cabergoline

but had prior treatment went on to achieve biochemical control by study end, suggesting these cases may have been more complex.

Although there are a number of published studies based on acromegaly registries worldwide (e.g., [13–21]), only a few such studies have reported on results for the US acromegaly population [22–26]. The current study supplements the literature by providing a description of treatment patterns based on an ongoing US acromegaly registry.

The results from this study indicate that a higher proportion of acromegaly patients that present de novo, uncontrolled and untreated, to a specialized pituitary center may achieve disease remission compared to acromegaly patients that present uncontrolled and previously treated. These data suggest that the patients that are uncontrolled and previously treated at presentation may be more treatment resistant and have more complex management requirements than those that present untreated. It is possible that the previously treated patients are

referred to a specialized pituitary center due to failing treatment elsewhere. The complexity of previously treated cases was underscored in this study by a somewhat higher proportion of these patients presenting with use of antihypertensive medications (26.5% vs. 22.5%) and with hypothyroidism (17.6% vs. 10%) indicating a potentially higher degree of hypopituitarism; they were also slightly older (mean age 50.1 versus 44.7 years). The management complexity of these patients was also indicated by an overall longer follow-up time period versus those that presented untreated (median follow-up period of 7.8 years vs. 4.2 years). These patients may have had a longer duration of the disease that was left uncontrolled and untreated, manifesting in higher rates of comorbidities.

Conversely, these results also show that even among uncontrolled patients that previously received treatment for acromegaly, such as pituitary surgery, further disease management at a specialized pituitary center results in improved biochemical control in up to 50% of patients. These improvements are likely associated with access to successful repeat pituitary surgery or specialized tailoring of medical therapy for patients not suited for surgery. Specifically, in this study the use of medical therapies and surgeries, including pegvisomant and repeat surgeries by an experienced neurosurgeon led to an improvement in disease control in most patients presenting to the center. Finally, these center-specific findings suggest that for some difficult-to-treat acromegaly patients, achieving biochemical control even at a specialized pituitary center may be challenging with currently available treatment options.

Patients who remained uncontrolled despite maximal surgical and medical treatment were considered for radiosurgery or radiotherapy. Risks and benefits of these therapies were weighed in all cases, and in all cases presented here, patients did not receive radiation during the treatment period described. In general, the approach towards patients with acromegaly at this center ascribes radiation to a lower treatment priority than surgery or medication, and weighs heavily the risks associated with radiation treatment [9, 10].

This study provided a large data set on acromegaly patients treated at a specialized pituitary center, thereby filling the need for more data on observed long-term treatment outcomes for acromegaly in the US. The study included detailed medical chart information across a lengthy follow-up period, enabling tracking of treatment patterns and associated clinical outcomes. The study had limitations. The small sample size was limited in power to conduct statistical tests to assess significant differences between cohorts in the study sample. It is possible that results vary across centers. Future studies should compare the outcomes of acromegaly patients treated at different centers. Patients examined in this study likely represent cases with complex acromegaly, referred for specialized tertiary or quaternary care. The study reflects care over more than two decades. Acromegaly management has changed significantly over that time. Since this study was completed, some patients may have achieved control. Other limitations include those that are typical of observational studies and registries, such as lack of randomized-placebo controlled study design, which would have ensured strict criteria such as medication titration protocols and treatment adherence.

Conclusions

Treatment outcomes for biochemically-uncontrolled acromegaly patients improve with directed care, particularly for those that initially present untreated. Patients often require multiple modalities of treatment, many of which are offered at specialized pituitary centers. Despite care at such a center, some patients did not achieve biochemical control with currently available methods of treatment, showing a clear unmet need for additional treatment options. Future research should consider that

in any evaluation of a clinical practice, treatment decisions and outcomes are not only guided by physicians' clinical management decisions and preferences, but also by patients' access to care (such as insurance), preferences, and treatment compliance.

Abbreviations
CSMC: Cedars-Sinai Medical Center; GH: Growth hormone; IGF: Insulin-like growth factor; SD: Standard deviations; SRLs: Somatostatin receptor ligands; ULN: Upper limit of normal

Acknowledgements
Not applicable

Funding
This study was funded by Novartis Pharmaceuticals Corporation. The funder reviewed the manuscript.

Authors' contributions
JDC, MSB, DC, EC, AM, QS, MPN, and VB all met the ICMJE criteria for authorship. JDC, MSB, DC, EC, AM, QS, MPN, and VB were involved in the design of the study, interpretation of results, and writing of the manuscript. Additionally, JDC, AM, and VB participated in data acquisition and EC conducted the statistical analyses. All authors read and approved the final manuscript.

Competing interests
Vivien Bonert, John D. Carmichael, and Adam Mamelak were responsible for overseeing this study at Cedars-Sinai Medical Center, which received funding for this research. Maureen Neary and Qayyim Said are employees of Novartis Pharmaceuticals Corporation. Michael S. Broder, Eunice Chang, and Dasha Cherepanov are employees of Partnership for Health Analytic Research, LLC, a health services research company paid by Novartis to conduct this research. Dr. John D. Carmichael is currently located at the University of Southern California (USC) Pituitary Center at the Keck School of Medicine of USC.

Author details
[1]Pituitary Center, Cedars-Sinai Medical Center, 8700 Beverly Blvd, Los Angeles, CA 90048, USA. [2]Partnership for Health Analytic Research, LLC, 280 S. Beverly Dr., Suite 404, Beverly Hills, CA 90212, USA. [3]Health Economics and Outcomes Research, Novartis Pharmaceuticals Corporation, One Health Plaza, East Hanover, NJ 07936, USA. [4]Global Oncology Market Access and Policy, Novartis Pharmaceuticals Corporation, One Health Plaza, East Hanover, NJ 07936, USA.

References
1. Melmed S. Medical progress: Acromegaly. N Engl J Med. 2006;355(24):2558–73. Review. Erratum in: N Engl J Med. 2007 Feb 22;356(8):879.
2. Chanson P, Salenave S. Acromegaly. Orphanet J Rare Dis. 2008;3:17.
3. Gittleman H, Ostrom QT, Farah PD, Ondracek A, Chen Y, Wolinsky Y, et al. Descriptive epidemiology of pituitary tumors in the United States, 2004-2009. J Neurosurg. 2014;121(3):527–35.
4. Agustsson TT, Baldvinsdottir T, Jonasson JG, Olafsdottir E, Steinthorsdottir V, Sigurdsson G, et al. The epidemiology of pituitary adenomas in Iceland, 1955-2012: a nationwide population-based study. Eur J Endocrinol. 2015;173(5):655–64.
5. Chanson P, Salenave S, Kamenicky P, Cazabat L, Young J. Pituitary tumours: acromegaly. Best Pract Res Clin Endocrinol Metab. 2009;23(5):555–74.
6. Daly AF, Rixhon M, Adam C, Dempegioti A, Tichomirowa MA, Beckers A. High prevalence of pituitary adenomas: a cross-sectional study in the province of Liege, Belgium. J Clin Endocrinol Metab. 2006;91(12):4769–75.
7. Fernandez A, Karavitaki N, Wass JA. Prevalence of pituitary adenomas: a community-based, cross-sectional study in Banbury (Oxfordshire, UK). Clin Endocrinol. 2010;72(3):377–82.

8. Giustina A, Chanson P, Kleinberg D, Bronstein MD, Clemmons DR, Klibanski A, et al. Expert consensus document: a consensus on the medical treatment of acromegaly. Nat Rev Endocrinol. 2014;10(4):243–8.

9. Katznelson L, Laws ER Jr, Melmed S, Molitch ME, Murad MH, Utz A, et al. Acromegaly: an endocrine society clinical practice guideline. J Clin Endocrinol Metab. 2014;99(11):3933–51.

10. Melmed S, Colao A, Barkan A, Molitch M, Grossman AB, Kleinberg D, et al. Guidelines for acromegaly management: an update. J Clin Endocrinol Metab. 2009;94(5):1509–17.

11. Carmichael JD, Bonert VS, Nuño M, Ly D, Melmed S. Acromegaly clinical trial methodology impact on reported biochemical efficacy rates of somatostatin receptor ligand treatments: a meta-analysis. J Clin Endocrinol Metab. 2014;99(5):1825–33.

12. Colao A, Auriemma RS, Pivonello R, Kasuki L, Gadelha MR. Interpreting biochemical control response rates with first-generation somatostatin analogues in acromegaly. Pituitary. 2016;19(3):235–47.

13. Arosio M, Reimondo G, Malchiodi E, Berchialla P, Borraccino A, De Marinis L, et al. Predictors of morbidity and mortality in acromegaly: an Italian survey. Eur J Endocrinol. 2012;167(2):189–98.

14. Bex M, Abs R, T'Sjoen G, Mockel J, Velkeniers B, Muermans K, et al. AcroBel–the Belgian registry on acromegaly: a survey of the 'real-life' outcome in 418 acromegalic subjects. Eur J Endocrinol. 2007;157(4):399–409.

15. Dal J, Feldt-Rasmussen U, Andersen M, Kristensen LØ, Laurberg P, Pedersen L, et al. Acromegaly incidence, prevalence, complications and long-term prognosis: a nationwide cohort study. Eur J Endocrinol. 2016;175(3):181–90.

16. Delemer B, Chanson P, Foubert L, Borson-Chazot F, Chabre O, Tabarin A, et al. Patients lost to follow-up in acromegaly: results of the ACROSPECT study. Eur J Endocrinol. 2014;170(5):791–7.

17. Fieffe S, Morange I, Petrossians P, Chanson P, Rohmer V, Cortet C, et al. Diabetes in acromegaly, prevalence, risk factors, and evolution: data from the French Acromegaly registry. Eur J Endocrinol. 2011;164(6):877–84.

18. Holdaway IM, Rajasoorya RC, Gamble GD. Factors influencing mortality in acromegaly. J Clin Endocrinol Metab. 2004;89(2):667–74.

19. Portocarrero-Ortiz LA, Vergara-Lopez A, Vidrio-Velazquez M, Uribe-Diaz AM, García-Dominguez A, Reza-Albarrán AA, et al. The Mexican Acromegaly registry: clinical and biochemical characteristics at diagnosis and therapeutic outcomes. J Clin Endocrinol Metab. 2016;101(11):3997–4004.

20. Schöfl C, Franz H, Grussendorf M, Honegger J, Jaursch-Hancke C, Mayr B, et al. Long-term outcome in patients with acromegaly: analysis of 1344 patients from the German Acromegaly register. Eur J Endocrinol. 2012;168(1):39–47.

21. Sesmilo G, Gaztambide S, Venegas E, Picó A, Del Pozo C, Blanco C, et al. Changes in acromegaly treatment over four decades in Spain: analysis of the Spanish Acromegaly registry (REA). Pituitary. 2013;16(1):115–21.

22. Drange MR, Fram NR, Herman-Bonert V, Melmed S. Pituitary tumor registry: a novel clinical resource. J Clin Endocrinol Metab. 2000;85(1):168–74.

23. Katznelson L, Kleinberg D, Vance ML, Stavrou S, Pulaski KJ, Schoenfeld DA, et al. Hypogonadism in patients with acromegaly: data from the multi-centre acromegaly registry pilot study. Clin Endocrinol. 2001;54(2):183–8. Erratum in: Clin Endocrinol (Oxf) 2001 Nov;55(5):699. Stravou S [corrected to Stavrou S]

24. Nachtigall L, Delgado A, Swearingen B, Lee H, Zerikly R, Klibanski A. Changing patterns in diagnosis and therapy of acromegaly over two decades. J Clin Endocrinol Metab. 2008;93(6):2035–41.

25. Reyes-Vidal C, Fernandez JC, Bruce JN, Crisman C, Conwell IM, Kostadinov J, et al. Prospective study of surgical treatment of acromegaly: effects on ghrelin, weight, adiposity, and markers of CV risk. J Clin Endocrinol Metab. 2014;99(11):4124–32.

26. Swearingen B, Barker FG 2nd, Katznelson L, Biller BM, Grinspoon S, Klibanski A, et al. Long-term mortality after transsphenoidal surgery and adjunctive therapy for acromegaly. J Clin Endocrinol Metab. 1998;83(10):3419–26.

27. Carmichael JD, Bonert VS, Mirocha JM, Melmed S. The utility of oral glucose tolerance testing for diagnosis and assessment of treatment outcomes in 166 patients with acromegaly. J Clin Endocrinol Metab. 2009;94(2):523–7.

27

Two novel *LHX3* mutations in patients with combined pituitary hormone deficiency including cervical rigidity and sensorineural hearing loss

Khushnooda Ramzan[1*], Bassam Bin-Abbas[2], Lolwa Al-Jomaa[1], Rabab Allam[1], Mohammed Al-Owain[3,4†] and Faiqa Imtiaz[1†]

Abstract

Background: Congenital combined pituitary hormone deficiency (CPHD) is a rare heterogeneous group of conditions. CPHD-type 3 (CPHD3; MIM# 221750) is caused by recessive mutations in *LHX3*, a LIM-homeodomain transcription factor gene. The isoforms of LHX3 are critical for pituitary gland formation and specification of the anterior pituitary hormone-secreting cell types. They also play distinct roles in the development of neuroendocrine and auditory systems.

Case presentation: Here, we summarize the clinical, endocrinological, radiological and molecular features of three patients from two unrelated families. Clinical evaluation revealed severe CPHD coupled with cervical vertebral malformations (rigid neck, scoliosis), mild developmental delay and moderate sensorineural hearing loss (SNHL). The patients were diagnosed with CPHD3 based on the array of hormone deficiencies and other associated syndromic symptoms, suggestive of targeted *LHX3* gene sequencing. A novel missense mutation c.437G > T (p. Cys146Phe) and a novel nonsense mutation c. 466C > T (p. Arg156Ter), both in homozygous forms, were found. The altered Cys146 resides in the LIM2 domain of the encoded protein and is a phylogenetically conserved residue, which mediates LHX3 transcription factor binding with a zinc cation. The p. Arg156Ter is predicted to result in a severely truncated protein, lacking the DNA binding homeodomain.

Conclusions: Considering genotype/phenotype correlation, we suggest that the presence of SNHL and limited neck rotation should be considered in the differential diagnosis of CPHD3 to facilitate molecular diagnosis. This report describes the first *LHX3* mutations from Saudi patients and highlights the importance of combining molecular diagnosis with the clinical findings. In addition, it also expands the knowledge of *LHX3*-related CPHD3 phenotype and the allelic spectrum for this gene.

Keywords: *LHX3*, Pituitary hormone deficiency, Sensorineural hearing loss, Cysteine 146, Differential diagnosis

Background

Combined pituitary hormone deficiency (CPHD) refers to a rare heterogeneous group of conditions, which is characterized by true deficiency of at least two anterior pituitary hormones. CPHD has been linked with abnormalities in the genes encoding both signaling molecules and transcription factors, which have been shown to play a role in the development and maturation of the

---
* Correspondence: kramzan@kfshrc.edu.sa
†Equal contributors
[1]Department of Genetics, King Faisal Specialist Hospital and Research Centre, P.O.Box 3354, Riyadh 11211, Saudi Arabia
Full list of author information is available at the end of the article

pituitary gland. These genes include *HESX1*, *LHX3*, *LHX4*, *POU1F1*, *PROP1*, *SIX6*, *OTX2*, *PTX2*, *GLI2* and *SOX3* [1–3]. The pituitary phenotype caused by genetic defects in these genes may be isolated (pure pituitary phenotype) or may be associated with variable extrapituitary maifestations (syndromic CPHD) [4]. Clinical presentation is variable, depending on the type and severity of deficiencies and at the age of diagnosis. If untreated, main symptoms usually include short stature, cognitive alterations or delayed puberty. CPHD is related to significant morbidity, especially hypoglycemia and its consequences in newborns. Treatment should be started immediately and a strict specialized follow-up is necessary [5]. Here, we describe the clinical, endocrinological, radiological and molecular features of three new cases of *LHX3*-related CPHD3.

Mutations in the *LHX3* gene (MIM# 600577), located on chromosome 9q34.3, underlie combined pituitary hormone deficiency type 3 (CPHD3, MIM# 221750). The encoded protein (Uniprot: Q9UBR4) is a LIM-homeodomain (LIM-HD) transcription factor, which features two amino-terminal LIM domains (cysteine-rich zinc-binding domain) and a centrally-located DNA-binding homeodomain [6]. In addition, the LHX3 protein also possesses a carboxyl terminus that includes the major trans-activation domain. Alternative splicing generates two isoforms, LHX3a and LHX3b, which are 397 and 402 amino acids long, respectively. These isoforms possess identical LIM domains, homeodomains and carboxyl termini but possess different amino-termini and differentially activate pituitary gene targets [7, 8].

Typically, genetically-confirmed CPHD3 patients with homozygous *LHX3* mutations present with hypopituitarism including deficiencies in the growth hormone (GH), thyroid stimulating hormone (TSH), prolactin (PRL), leutinizing hormone (LH), follicular stimulating hormone (FSH) and abnormal pituitary morphology. Adrenocorticotrophic hormone (ACTH) deficiency, cervical abnormalities with or without restricted neck rotation and sensorineural hearing loss (SNHL) has also been reported in a subset of these patients. The phenotypes in three patients (aged 2–11 year) in this report include CPHD, rigid cervical spine, restricted neck rotation, scoliosis, mild developmental delay and congenital hearing impairment. Targeted sequencing of the *LHX3* gene revealed two novel recessive variants in these patients. Finally, we surveyed the functional consequences of these mutations.

Case presentation

We ascertained three patients with syndromic symptoms associated with CPHD. An informed written consent was used to recruit the patients and their family members. All affected patients underwent detailed examination at the departments of clinical genetics and pediatrics of King Faisal Specialist Hospital and Research Centre, Riyadh, Saudi Arabia. Laboratory testing, radiological investigation (X-ray) and audiologic assessments were performed. Pituitary examination was made by multisequential multiplanar magnetic resonance imaging (MRI) by applying standard scanning protocols [9]. The hormonal tests were measured by radioimmunoassay techniques by Roche Diagnostics, USA. Hormonal evaluation included basal levels for GH response to glucagon stimulation, TSH, PRL, LH, FSH, cortisol, ACTH and free thyroxine (FT4) levels. Growth biochemical markers including insulin growth factor 1 (IGF1) and insulin

growth factor binding protein 3 (IGFBP3) were also assessed. The diagnoses of hormonal deficiencies were established using the normal range as cutoff limits: Basal GH (>10 µg/L), TSH (0.27–4.2 mU/L), PRL (2.5–15 µg/L), LH (0.1–3.3 U/L), FSH (0.1–7 U/L), ACTH (5–60 ng/L), cortisol (190–750 nmol/L), FT4 (12–22 pmol/L), IGF1 (115–498 ng/L) and IGFBP3 (0.7–3.6 mg/L).

Cases

Patient 1, Family 1

This boy (II:2, Fig. 1a) was a product of an uneventful pregnancy and normal vaginal delivery at 39 weeks of gestation, whose healthy consanguineous parents had previously lost a daughter in infancy probably because of the same condition. At birth, he was noted to have a micropenis with a stretched penile length of 1.8 cm and undescended testes. Other dysmorphic features included short webbed neck with limited rotation and triangular face. During hypoglycemic attack at the 3rd month of the life, ACTH and GH deficiencies were diagnosed. Later TSH and gonadotropin deficiencies were also found (see Table 1). Both TSH and FT4 were low suggesting central hypothyroidism. MRI of pituitary gland showed a small cystic lesion replacing the adenohypophysis of the pituitary gland representing developmental cystic abnormality. The pituitary stalk was present with normally placed neurohypophysis. Skeletal survey showed closure of sagittal suture causing dolichocephaly and hypoplasia of the facial bones. Thyroxine (25 µg daily), hydrocortisone (2.5 mg twice daily) and subcutaneous injections for GH (0.035 mg/kg/day) were initiated to normalize glycemia and to improve somatic growth at the 5th month of age. His height was 107 cm at age of 7 years (on the 5th percentile, –2SD). Testosterone therapy was given at a dose of 25 mg monthly for 3 months, which improved penile length to 3.1 cm. He also had moderate SNHL at the age of 2 years.

Patient 2, Family 2

The proband (II:2, Fig. 1b) of family 2 is the second child of healthy first degree parents, born via normal vaginal delivery at 39 weeks of gestation. He was initially evaluated in a local hospital for mild hypoglycemic attacks which were associated with jitteriness and irritability. He was first seen at our clinic at age of 2 years. He was clinically normal, apart from an abnormal head tilt secondary to abnormal neck posturing. His height was -3SD and he had a stretched penile length of 0.5 cm (–5.3 SD) with non-palpable testes. The patient had craniosynostosis causing plagiocephaly. Hypopituitarism was confirmed (Table 1). An MRI of his pituitary gland showed a small rudimentary adenohypophysis and a normal pituitary stalk present with normally placed neurohypophysis. A skeletal survey showed closure of sagittal

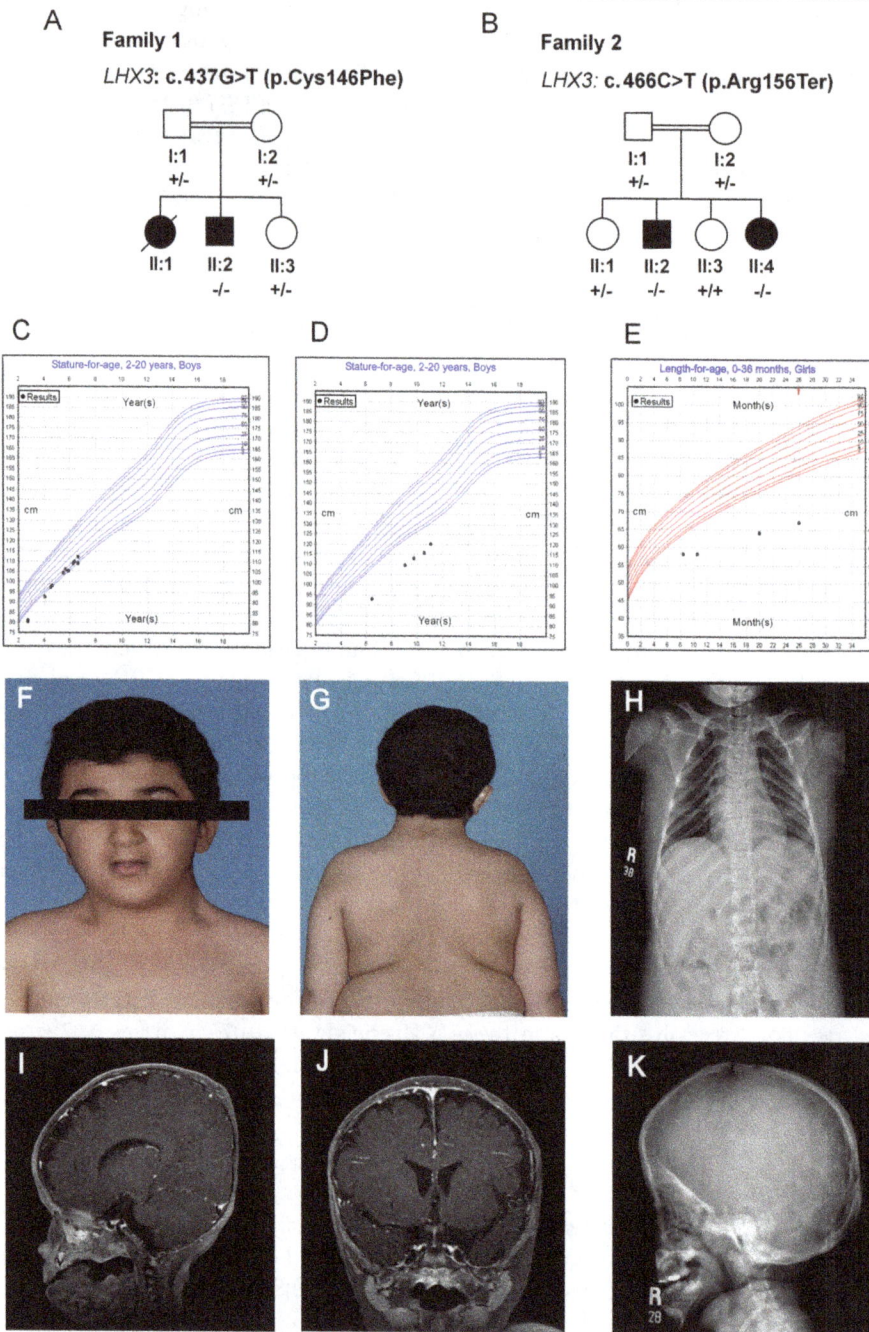

Fig. 1 Family pedigrees, genotypes, growth charts for patients and clinical presentation. **a, b** Pedigrees of the families studied with CPHD3 demonstrating the recessive inheritance pattern. *Filled symbols* indicate affected individuals. The respective genotype is indicated below each individual. Symbols are: + for wild type allele;—for mutated allele. **c, d, e** Representative growth chart for Patients II:2 (Family 1), II:2 (Family 2) and II:4 (Family 2) showing reduced growth velocity for all patients and reduced response for patient 2 and 3 compared to patient 1. Affected patient 2 (II:2 from family 2) showing **f** neck rotation, **g** scoliosis and **h** lower thoracic scoliosis by spine x-ray. **i, j** Multisequential multiplanar brain MRI reveals pituitary gland hypoplasia for patient II:2 from family 1 **i** coronal view **j** sagittal view **k** skull x-ray demonstrates an increased anterior-posterior diameter of calvarium suggestive of dolicocephaly

suture causing dolichocephaly and thoracic scoliosis. L-thyroxine (50 mcg daily), hydrocortisone (2.5 mg twice daily) and GH injections (0.035 mg/kg/day) were initiated. Orchipexy was performed at the age of 2.5 years. Testosterone therapy (25 mg monthly) was given for 3 months which improved penile length to 1.5 cm. Two other testosterone courses were given at the age of 5 years and 10 years with a partial improvement in penile length to 3 cm. Bilateral moderate SNHL was also found at the age of 3 years. His growth improved in response to GH

Table 1 Clinical data for three patients with novel *LHX3* mutations

	Patient 1 (II:2, Family 1)	Patient 2 (II:2, Family 2)	Patient 3 (II:4, Family 2)
Age, years	7	11	2
Gestational age, weeks	39	39	39
Birth weight, kg (SD)	3.2 (0SD)	3 (− 0.7SD)	2.9 (− 0.7SD)
Birth length, cm (SD)	45 (−2.5SD)	NA	46 (−1.8SD)
Age of onset, months	3	2	2
Initial manifestation hypopituitarism	+	+	+
Basal GH µg/L (>10)	<0.2	<0.5	<0.5
TSH mU/L (0.27–4.2)	0.02	0.04	0.4
PRL µg/L (2.5–15)	0.1	0.1	NA
LH U/L (0.1–3.3)	<0.1	<0.1	<0.1
FSH U/L (0.1–7)	<0.1	<0.1	<0.1
ACTH ng/L (5–60)	6	8	16
cortisol nmol/L (190–750)	70	62	102
FT4 pmol/L (12–22)	4.4	9.3	10.3
IGF1 ng/L (115–498)	<25	<25	NA
IGFBP3 mg/L (0.7–3.6)	<0.5	<0.3	NA
Hypolplastic pituitary gland	+	+	-
Limited neck rotation	+	+	-
SNHL	+	+	+
Developmental delay (Mild)	+	+	+
Other findings	Dolichocephaly, Hypolasia of facial bones, frontal bossing, short webbed neck	Dolichocephaly, Thoracic scoliosis, squint	None
Mutation Identified	c.437G > T (p. Cys146Phe) Homozygous	c.466C > T (p. Arg156Ter) Homozygous	
Type of mutation	Missense mutation	Nonsense	
Effect on protein	Location a well-established domain	Null mutation	
Computation (in silico) predictive analysis	"Damaging"	"Damaging"	
Population data	Not annotated as polymorphism	Not annotated as polymorphism	
Functional data	Located in functional domain	Located in functional domain	
Allelic and family segregation data	Recessive mutation and strong segregation	Recessive mutation and strong segregation	
Other Evidence	Relevant to patient's phenotype	Relevant to patient's phenotype	
Variant classification (ACMG)	Likely pathogenic	Pathogenic	

NA not available

treatment; he had a growth velocity of 3–4 cm per year. His height was 110 cm at the age of 10 years (−4SD). The prescribed dose for GH injections was 0.035 mg/kg/day; however the patient was not compliant with treatment, which negatively affected the growth velocity and the ultimate height at the age of 10 years.

Patient 3, Family 2
The younger sister (II:4, Fig. 1b) of the patient 2 was born via normal vaginal delivery at 39 weeks of gestation. Her birth weight (2.9 kg) and birth length (46 cm) was adequate for gestational age. She also presented with jitteriness secondary to hypoglycemia at 2nd month of age and was suspected to have hypopituitarism (Table 1), because her older brother had been diagnosed with the same condition before. Treatment thyroxine, hydrocortisone and GH injections were started. She has moderate SNHL and a normal skeletal survey. Magnetic resonance imaging showed a normal pituitary gland. Clinical features and hormonal levels for all three affected patients are summarized in Table 1.

Genetic analyses
Genomic DNA extraction was carried out using PURE-GENE DNA Extraction Kit according to manufacturer's instructions (Gentra Systems, Minneapolis, MN) from

the venous blood samples collected from each subject. All exons and adjacent exon-intron boundaries of the both *LHX3* transcripts were amplified in Veriti® 96-Well Fast Thermal Cycler (Applied Biosystems, Foster City, CA) using HotStar Taq DNA Polymerase (Qiagen, Germantown, MD). Primers were designed by the use of Primer3 web based server (http://frodo.wi.mit.edu/primer3/; sequences of primers used for PCR amplification are listed in Table 2). The PCR products were sequenced by dye termination sequencing using BigDye® Terminator Cycle Sequencing v3.1 Kit and ABI Prism 3730 Genetic Analyzer (Applied Biosystems, Inc., Foster City, CA, USA). Sequence analysis was performed using the SeqMan 6.1 module of the Lasergene (DNA Star Inc. WI, USA) software package and the results were compared with reference sequence. Accession numbers: Nucleotide and amino acid numbering are for *LHX3*, variant 2 (also known as isoform b) and correspond to NCBI reference sequence accession number NM_014564.3 for the cDNA and NP_055379.1 for the protein.

In silico prediction and pathogenicity assessment

For interpretation of the identified sequence variants as per ACMG guidelines, PolyPhen2 (Polymorphism phenotyping; http://genetics.bwh.harvard.edu/pph2/), SIFT (Sorting Intolerant From Tolerant; http://sift.jcvi.org/) and MutationTaster (http://www.mutationtaster.org/) were used for pathogenicity assessment [10]. Project HOPE ([11]; http://www.cmbi.ru.nl/hope/) was used to predict the possible structural changes in the mutant protein using a normal LHX3 structure (PDB-file: 2JTN). The sequences form the *Homo Sapiens* LHX3 protein and homologous proteins from other eukaryotic species were obtained from the National Center for Biotechnology Information (NCBI; http://www.ncbi.nlm.-nih.gov/). A multiple alignment between these proteins was performed using Clustal Omega (http://www.ebi.ac.uk/Tools/msa/clustalo/).

Results

Sanger sequencing of *LHX3* gene in the affected boy (II:2 from pedigree, Fig. 1a) from the first consanguineous family led us to the identification of a homozygous

nucleotide change (c.437G > T), resulting in a cysteine-to-phenylalanine substitution at 146 amino acid of the encoded protein (p. Cys146Phe) (Fig. 2a). In the two sibs (II:2 & II:4 from pedigree, Fig. 1b) from the second family, we identified homozygosity for a single base exchange (c.466C > T). At the protein level, this transition predicts change of amino acid 156 from arginine to a stop codon (p. Arg156Ter) (Fig. 2b). Parents and siblings of the affected patients were all healthy and show no signs or symptoms related to the disorder. In addition, they were either heterozygous or wild type for the identified mutations (Fig. 1a and b). p. Cys146Phe is predicted to be "damaging" based on PolyPhen2, SIFT and MutationTaster. p. Arg156Ter is also predicted to be "disease causing" by MutationTaster. Both the alterations were not annotated in either dbSNP [12], the 1000 Genomes Project database [13], or Exome Aggregation Consortium (ExAC) [14] and were absent in 400 normal chromosomes of ethnically matched controls, precluding that these represented benign or more common polymorphisms.

The identified p. Cys146Phe substitution resides in the LIM2 domain of the LHX3 protein (Q9UBR4). LIM domain is recognized as a tandem zinc-finger (Znf) structure that functions as a modular protein-binding interface and LIM homeodomain proteins have been shown to play roles in cytoskeletal organization, organ development, cell adhesion, cell motility and signal transduction [15, 16]. Znf motif mostly contain a pattern of cysteine and histidine residues that coordinately bind to zinc ions at the base of each of the two 'fingers', but in some cases they bind other metals such as iron, or no metal at all [17]. The cysteine at position 146 is a zinc ligating residue, involved in binding with the zinc cation (Fig. 2c). A three-dimensional-structure prediction analysis for p. Cys146Phe mutation by project HOPE predicts that the mutant residue (phenylalanine) will probably not fit in place of the smaller size wild-type cysteine residue which is buried in the core of the protein and will thus disturb the possible rearrangements of surrounding residues. In addition, the replacement of cysteine at p.146 will disrupt the putative interaction with zinc cation, thus affecting biological activity of LHX3. This cysteine is entirely conserved in LHX3

Table 2 Sequences of oligonucleotide primers used for PCR amplification

Primer	Sense Strand	Antisense Strand
*LHX3*_Exon 1a	5'- CAACCCAGCCAGGGAG - 3'	5'- GTTTCCATCTCTGTGTCCCG - 3'
*LHX3*_ Exon 1b	5'- CCCGGAGTCGCTTGGAC - 3'	5'- GCCCAGATCCTCTAGCTCC - 3'
*LHX3*_ Exon 2	5'- CAGCCCTGAGTCCTGTGG - 3'	5'- TGATTGTGAGGGGAGGAGTC - 3'
*LHX3*_ Exon 3	5'- CGGACAGAGCCTTCCTC - 3'	5'- GGAGAGAATTTCCCCGGAC - 3'
*LHX3*_ Exon 4 + 5	5'- CTTCCGAGAAGCCTGTG - 3'	5'- TCCATGGGAAATTCAGATCC - 3'
*LHX3*_ Exon 6	5'- CTGCAGGATGGGACTCTG - 3'	5'- CACCAGCCCTCCCTTGAC - 3'

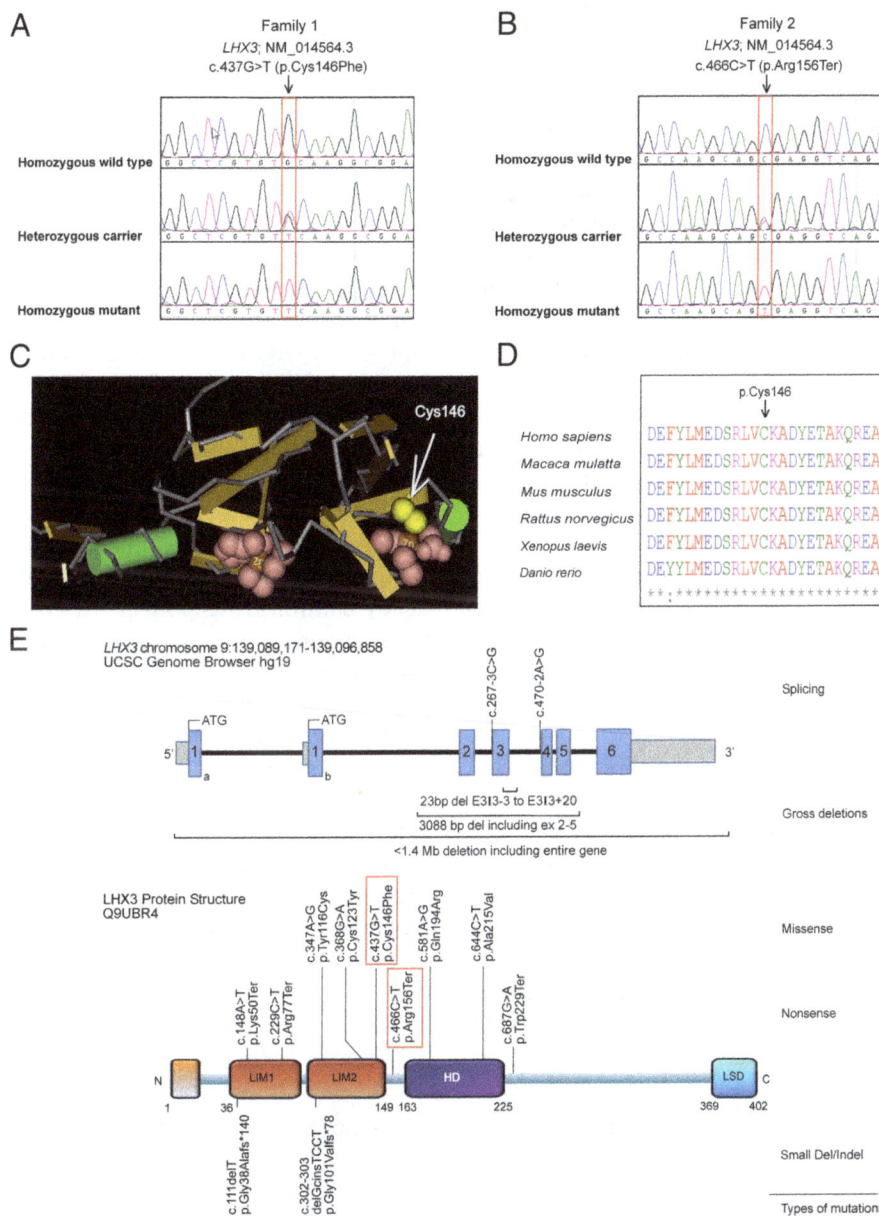

Fig. 2 Identification of two novel mutations in *LHX3*. **a** Sequencing chromatogram indicating the homozygous wild type, heterozygous carrier and homozygous mutant forms. Homozygous c.437 G > T (p. Cys146Phe) mutation is identified in affected individual (II:2, family 1). **b** Homozygous c.466 C > T (p. Arg156Ter) mutation is identified in affected individuals (II:2 & II:4, family 2). Nucleotide and amino acid numbering correspond to NM_014564.3 for the cDNA and NP_055379.1 for the protein. Nucleotides were numbered using A of the ATG translation initiation codon as +1 nucleotide of the coding sequence. Mutations are highlighted (*arrow*). **c** Ribbon/Cartoon-presentation of zinc finger motif of the LHX3 consisting of α-helix (*green*) and β-sheets (*brown*). The Zn binding residues of LIM domains are highly conserved; cysteine at position 146 (*yellow*) is a zinc ligating residue, involved in binding with the zinc cation (brown). **d** The multiple-sequence alignment was generated with the Clustal Omega Multiple Sequence Alignment tool and depicts conservation of the crucial p. Cys146 residue during evolution. *Asterisk* (*) indicates positions which have a single, fully conserved residue. *Colon* (:) indicates conservation between groups of strongly similar properties - scoring > 0.5. **e** *LHX3* mutations associated with combined pituitary hormone deficiency. Schematic representation of intron-exon structure of *LHX3* gene, domain graph of the encoded protein (Uniprot identifier: Q9UBR4), and the genetic variants. Exons are designated as *boxes* 1–6 and introns are shown by *thin lines*. A full-length wild type LHX3 protein is shown, with its N-terminus and C-terminus. Alternative splicing generates two isoforms, LHX3a and LHX3b, which are 397 and 402 amino acids long respectively. The isoforms differ only in the amino-terminal domains. Other known functional domains are following: LIM domains (LIM); homeodomain (HD), and carboxyl trans-activation domain (LSD). Novel variants identified in our study are *boxed in red* alongside previously reported variants in HGMD database [28]. The mutations are grouped according to canonical classes and further identified by their amino acid changes

proteins in homologous sequences (Fig. 2d). It is part of the amino acid sequence 'signature' that defines the LIM domains proteins [18], indicating that the Cys146 residue is critical to overall LHX3 function. The identified nonsense mutation p. Arg156Ter is predicted to result in a premature stop codon, loss of entire DNA-binding homeodomain and carboxyl terminus causing the production of short, inactive LHX3 protein or non-sense mediated decay of the aberrant mRNA. Mutant LHX3 proteins lacking a homeodomain do not bind DNA and thus do not induce transcription from pituitary genes. A complete loss of function is assumed with this homozygous mutation.

Hence, the factors that p. Arg156Ter being a null variant and critical location of p. Cys146Phe in a well-established domain, their absence in population data/controls, computational evidence, segregation analysis and relevance to the patients phenotype, led us to classify these allelic variants; p. Arg156Ter and p. Cys146Phe as "pathogenic" and "likely pathogenic" respectively, according to the recommendations of ACMG guidelines [10] for the interpretation of sequence variants (see Table 1).

Discussion and conclusions

Pituitary organogenesis is a highly complex process and tightly regulated cascade of several transcription activators and repressors, and signaling molecules [19, 20]. Anterior pituitary ontogenesis begins early around embryonic day (E) 7.5, corresponding to the first visualization of the pituitary placode. Briefly, during the early stage of pituitary development, which corresponds to E6.5-10.5 in mice, the extrinsic signaling pathways are activated, including bone morphogenetic protein (BMP2,

BMP4), fibroblast growth factor (FGF8, 10 and 18), Sonic Hedgehog (SHH) and wingless (WNT4) pathways [21]. Within the developing Rathke's pouch and anterior pituitary, a number of transcription factors are involved in a timely manner during the steps of differentiation; early acting such as paired homeodomain transcription factors (HESX1, PITX1, PITX2), LIM homeobox (LHX3, LHX4) or late-acting such as PROP1 (prophet of Pit-1) and POU1F1 (previously called PIT-1) [22]. *Lhx3* gene expression is detected in the developing nervous system and Rathke's pouch at approximately E9 [6]. By E12, POU1F1 synergistically partners with PITX1 and PITX2 for the differentiation of specific pituitary-specific cell types; thyrotropes, lactotropes and somatotropes [23]. The gonadotrope and thyrotropic precursors are activated by zinc-finger transcription factor, GATA2 in response to inductive interaction of LHX3 and BMP2 signaling [20]. Terminal differentiation of the pituitary completes at approximately E17 in response to the tightly controlled temporospatial gradient expression of transcription factor [7, 24]. A simplified scheme of expression of the transcription factors is given in Fig. 3. In *Lhx3* null mutant mice, Rathke's pouch is initially formed but then fails to grow resulting in either stillbirth or death shortly following birth, thus providing a genetic paradigm for the study of pituitary development [25]. LHX3 is known to plays an essential role in the proper development of the spinal motoneurons (which likely explains neck rotation anomalies in human with *LHX3* mutation) and is also expressed in the auditory system [4, 26, 27]. Only a small number of studies have previously reported the clinical phenotype and genetic basis of *LHX3* patients (Human Gene Mutation Database

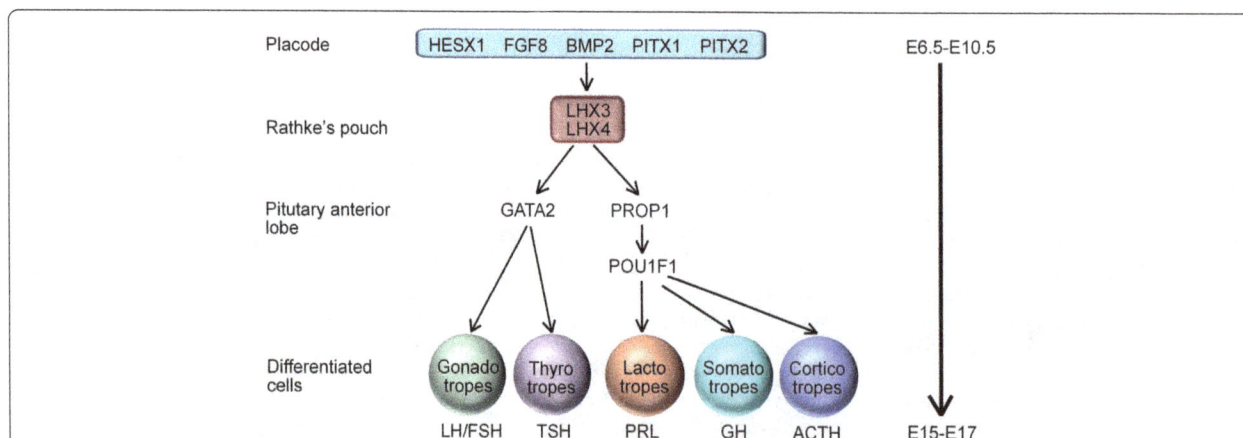

Fig. 3 A simplified scheme of the development cascade representing the main transcription factors expression during pituitary development (adapted from de Moraes et al. [20]). Pituitary cell lineages are determined by the activation or repression of each transcription factor. LHX3 participates in the pituitary cell differentiation and maturation process. The anterior pituitary consists of five distinct cell types. These cells and their specific hormones are lactotropes, which produce PRL; somatotropes, which produce GH; gonadotropes, which produce LH and FSH; corticotropes, which produce ACTH; and thyrotropes, which produce TSH. Any mutation that alters the length, quality or quantity of any gene involved in the development cascade will result in pituitary development failure

Two novel LHX3 mutations in patients with combined pituitary hormone deficiency including cervical...

193

[28]). Together with two novel mutations identified in our study, there are now 16 different *LHX3* variants (Fig. 2e) in patients with CPHD3 phenotype as detailed in Table 3. The clinical phenotypes of human *LHX3* mutations encompass a varied presentation. The earliest descriptions of *LHX3* mutations were associated with panhypopituitarism without ACTH deficiency or any extrapituitary phenotypes [29]. Later, a rigid cervical spine with limited head rotation, mental retardation and MRI findings of a hypodense lesion in the pituitary was also reported in addition to CPHD [30]. Four homozygous *LHX3* mutations with CPHD, with or without limited neck rotation were identified in a cohort of 366 patients with hypopituitarism or CPHD. Hearing status in these patients was not documented to be either normal or with any hearing deficit [31]. Bilateral SNHL was first associated as an additional CPHD3 phenotype in the four patients with CPHD, severe pituitary hypoplasia, ACTH deficiency and skeletal abnormalities [32]. The occurrence of SNHL was explained by expression of *LHX3* in a pattern overlapping that of *SOX2* in the sensory epithelium of developing inner ear [32]. Later, six patients from a same genealogy with CPHD, restricted neck rotation, scoliosis and congenital hearing impairment were described to harbor a recessive novel splice acceptor site mutation [33]. More recently, a complete loss of function mutation is associated with CPHD including ACTH deficiency, short neck and SNHL [5].

Compound heterozygous *LHX3* defects in a nonconsanguineous patient with syndromic CPHD, severe scoliosis and normal intelligence and a novel homozygous mutation p.T194R were recently reported [34, 35].

A candidate-gene approach was used on the basis of documented pituitary abnormalities, restricted neck rotation and SNHL, *LHX3* gene was then sequenced. Herein, we characterize two novel mutations in three patients from two unrelated Saudi consanguineous families. The three patients presented with early infantile hypoglycemia and deficiency of all anterior pituitary hormones including ACTH. Two of the affected patients also displayed rigidity of the cervical spine and short neck with limited rotation. Clinically, there was no evidence of cardiac defects or skin manifestations as reported earlier in some reports [32, 34]. Birth length in one of our patients was slightly below the mean centile for gestational age, which supports earlier findings that IGFs are necessary for that period but the severe deficiency interacts with intrauterine longitudinal growth [33]. Hearing impairment was noticed for all three affected at the age of 2–3 years, audiologic assessment later confirmed moderate SNHL that was partially managed with hearing aids and all had receptive and expressive language delay. Perinatal mortality has been reported in other families with *LHX3* mutations; our study family 1 had a baby girl who died at an early age probably due to the similar phenotype. Both the male

Table 3 *LHX3* mutations in patients with CPHD3 phenotype

No.	Mutation	Amino acid change	Mutation Type	Reference	
				Authors	Journal [Reference No]
1	c.148A > T	Lys50Ter	Nonsense	Rajab A et al.	Hum Mol Genet 2008 [32]
2	c.229C > T	Arg77Ter	Nonsense	Bonfig W et al.	Eur J Pediatr 2011 [5]
3	c.347A > G	Tyr116Cys	Missense	Netchine I et al.	Nat Genet 2000 [29]
4	c.368G > A	Cys123Tyr	Missense	Sobrier M et al.	J Clin Endocrinol Metab 2012 [35]
5	c.437G > T	Cys146Phe	Missense	Ramzan K et al.	BMC Endocr Disord
6	c.466C > T	Arg156Ter	Nonsense	Ramzan K et al.	BMC Endocr Disord
7	c.581A > G	Gln194Arg	Missense	Bechtold-Dalla Pozza S et al.	Horm Res Paediatr 2012 [34]
8	c.644C > T	Ala215Val	Missense	Pfaeffle R et al.	J Clin Endocrinol Metab 2007 [31]
9	c.687G > A	Trp229Ter	Nonsense	Pfaeffle R et al.	J Clin Endocrinol Metab 2007 [31]
10	c.267-3C > G		Splicing	Sobrier M et al.	J Clin Endocrinol Metab 2012 [35]
11	c.470-2 A > G		Splicing	Kristrom B et al.	J Clin Endocrinol Metab 2009 [33]
12	c.111delT	Gly38Alafs*140	Deletion	Bhangoo A et al.	J Clin Endocrinol Metab 2006 [30]
13	c.302_303delG CinsTCCT	Gly101Valfs*78	Small indel	Pfaeffle R et al.	J Clin Endocrinol Metab 2007 [31]
14	<1.4 Mb incl. entire gene		Gross deletion	Pfaeffle R et al.	J Clin Endocrinol Metab 2007 [31]
15	23 bp E3I3-3 to E3I3 + 20		Gross deletion	Netchine I et al.	Nat Genet 2000 [29]
16	3088 bp incl. ex. 2-5		Gross deletion	Rajab A et al.	Hum Mol Genet 2008 [32]

Nucleotide and amino acid numbering are based on *LHX3*, variant 2 (also known as isoform b) and correspond to NCBI reference sequence accession number NM_014564.3 for the cDNA and NP_055379.1 for the protein. Nucleotide numbering commenced with the A of the ATG translation initiation codon as +1 patients had markedly delayed pubertal development and micropenis symptom, which can thus facilitate the diagnosis in case of a male child. Short neck and neonatal hypoglycemia may be overlooked in neonatal cases, but the prolonged jaundice and hypothyroidism should lead to the diagnosis of CPHD.

The incidence of reported mutations in *LHX3* gene remains low. Clinical, hormonal and radiological work-up is very important to better determine which transcription factor should be screened. We suggest that the presence of SNHL and limited neck rotation be considered in the differential diagnosis of CPHD3 to facilitate molecular diagnosis. The identification of a *LHX3* mutation at an early age is likely to be beneficial for patients to start an appropriate replacement of hormone deficiencies, auditory testing to allow regular speech development, counseling for limitations of cervical mobility and development of scoliosis, and for continual monitoring of these patients. The importance to characterize the patients with CPHD should be emphasized to physicians and researchers to help the genetic screening of patients, and to assist genetic counseling and prenatal diagnosis.

Abbreviations
ACTH: Adrenocorticotrophic hormone; CPHD: Combined pituitary hormone deficiency; FSH: Follicular stimulating hormone; FT4: Free thyroxine; GH: Growth hormone; IGF1: Insulin growth factor 1; IGFBP3: Insulin growth factor binding protein 3; LH: Leutinizing hormone; LIM-HD: LIM-homeodomain; MRI: Magnetic resonance imaging; PRL: Prolactin; SNHL: Sensorineural hearing loss; TSH: Thyroid stimulating hormone; Znf: Zinc-finger

Acknowledgement
The authors thank patients and their families for their participation. We also thank the sequencing core facilities for their technical help.

Funding
This work was funded and supported in part by King Faisal Specialist Hospital and Research Centre (RAC#2100001) and the King Salman Centre for Disability Research (KSCDR #85722).

Authors' contributions
KR was primarily responsible for the molecular genetic studies, data interpretation, drafting and finalizing the manuscript; BB and MO were primarily responsible for clinical support, clinical evaluation and sample collection; BB and MO also participated in editing of the manuscript; RA assisted in carrying out molecular genetic studies; LA coordinated the study. FI provided oversight for the project and final editing of the manuscript. All authors read and approved the final manuscript.

Competing interests
The authors declare that they have no competing interests.

Author details
[1]Department of Genetics, King Faisal Specialist Hospital and Research Centre, P.O.Box 3354, Riyadh 11211, Saudi Arabia. [2]Department of Pediatrics, King Faisal Specialist Hospital and Research Centre, Riyadh, Saudi Arabia. [3]Department of Medical Genetics, King Faisal Specialist Hospital and Research Centre, Riyadh, Saudi Arabia. [4]College of Medicine, Alfaisal University, Riyadh, Saudi Arabia.

References
1. Kelberman D, Dattani MT. Hypothalamic and pituitary development: novel insights into the aetiology. Eur J Endocrinol. 2007;157 Suppl 1:3–14.
2. Diaczok D, Romero C, Zunich J, Marshall I, Radovick S. A novel dominant negative mutation of OTX2 associated with combined pituitary hormone deficiency. J Clin Endocrinol Metab. 2009;93:4351–8.
3. Romero CJ, Pine-Twaddell E, Radovick S. Novel mutations associated with combined pituitary hormone deficiency. J Mol Endocrinol. 2011;46:R93–R102.
4. Kelberman D, Dattani MT. The role of transcription factors implicated in anterior pituitary development in the aetiology of congenital hypopituitarism. Ann Med. 2006;38:560–77.
5. Bonfig W, Krude H, Schmidt H. A novel mutation of LHX3 is associated with combined pituitary hormone deficiency including ACTH deficiency, sensorineural hearing loss, and short neck-a case report and review of the literature. Eur J Pediatr. 2011;170:1017–21.
6. Bach I, Rhodes SJ, Pearse 2nd RV, Heinzel T, Gloss B, Scully KM, Sawchenko PE, Rosenfeld MG. P-Lim, a LIM homeodomain factor, is expressed during pituitary organ and cell commitment and synergizes with Pit-1. Proc Natl Acad Sci U S A. 1995;92:2720–4.
7. Sloop KW, Meier BC, Bridwell JL, Parker GE, Schiller AM, Rhodes SJ. Differential activation of pituitary hormone genes by human Lhx3 isoforms with distinct DNA binding properties. Mol Endocrinol. 1999;13:2212–25.
8. West BE, Parker GE, Savage JJ, Kiratipranon P, Toomey KS, Beach LR, Colvin SC, Sloop KW, Rhodes SJ. Regulation of the follicle-stimulating hormone beta gene by the LHX3 LIM-homeodomain transcription factor. Endocrinology. 2004;145:4866–79.
9. Chaudhary V, Bano S. Imaging of pediatric pituitary endocrinopathies. Indian J Endocrinol Metab. 2012;16:682–91.
10. Richards S, Aziz N, Bale S, Bick D, Das S, Gastier-Foster J, Grody WW, Hegde M, Lyon E, Spector E, Voelkerding K, Rehm HL, ACMG Laboratory Quality Assurance Committee. Standards and guidelines for the interpretation of sequence variants: a joint consensus recommendation of the American College of Medical Genetics and Genomics and the Association for Molecular Pathology. Genet Med. 2015;17:405–24.
11. Venselaar H, Te Beek TA, Kuipers RK, Hekkelman ML, Vriend G. Protein structure analysis of mutations causing inheritable diseases. An e-Science approach with life scientist friendly interfaces. BMC Bioinf. 2010;11:548.
12. Database of Single Nucleotide Polymorphisms (dbSNP). Bethesda: National Center for Biotechnology Information, National Library of Medicine; (dbSNP Build ID: 138). http://www.ncbi.nlm.nih.gov/SNP/. Accessed 14 Feb 2017.
13. 1000 Genome projects. http://browser.1000genomes.org/. Accessed 14 Feb 2017.
14. Exome Aggregation Consortium (ExAC). http://exac.broadinstitute.org/. Accessed 14 Feb 2017.
15. Bhati M, Lee C, Nancarrow AL, Lee M, Craig VJ, Bach I, Guss JM, Mackay JP, Matthews JM. Implementing the LIM code: the structural basis for cell type-specific assembly of LIM-homeodomain complexes. EMBO J. 2008;27:2018–29.
16. Matthews JM, Bhati M, Lehtomaki E, Mansfield RE, Cubeddu L, Mackay JP. It takes two to tango: the structure and function of LIM, RING, PHD and MYND domains. Curr Pharm Des. 2009;15:3681–96.
17. Perez-Alvarado GC, Miles C, Michelsen JW, Louis HA, Winge DR, Beckerle MC, Summers MF. Structure of the carboxy-terminal LIM domain from the cysteine rich protein CRP. Nat Struct Biol. 1994;1:388–98.
18. Kadrmas JL, Beckerle MC. The LIM domain: from the cytoskeleton to the nucleus. Nat Rev Mol Cell Biol. 2004;5:920–31.
19. Prince KL, Walvoord EC, Rhodes SJ. The role of homeodomain transcription factors in heritable pituitary disease. Nat Rev Endocrinol. 2011;7:727–37.
20. de Moraes DC, Vaisman M, Conceicao FL, Ortiga-Carvalho TM. Pituitary development: a complex, temporal regulated process dependent on specific transcriptional factors. J Endocrinol. 2012;215:239–45.
21. Gleiberman AS, Fedtsova NG, Rosenfeld MG. Tissue interactions in the induction of anterior pituitary: role of the ventral diencephalon, mesenchyme, and notochord. Dev Biol. 1999;213:340–53.

22. Dattani MT. Growth hormone deficiency and combined pituitary hormone deficiency: does the genotype matter? Clin Endocrinol (Oxf). 2005;63:121–30.

23. Simmons DM, Voss JW, Ingraham HA, Holloway JM, Broide RS, Rosenfeld MG, Swanson LW. Pituitary cell phenotypes involve cell-specific Pit-1 mRNA translation and synergistic interactions with other classes of transcription factors. Genes Dev. 1990;4:695–711.

24. Seidah NG, Barale JC, Marcinkiewicz M, Mattei MG, Day R, Chrétien M. The mouse homeoprotein mLIM-3 is expressed early in cells derived from the neuroepithelium and persists in adult pituitary. DNA Cell Biol. 1994;13:1163–80.

25. Sheng HZ, Zhadanov AB, Mosinger Jr B, Fujii T, Bertuzzi S, Grinberg A, Lee EJ, Huang SP, Mahon KA, Westphal H. Specification of pituitary cell lineages by the LIM homeobox gene Lhx3. Science. 1996;272:1004–7.

26. Tsuchida T, Ensini M, Morton SB, Baldassare M, Edlund T, Jessell TM, Pfaff SL. Topographic organization of embryonic motor neurons defined by expression of LIM homeobox genes. Cell. 1994;79:957–70.

27. Sharma K, Sheng HZ, Lettieri K, Li H, Karavanov A, Potter S, Westphal H, Pfaff SL. LIM homeodomain factors Lhx3 and Lhx4 assign subtype identities for motor neurons. Cell. 1998;95:817–28.

28. The Human Gene Mutation Database, http://www.hgmd.cf.ac.uk. Accessed 14 Feb 2017.

29. Netchine I, Sobrier ML, Krude H, Schnabel D, Maghnie M, Marcos E, Duriez B, Cacheux V, Moers A, Goossens M, Grüters A, Amselem S. Mutations in LHX3 result in a new syndrome revealed by combined pituitary hormone deficiency. Nat Genet. 2000;25:182–6.

30. Bhangoo AP, Hunter CS, Savage JJ, Anhalt H, Pavlakis S, Walvoord EC, Ten S, Rhodes SJ. Clinical case seminar: a novel LHX3 mutation presenting as combined pituitary hormonal deficiency. J Clin Endocrinol Metab. 2006;91:747–53.

31. Pfaeffle RW, Savage JJ, Hunter CS, Palme C, Ahlmann M, Kumar P, Bellone J, Schoenau E, Korsch E, Brämswig JH, Stobbe HM, Blum WF, Rhodes SJ. Four novel mutations of the LHX3 gene cause combined pituitary hormone deficiencies with or without limited neck rotation. J Clin Endocrinol Metab. 2007;92:1909–19.

32. Rajab A, Kelberman D, de Castro SC, Biebermann H, Shaikh H, Pearce K, Hall CM, Shaikh G, Gerrelli D, Grueters A, Krude H, Dattani MT. Novel mutations in LHX3 are associated with hypopituitarism and sensorineural hearing loss. Hum Mol Genet. 2008;17:2150–9.

33. Kristrom B, Zdunek AM, Rydh A, Jonsson H, Sehlin P, Escher SA. A novel mutation in the LIM homeobox 3 gene is responsible for combined pituitary hormone deficiency, hearing impairment, and vertebral malformations. J Clin Endocrinol Metab. 2009;94:1154–61.

34. Bechtold-Dalla Pozza S, Hiedl S, Roeb J, Lohse P, Malik RE, Park S, Durán-Prado M, Rhodes SJ. A recessive mutation resulting in a disabling amino acid substitution (T194R) in the LHX3 homeodomain causes combined pituitary hormone deficiency. Horm Res Paediatr. 2012;77:41–51.

35. Sobrier ML, Brachet C, Vie-Luton MP, Perez C, Copin B, Legendre M, Heinrichs C, Amselem S. Symptomatic heterozygotes and prenatal diagnoses in a nonconsanguineous family with syndromic combined pituitary hormone deficiency resulting from two novel LHX3 mutations. J Clin Endocrinol Metab. 2012;97:E503–509.

Permissions

All chapters in this book were first published in ED, by BioMed Central; hereby published with permission under the Creative Commons Attribution License or equivalent. Every chapter published in this book has been scrutinized by our experts. Their significance has been extensively debated. The topics covered herein carry significant findings which will fuel the growth of the discipline. They may even be implemented as practical applications or may be referred to as a beginning point for another development.

The contributors of this book come from diverse backgrounds, making this book a truly international effort. This book will bring forth new frontiers with its revolutionizing research information and detailed analysis of the nascent developments around the world.

We would like to thank all the contributing authors for lending their expertise to make the book truly unique. They have played a crucial role in the development of this book. Without their invaluable contributions this book wouldn't have been possible. They have made vital efforts to compile up to date information on the varied aspects of this subject to make this book a valuable addition to the collection of many professionals and students.

This book was conceptualized with the vision of imparting up-to-date information and advanced data in this field. To ensure the same, a matchless editorial board was set up. Every individual on the board went through rigorous rounds of assessment to prove their worth. After which they invested a large part of their time researching and compiling the most relevant data for our readers.

The editorial board has been involved in producing this book since its inception. They have spent rigorous hours researching and exploring the diverse topics which have resulted in the successful publishing of this book. They have passed on their knowledge of decades through this book. To expedite this challenging task, the publisher supported the team at every step. A small team of assistant editors was also appointed to further simplify the editing procedure and attain best results for the readers.

Apart from the editorial board, the designing team has also invested a significant amount of their time in understanding the subject and creating the most relevant covers. They scrutinized every image to scout for the most suitable representation of the subject and create an appropriate cover for the book.

The publishing team has been an ardent support to the editorial, designing and production team. Their endless efforts to recruit the best for this project, has resulted in the accomplishment of this book. They are a veteran in the field of academics and their pool of knowledge is as vast as their experience in printing. Their expertise and guidance has proved useful at every step. Their uncompromising quality standards have made this book an exceptional effort. Their encouragement from time to time has been an inspiration for everyone.

The publisher and the editorial board hope that this book will prove to be a valuable piece of knowledge for researchers, students, practitioners and scholars across the globe.

List of Contributors

Xianbin Zhang, Haidong Bao, Jing Zhang, Zhongyu Wang and Peng Gong
Department of Hepatobiliary Surgery, the First Affiliated Hospital of Dalian Medical University, Zhongshan Road No. 222, Dalian 116011, Liaoning Province, China

Li Ma
Department of Epidemiology, Dalian Medical University, Dalian 116044, Liaoning Province, China

Faheem G Sheriff, William P Howlett and Kajiru G Kilonzo
Kilimanjaro Christian Medical Centre, Moshi, Tanzania

Yukihiro Goto, Kazunori Tatsuzawa, Kazuyasu Aita, Yuichi Furuno, Takuya Kawabe, Kei Ohwada, Hiroyasu Sasajima and Katsuyoshi Mineura
Department of Neurosurgery, Kyoto Prefectural University Graduate School of Medicine, Kawaramachi-Hirokoji, Kamigyo-ku, Kyoto 602-8566, Japan

Mehtap Evran, Murat Sert and Tamer Tetiker
Department of Internal Medicine, Division of Endocrinology, Balcali Hospital, Cukurova University Medical Faculty, 01330 Adana, Turkey

Viveka P. Jyotsna
Department of Endocrinology and metabolism, All India Institute of Medical Sciences, Room No. 305, Third Floor, Biotechnology Building, New Delhi, India

Ekta Malik, Shweta Birla and Arundhati Sharma
Department of Anatomy, All India Institute of Medical Sciences, New Delhi, India

Steffen Kristian Fleck, Christian Rosenstengel, Marc Matthes and Henry Werner Siegfried Schroeder
Department of Neurosurgery, University Medicine Greifswald, Ferdinand-Sauerbruch-Strasse, 17475 Greifswald, Germany

Henri Wallaschofski, Matthias Nauck and Christin Spielhagen
Institute of Clinical Chemistry and Laboratory Medicine, University Medicine Greifswald, Ferdinand-Sauerbruch-Strasse, 17475 Greifswald, Germany

Thomas Kohlmann
Institute of Community Medicine, University Medicine Greifswald, Ferdinand-Sauerbruch-Strasse, 17475 Greifswald, Germany

Doris T. Chan, Andrea O. Y. Luk, W. Y. So, Alice P. S. Kong, Francis C. C. Chow and Ronald C. W. Ma
Department of Medicine and Therapeutics, The Chinese University of Hong Kong, Prince of Wales Hospital, Shatin, Hong Kong

Anthony W. I. Lo
Department of Anatomical and Cellular Pathology, The Chinese University of Hong Kong, Prince of Wales Hospital, Shatin, Hong Kong

Ayako Kumabe, Tsuneaki Kenzaka, Yoshioki Nishimura and Masami Matsumura
Division of General Internal Medicine, Jichi Medical University Hospital, 3311-1 Yakushiji, Shimotsuke, Tochigi 329-0498, Japan

Masaki Aikawa and Masaki Mori
Department of Internal Medicine, Division of Hematology, Jichi Medical University, Shimotsuke, Japan

George C. Nikou
Medicine, Laiko University Hospital, Athens, Greece

Kalliopi Pazaitou-Panayiotou
Unit of Endocrinology and Endocrine Oncology, Theagenio Cancer Hospital, Thessaloniki, Greece

Dimitrios Dimitroulopoulos
Gastroenterology Department, Agios Savas Cancer Hospital, Athens, Greece

Georgios Alexandrakis
Gastroenterology Department, NIMTS Hospital, Athens, Greece

Pavlos Papakostas
Oncology Department, Hippokrateion Hospital, Athens, Greece

Michalis Vaslamatzis
Oncology Department, Evangelismos Hospital, Athens, Greece

Philippos Kaldrymidis
Department of Endocrinology, Metaxa Cancer Hospital, Piraeus, Greece

Vyron Markussis
Ipsen epe, Athens, Greece

Anna Koumarianou
Hematology-Oncology Unit, Fourth Department of Internal Medicine, Attikon University Hospital, Medical School, National and Kapodestrian University of Athens, Rimini 1, 12462, Haidari, Athens, Greece

Xin-Wei Qiao, Yu-Li Song and Chong-Mei Lu
Department of Gastroenterology, Peking Union Medical College Hospital, Peking Union Medical College, Chinese Academy of Medical Sciences, Beijing 100730, People's Republic of China

Ling Qiu
Department of Clinical Laboratory, Peking Union Medical College Hospital, Peking Union Medical College, Chinese Academy of Medical Sciences, Beijing 100730, People's Republic of China

Yuan-Jia Chen
Department of Gastroenterology, Peking Union Medical College Hospital, Peking Union Medical College, Chinese Academy of Medical Sciences, Beijing 100730, People's Republic of China
Key Laboratory of Endocrinology (Ministry of Health), Department of Endocrinology, Peking Union Medical College Hospital, Peking Union Medical College, Chinese Academy of Medical Sciences, Beijing 100730, People's Republic of China

Chang-Ting Meng, Zhao Sun and Chun-Mei Bai
Department of Oncology, Peking Union Medical College Hospital, Peking Union Medical College, Chinese Academy of Medical Sciences, Beijing 100730, People's Republic of China

Da-Chun Zhao
Department of Pathology, Peking Union Medical College Hospital, Peking Union Medical College, Chinese Academy of Medical Sciences, Beijing 100730, People's Republic of China

Tai-Ping Zhang
Department of Surgery, Peking Union Medical College Hospital, Peking Union Medical College, Chinese Academy of Medical Sciences, Beijing 100730, People's Republic of China

Yu-Pei Zhao
Key Laboratory of Endocrinology (Ministry of Health), Department of Endocrinology, Peking Union Medical College Hospital, Peking Union Medical College, Chinese Academy of Medical Sciences, Beijing 100730, People's Republic of China
Department of Surgery, Peking Union Medical College Hospital, Peking Union Medical College, Chinese Academy of Medical Sciences, Beijing 100730, People's Republic of China

Yu-Hong Wang and Jie Chen
Department of Gastroenterology, The First Affiliated Hospital of Sun Yat-sen University, Guangzhou 510000, People's Republic of China

Yu-hong Wang, Jin-hui Wang, Min-hu Chen and Jie Chen
Department of Gastroenterology, The First Affiliated Hospital of Sun Yat-sen University, 58 Zhongshan II Road, Guangzhou, People's Republic of China

Yuan Lin and Ling Xue
Department of Pathology, The First Affiliated Hospital of Sun Yat-sen University, 58 Zhongshan II Road, Guangzhou, People's Republic of China

Katarina Edfeldt, Per Hellman, Gunnar Westin and Peter Stalberg
Department of Surgical Sciences, Uppsala University, Uppsala University Hospital, Entrance 70, 1 tr, SE-75185 Uppsala, Sweden

Surya Panicker Rajeev and Steffan McDougall
Department of Obesity and Endocrinology, University Hospital Aintree, Liverpool L9 7AL, UK

Monica Terlizzo
Department of Pathology, University Hospital Aintree, Liverpool L9 7AL, UK

Daniel Palmer
Department of Molecular and Clinical Cancer Medicine, Institute of Translational Medicine, University of Liverpool, Liverpool L69 3BX, UK

Christina Daousi and Daniel J Cuthbertson
Department of Obesity and Endocrinology, University Hospital Aintree, Liverpool L9 7AL, UK
Department of Obesity and Endocrinology, Institute of Ageing and Chronic Disease, University of Liverpool, Liverpool L69 3BX, UK

Jana Breitfeld, Susanne Martens, Peter Kovacs and Anke Tönjes
Department of Medicine, University of Leipzig, Liebigstrasse 20, Leipzig 04103, Germany
IFB Adiposity Diseases, University of Leipzig, Philipp-Rosenthal-Str. 27, Leipzig 04103, Germany

Jürgen Klammt, Marina Schlicke and Roland Pfäffle
Hospital for Children & Adolescents, University of Leipzig, Liebigstrasse 22, Leipzig 04103, Germany

Kerstin Krause, Kerstin Weidle, Dorit Schleinitz and Michael Stumvoll
Department of Medicine, University of Leipzig, Liebigstrasse 20, Leipzig 04103, Germany

Dagmar Führer
Department of Endocrinology, University of Essen, Hufelandstraße 55, Essen 45147, Germany

Mirjana Kocova, Elena Kochova and Elena Sukarova-Angelovska
Department of Endocrinology and Genetics, University Pediatric Clinic, Vodnjanska 17, 1000 Skopje, Macedonia

S Ramkumar, Atul Dhingra, VP Jyotsna and Mohd. Ashraf Ganie
Department of Endocrinology and Metabolism, All India Institute of Medical Sciences, Ansari Nagar, New Delhi 110029, India

Chandan J Das
Departments of Radiology, All India Institute of Medical Sciences, New Delhi, India

Amlesh Seth
Departments of Urology, All India Institute of Medical Sciences, New Delhi, India

Mehar C Sharma
Departments of Pathology, All India Institute of Medical Sciences, New Delhi, India

Chandra Sekhar Bal
Departments of Nuclear Medicine, All India Institute of Medical Sciences, New Delhi, India

Aoife Garrahy
Division of Endocrinology, Beaumont Hospital, Dublin, Ireland

Amar Agha
Division of Endocrinology, Beaumont Hospital, Dublin, Ireland
RCSI Medical School, Dublin, Ireland

Xianbin Zhang
The First Affiliated Hospital of Dalian Medical University, Zhongshan 222, Dalian 116011, China
Institute for Experimental Surgery, Rostock University Medical Center, Schillingallee 69a, 18057 Rostock, Germany

Jiaxin Song and Lili Lu
Department of Epidemiology, Dalian Medical University, Lvshun West 9, Dalian 116044, China

Peng Liu, Mohammad Abdul Mazid and Yuru Shang
The First Affiliated Hospital of Dalian Medical University, Zhongshan 222, Dalian 116011, China

Yushan Wei
Department of Evidence-based Medicine and Statistics, the First Affiliated Hospital of Dalian Medical University, Zhongshan 222, Dalian 116011, China

Peng Gong
Department of General Surgery, the Shenzhen University General Hospital and Shenzhen University School of Medicine, Xueyuan 1098, Shenzhen 518055, China

Li Ma
Department of Epidemiology, Dalian Medical University, Lvshun West 9, Dalian 116044, China
Department of Epidemiology, Dalian Medical University, Zhongshan Road 222, Dalian 116011, China

Meng Zhang, Ping Zhao, Xiaodan Shi, Lianfeng Zhang and Lin Zhou
Department of Gastroenterology, the First Affiliated Hospital of Zhengzhou University, No.1, East Jianshe Road, Zhengzhou 450052, China

Ahong Zhao
Department of Pathology, the First Affiliated Hospital of Zhengzhou University, No.1, East Jianshe Road, Zhengzhou 450052, China

Lian Duan, Huijuan Zhu and Feng Gu
Key Laboratory of Endocrinology, Ministry of Health; Department of Endocrinology, Peking Union Medical College Hospital, Peking Union Medical College and Chinese Academy of Medical Sciences, Beijing 100730, China

Bing Xing
Department of Neurosurgery, Peking Union Medical College Hospital, Peking Union Medical College and Chinese Academy of Medical Sciences, Beijing 100730, China

Kirstie Lithgow and Gregory A. Kline
Division of Endocrinology, Department of Medicine, Cumming School of Medicine, University of Calgary, 1820 Richmond Rd SW, Calgary, AB T2T 5C7, Canada

Alex Chin
Clinical Biochemistry, Calgary Laboratory Services and Department of Pathology and Laboratory Medicine, Cumming School of Medicine, University of Calgary, 9, 3535 Research Road NW, Calgary, AB T2L 2K8, Canada

Chantel T. Debert
Division of Physical Medicine and Rehabilitation, Department of Clinical Neuroscience Cumming School of Medicine, University of Calgary, 2500 University Dr. NW, Calgary, AB T2N 1N4, Canada

John D. Carmichael, Adam Mamelak and Vivien Bonert
Cedars-Sinai Medical Center, 8700 Beverly Blvd, Los Angeles, CA 90048, USA

Michael S. Broder, Dasha Cherepanov and Eunice Chang
Partnership for Health Analytic Research, LLC, 280 S. Beverly Dr., Suite 404, Beverly Hills, CA 90212, USA

Qayyim Said and Maureen P. Neary
Novartis Pharmaceuticals Corporation, One Health Plaza, East Hanover, NJ 07936-1080, USA

Jie Yu, Fan Ping, Huabing Zhang, Wei Li, Tao Yuan, Yong Fu, Kai Feng, Weibo Xia, Lingling Xu and Yuxiu Li
Department of Endocrinology, Chinese Academy of Medical Sciences and Peking Union Medical College, Peking Union Medical College Hospital, Beijing, China

A. Ciresi, S. Radellini, V. Guarnotta and C. Giordano
Section of Endocrinology, Diabetology and Metabolic Diseases, Biomedical Department of Internal and Specialist Medicine (DIBIMIS), University of Palermo, Piazza delle Cliniche 2, 90127 Palermo, Italy

Mariasmeralda Caliri, Valentina Verdiani, Massimo Mannelli and Alessandro Peri
Endocrine Unit, Department of Experimental and Clinical Biomedical Sciences "Mario Serio", University of Florence, Careggi University Hospital, Florence, Italy

Edoardo Mannucci and Carlo Maria Rotella
Diabetology Unit, Department of Experimental and Clinical Biomedical Sciences "Mario Serio", University of Florence, Careggi University Hospital, Florence, Italy

Vittorio Briganti
Division of Nuclear Medicine, Careggi University Hospital, Florence, Italy

Luca Landoni and Alessandro Esposito
General and Pancreatic Surgery Department, The Pancreas Institute-University of Verona Hospital Trust, Verona, Italy

Giulia Burato
Department of Pathology and Diagnostics, University of Verona Hospital Trust, Verona, Italy

John D. Carmichael, Adam Mamelak and Vivien Bonert
Pituitary Center, Cedars-Sinai Medical Center, 8700 Beverly Blvd, Los Angeles, CA 90048, USA

Michael S. Broder, Dasha Cherepanov and Eunice Chang
Partnership for Health Analytic Research, LLC, 280 S. Beverly Dr., Suite 404, Beverly Hills, CA 90212, USA

Qayyim Said
Health Economics and Outcomes Research, Novartis Pharmaceuticals Corporation, One Health Plaza, East Hanover, NJ 07936, USA

Maureen P. Neary
Global Oncology Market Access and Policy, Novartis Pharmaceuticals Corporation, One Health Plaza, East Hanover, NJ 07936, USA

Khushnooda Ramzan, Lolwa Al-Jomaa, Rabab Allam and Faiqa Imtiaz
Department of Genetics, King Faisal Specialist Hospital and Research Centre, Riyadh 11211, Saudi Arabia

Bassam Bin-Abbas
Department of Pediatrics, King Faisal Specialist Hospital and Research Centre, Riyadh, Saudi Arabia

Mohammed Al-Owain
Department of Medical Genetics, King Faisal Specialist Hospital and Research Centre, Riyadh, Saudi Arabia
College of Medicine, Alfaisal University, Riyadh, Saudi Arabia

Index

www.ingramcontent.com/pod-product-compliance
Lightning Source LLC
Chambersburg PA
CBHW082022190326
41458CB00010B/3245